CLINICAL EXERCISES IN INTERNAL MEDICINE

VOLUME 1

THYROID DISEASE

JOEL I. HAMBURGER, M.D., F.A.C.P.

Northland Thyroid Laboratory,
Southfield, Michigan

1978

W. B. SAUNDERS COMPANY · Philadelphia · London · Toronto

W. B. Saunders Company: West Washington Square
Philadelphia, PA   19105

1 St. Anne's Road
Eastbourne, East Sussex BN21 3UN, England

1 Goldthorne Avenue
Toronto, Ontario M8Z 5T9, Canada

Thyroid Disease   ISBN   0-7216-4485-6

Last digit is the print number: 9   8   7   6   5   4   3   2   1

To Hilda

PREFACE

Clinical Exercises in Internal Medicine: Thyroid Disease is not a textbook or a substitute for a textbook. Rather, it is a teaching device which has the objective of bridging the gap between didactic instruction and clinical practice. Self-assessment sections constitute the core of the book. I would like to emphasize that the case records are those of real patients, and the dilemmas the reader is asked to consider are the very ones faced by the author. However, the reader has the important advantage of having followup information available. Thus he or she is able to compare his or her solutions with mine. Since thyroid problems often take many years to evolve, the result that may be apparent soon after a given treatment may differ considerably from the result that is ultimately achieved. Hence, to become an experienced clinical thyroidologist requires many years. This book attempts to compress those years into a volume which can be digested in a few days, more or less.

Since these patients are real and their problems are real, it should not be surprising that the actions I chose at the time were not necessarily those that I might now prefer. After all, one is not born with clinical experience and will rarely have the opportunity to acquire very much while in training. The mastery of clinical skills is a slow process that should not cease until the physician stops caring for patients.

Furthermore, the reader should not approach the self-assessment challenges with the idea that the purpose is to select the "right" answer. Should he do so, he will be disappointed to find that more than one answer may have merit in some cases, and that what is called for is not so much selection as analysis. The goal of this volume is to encourage an analytical approach to the consideration of alternative methods for dealing with thyroid problems. Experts may differ on therapeutic decisions, but all should agree that the best decision is most likely to result from a careful consideration of the advantages and disadvantages of possible alternatives.

The didactic portions which precede each of the self-assessment sections should be viewed as introductory material containing the more valuable clinical lessons I have learned over the years. It is not intended that these portions of the text cover all aspects of thyroidology comprehensively; there are a number of reference volumes available for this purpose. This book is structured to advance the reader (who presumably has a basic knowledge of the subject and some clinical experience) relatively quickly through basic principles of pathophysiology, clinical diagnosis, laboratory diagnosis, and therapy to the application of these principles in selected clinical problems. The reader will soon appreciate that certain concepts are presented repetitively. These are points which I consider both important and inadequately emphasized in the literature. It is my intention that no one who reads this volume will continue to be unfamiliar with these concepts.

References are listed, and the principal messages (as I see them) of the references are noted. In some instances, serial references are employed to show how certain important concepts have evolved in the literature.

In sum, I expect that this book will serve as a modern clinical learning source for students and practitioners who are interested in improving clinical skills that are important for the accurate and efficient diagnosis and treatment of thyroid patients. I trust that it will prove both instructive and fun to read.

NOTE: For all case studies the normal ranges for laboratory values are those cited in Table 1–1 unless otherwise noted.

ACKNOWLEDGMENTS

My appreciation is extended to Mrs. Hanica Ullmann, Ph.D. candidate, Instructor of English Literature, Wayne State University, Detroit, Michigan, for her review of the manuscript which greatly improved its readability.

I am particularly indebted to Dr. J. Martin Miller, my teacher and friend of many years, for taking the time to review this book just prior to publication. Among his perceptive observations are two that deserve comment.

Dr. Miller correctly noted that the high frequency with which lymphoepithelial goiter (better known to most as Hashimoto's disease) is seen in clinical practice is in stark contrast with the limited reference to the condition in this book. This reflects my experience that the clinically relevant aspects of the disease are expressed in terms of goiter (usually diffuse but occasionally nodular) and hypothyroidism. The problem is therefore dealt with primarily in the chapters on simple goiter and hypothyroidism. The immunologic features of the disease which have received so much attention in the literature have little importance from the standpoint of management.* Furthermore, there are few therapeutic problems in Hashimoto's disease, and the treatment is generally rather straightforward. Hence, I simply do not have very much to say about it. Nevertheless, the reader should have no doubt that Hashimoto's disease is indeed one of the more common afflictions of the thyroid gland seen in clinical practice.

Dr. Miller also correctly observed that although a self-assessment section might be expected to assess the reader's comprehension of the preceding didactic material, in this book such is not necessarily the case. Here the self-assessment sections are not supplemental to the text; on the contrary, they are the text. They assess the reader's total fund of knowledge and experience with thyroid patients by means of problems which are generally of more than elementary difficulty. The didactic

---

*For the latest on autoimmunity in the thyroid read:

1. Allison AC: Self-tolerance and autoimmunity in the thyroid. *New Eng J Med* 295:821–827, 1976.
2. Volpé R: The role of autoimmunity in hypoendocrine and hyperendocrine function with special emphasis on autoimmune thyroid disease. *Ann Intern Med* 87:86–99, 1977.

portions serve to highlight certain principles which will be exemplified by the cases; but mastery of these lessons will not be enough to permit the reader to appreciate all the points illustrated by the cases. However, this is not important. The reader who diligently spends the time to think through each of these problems and then compares his judgments with mine, should find that he or she has not only expanded his clinical horizons but also has had some fun in doing it.

My associates Drs. Donald A. Meier, Sheldon S. Stoffer, Charles I. Taylor, and Michael Garcia contributed greatly to this effort by providing cases for the self-assessment sections, suggesting many improvements in the text, and proofreading extensively.

Dolores Stachura and Tina Eller, our secretaries, deserve special commendations for bearing with good grace the tedium of endless re-typing and proofreading of the material.

DEFINITIONS
AND
ABBREVIATIONS

Certain terms commonly encountered in the literature on thyroid disease are used rather loosely by some physicians (e.g., adenoma, nodule), but in this volume these terms will be used precisely as defined. Other terms will be defined because they might not be familiar to many physicians.

Abbreviations are a standard practice in scientific literature and serve the dual purpose of reducing the size of a book and permitting more rapid reading of the material. However, unfamiliar abbreviations may constitute a hindrance to the reader's comprehension. Therefore, I have included a list of abbreviations in this section.

The following guidelines have been employed with respect to abbreviations:

1. Abbreviations familiar to all scientists (e.g., cm, mm, etc.) are used throughout the text without definition.

2. Abbreviations peculiar to thyroidology, although familiar to all physicians, will be defined in this glossary but not necessarily in the text.

3. Abbreviations used by me alone are defined here and in each section of the text where they are employed.

DEFINITIONS

ADENOMA, THYROID: A discrete thyroid mass which fulfills the histologic or pathophysiologic criteria for a benign neoplasm.

COLLOID GOITER: I dislike this term because it is often employed to imply some profound understanding of pathophysiologic mechanisms, whereas actually the term is meaningless. All goiters have colloid — so what? This term carries with it no specific diagnostic or therapeutic implications. For these reasons I use the term "simple goiter" as defined below. I consider the latter preferable because it implies no in-depth analysis or understanding of pathophysiology and because for most patients the further study necessary to define the underlying abnormal mechanism will not be useful in determining the treatment.

DYSHORMONOGENESIS: Defective synthesis or secretion of thyroid hormone resulting from insufficient activity of one or more essential enzymes. Dyshormonogenesis may be compensated or decompensated.

> COMPENSATED: Because of compensatory hyperplasia of the thyroid, a normal output of thyroid hormone may be maintained, and the patient is euthyroid.

> DECOMPENSATED: In spite of thyroidal compensatory hyperplasia, output of thyroid hormone is subnormal, and the patient is hypothyroid.

GRAVES' DISEASE: A syndrome of which the principal features are hyperthyroidism, diffuse goiter, and ophthalmopathy. However, not all of these features need be present in any given patient at any given time. For example, it is proper to speak of euthyroid Graves' disease as a stage in the evolution of the illness during which the patient may not have hyperthyroidism but only goiter or ophthalmopathy.

HYPERTHYROIDISM (THYROTOXICOSIS): The clinical syndrome resulting from the delivery of an excessive quantity of thyroid hormone to the patient, regardless of the source of the hormone.

HYPOTHYROIDISM: The clinical syndrome resulting from the lack of an adequate supply of thyroid hormone.

IMAGE: A pictorial representation of the thyroid gland produced after the administration of a radioactive tracer which is selectively concentrated by the thyroid. This term is preferable to "scan," because images are now more often obtained by means of gamma cameras (stationary devices) than by rectilinear scanners.

MYXEDEMA: This term is often used synonymously with hypothyroidism, but in general it should be restricted to indicate a severe deficiency state.

NEOPLASM: A new growth, benign *or* malignant.

NODULE, THYROID: Any discrete thyroid mass whether neoplastic or non-neoplastic, detectable by *physical examination.*

SIMPLE GOITER: A generalized enlargement of the thyroid gland, whether smooth, irregular, or nodular, in an euthyroid patient who presents no evidence of abnormal hormonal secretory activity.

ABBREVIATIONS

AFTA:	Autonomously functioning thyroid adenoma
AST:	Acute suppurative thyroiditis
ATD:	Antithyroid drugs
BEI:	Butanol-extractable iodine
BMR:	Basal metabolic rate
DIT:	Diiodotyrosine
DT_4:	Dextrothyroxine
EKG:	Electrocardiogram
ENT:	Extranodular thyroid tissue

ESR:	Erythrocyte sedimentation rate
FTI:	Free thyroxine index
I:	Iodide
^{131}I:	The isotope of iodine most widely employed for thyroid function testing and therapy
^{125}I:	An isotope of iodine used chiefly in testing
^{123}I:	A newly available isotope of iodine with a very short half-life which is advantageous for thyroid imaging
LATS:	Long-acting thyroid stimulator
LT_4:	Levothyroxine
μCi:	Microcurie
μg:	Micrograms
μU:	Microunit
mCi:	Millicurie
MIT:	Monoiodotyrosine
MNG:	Multinodular goiter
ng:	Nanograms
NG–NH:	No goiter–no hypothyroidism
PBI:	Protein-bound iodine
PII:	Plasma inorganic iodide
PTU:	Propylthiouracil
RAI:	Radioactive iodine uptake, the 24-hour value unless otherwise specified
RIA:	Radioimmunoassay
SAT:	Subacute thyroiditis
SD:	Standard deviation
SSKI:	Saturated solution of potassium iodide
ST_4:	Supplemental thyroid hormone
T_3:	Triiodothyronine
T_3(RIA):	A test which measures the serum concentration of T_3 by RIA
T_4:	Thyroxine
T_4(D):	A test which measures the serum concentration of T_4 by displacement, or competitive protein binding
T_4(RIA):	A test which measures the serum concentration of T_4 by RIA
TBG:	Thyroxine-binding globulin
TBG(S):	A test that estimates the saturation of TBG. Formerly (and still widely) referred to as the T_3 resin uptake test or T_3 test. The older term is less accurate because the test does not measure the serum T_3 concentration, and there is another test—the T_3(RIA) test—that does.
TBPA:	Thyroxine-binding prealbumin
Tc:	Technetium-99m
TDG:	Toxic diffuse goiter, hyperthyroidism of the Graves' type
TMNG:	Toxic multinodular goiter
TRG:	Toxic recurrent goiter (after previous thyroidectomy)
TRH:	Thyrotropin-releasing hormone
TSH:	Thyroid-stimulating hormone
TSH(RIA):	A test that measures the serum concentration of TSH by RIA

CONTENTS

CHAPTER 1

LABORATORY EVALUATION OF THE THYROID

PART I.   THYROID PHYSIOLOGY

A basic knowledge of thyroid physiology is essential to the understanding of laboratory methods. Figure 1–1 illustrates the important aspects of normal thyroid physiology.

IODINE METABOLISM

In the United States the dietary content of iodine varies from 70 to 300 μg daily. In the past, as a result of removal of iodine from the soil by glaciers, iodine deficiency goiters were common in the area of the Great Lakes. The advent of iodized salt and improved methods of food distribution and mineral fortification have almost eliminated iodine deficiency as a dietary problem in this country. Recently, an increased iodine content in commercially baked bread has been recognized in the United States.

Ingested iodine is reduced to iodide in the gastrointestinal tract. Absorption is virtually complete. It may take place throughout the gastrointestinal tract, but it is maximal in the small intestine. Ingested iodotyrosines, triiodothyronine (T_3), thyroxine (T_4), and iodinated radiographic contrast media are absorbed intact. Absorbed iodide has a volume of distribution numerically equal to about 35 per cent of the body weight and is confined largely to the extracellular space. The plasma inorganic iodide level is usually less than 1.0 μg per 100 ml except in the post-absorptive state. Iodide is cleared from the plasma chiefly by the kidneys and the thyroid, with renal clearance normally three to four times that of the thyroid. Renal clearance of iodide is closely related to glomerular filtration rate. There is no evidence of tubular secretion.

1

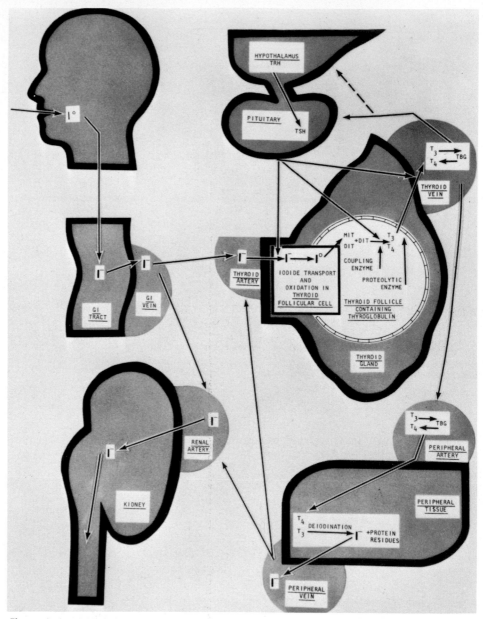

Figure 1–1. *Iodine metabolism.* Ingested iodine is reduced to iodide in the gastrointestinal tract and passes to the thyroid (about 20 per cent) or kidney (about 80 per cent). Thyroidal iodide is oxidized to iodine and utilized in the synthesis of T_3 and T_4 and the regulation of TSH. T_3 and T_4, bound principally to TBG, circulate to the tissues where they are metabolized, releasing iodide.

IODIDE TRANSPORT

Iodide enters the thyroid by active transport, an energy-dependent process which is augmented by thyroid-stimulating hormone (TSH). It then either is rapidly organified or remains free to diffuse passively from the thyroid back into the circulation. Transport of iodide from the plasma to the thyroid is subject to an autoregulatory mechanism which functions by inhibiting further transport of iodide as glandular iodide stores are increased. However, when iodide stores are depleted, iodide transport is enhanced. Thyroidal clearance of iodide is also related to the plasma inorganic iodide (PII) concentration. Within a range of 1 to 6 μg per 100 ml, acute changes in PII do not alter thyroidal iodide clearance significantly. Sharp reductions in PII below 1 μg per 100 ml will lead to an abrupt increase in thyroidal iodide clearance, whereas increases in PII over 6 μg per 100 ml will depress this clearance.

SYNTHESIS, STORAGE, AND SECRETION OF THE THYROID HORMONES

Figure 1–1 indicates the steps in the production of the thyroid hormones, beginning with the transport of iodide from the plasma into the thyroid follicular cell. Oxidation of iodide to iodine occurs under the influence of a peroxidase enzyme. At the colloid-cell interface iodide becomes incorporated in tyrosine components of thyroglobulin as either monoiodotyrosine (MIT) or diiodotyrosine (DIT). The ratio of MIT to DIT depends principally upon the availability of iodide and the rate at which hormonal synthesis is proceeding. The ratio may be altered by injury—inflammation or radiation—to the thyroid and also by some thyroid neoplasms. Coupling of MIT and DIT produces T_3, whereas two molecules of DIT combine to produce T_4. This coupling is enzymatically mediated. Under circumstances favoring MIT production, there may be a shift toward the production of T_3 rather than T_4. This may be a compensatory process in which the thyroid gland, which may be either deficient in iodide or functionally injured, shifts to the preferential production of a hormone which has relatively greater metabolic activity per molecule (i.e., T_3), thus possibly forestalling the development of hypothyroidism.

T_3 and T_4 are produced within the stored thyroglobulin of the follicular colloid. The thyroglobulin repository normally contains enough hormone to maintain the euthyroid state for 2 months without new synthesis. In response to TSH, the thyroglobulin molecule is split by proteases and peptidases into the component iodotyrosines and iodothyronines (T_3 and T_4). The iodotyrosines are enzymatically deiodinated, conserving iodide for reutilization in the synthesis of thyroid hormone. Normally, only negligible quantities of iodotyrosine are present in the circulation.

Although the thyroid hormonal secretion contains T_4 predominantly, since there is peripheral conversion of T_4 to T_3 and T_3 is more active, it seems likely that T_3 may actually be of greater importance than T_4 to the body economy. In fact, it has been suggested that T_4 actually serves only as a prohormone or precursor for T_3. However, the enthusiasm for this rather extreme view seems to be subsiding.

REGULATION OF THYROID FUNCTION

TSH (thyroid-stimulating hormone) is the principal regulator of thyroid function. Figure 1–1 presents diagrammatically the functional interrelationships between the hypothalamus, pituitary, and thyroid. It can be seen that TSH stimulates not only transport of iodide into the cell but also both synthesis and secretion of thyroid hormones. The action of TSH at the thyroid cell is mediated via activation of adenyl cyclase, with the subsequent generation of cyclic AMP. TSH secretion is provoked by low serum concentrations of thyroid hormone and is inhibited by high concentrations.

TRH (thyrotropin-releasing hormone) is a tripeptide secreted by the hypothalamus. It travels via the hypophyseal portal system to the pituitary to trigger TSH release. The recent identification of TRH has complicated our understanding of the interrelationships between the hypothalamus, pituitary, and thyroid. It still seems clear that the pituitary is the principal site for feedback response to altered plasma concentrations of the thyroid hormones, since qualitatively normal pituitary thyroid feedback relationships persist after inactivation of the hypothalamus. However, the recognition of children with tertiary (hypothalamic) hypothyroidism indicates that in some instances the absence of TRH may play a decisive role in the regulation of thyroid function. These patients had clinical and laboratory features of hypothyroidism without an elevation in serum TSH concentration. The thyroid glands were responsive to exogenous TSH, and the pituitaries released endogenous TSH in response to TRH.

It has been shown that TRH releases TSH in normal individuals, and an exaggerated release of TSH occurs in patients with primary hypothyroidism. However, the TRH-mediated TSH release is blunted not only by excessive thyroid hormone but also by replacement doses of thyroid hormone in patients who are euthyroid owing to such medication. It is difficult to explain these observations in terms of the usual endocrine feedback relationships. Therefore, the precise physiologic role of TRH under ordinary circumstances remains unclear.

The synthesis of TRH has given impetus to the development and evaluation of a number of testing procedures. Although the use of TRH permits the differentiation of tertiary from secondary hypothyroidism, the treatment is the same for both; hence, the added expense and inconvenience to the patient of the additional testing are of dubious value. It has been suggested that blunting of the TRH-induced TSH release may be a sensitive indicator of hyperthyroidism. Actually it is an indicator which is positive in many patients who have neither the clinical features of hyperthyroidism nor elevated serum concentrations of either of the thyroid hormones. With respect to the diagnosis of hyperthyroidism, it seems more likely that the blunted TRH–TSH response has the same clinical significance as that of an RAI which is nonsuppressible by T_3 (i.e., all hyperthyroid patients exhibit the phenomenon, but not all patients who exhibit the phenomenon have hyperthyroidism). An augmented release of TSH in response to TRH in patients with hypothyroidism may prove useful in the diagnosis of the early stages of this disease.

THYROID HORMONE-BINDING PROTEINS

Thyroid hormone circulates in the plasma largely bound to protein. The principal binding protein for both T_4 and T_3 is a globulin called thyroxine-binding globulin (TBG), which on electrophoresis migrates between the α-1 and α-2 globulins and is produced primarily in the liver. A second binding protein moves ahead of albumin electrophoretically and is called thyroxine-binding prealbumin (TBPA). TBPA is present in greater quantity than TBG but binds T_4 less strongly and T_3 very weakly; hence, it is less important physiologically than TBG. A relatively small proportion of circulating T_3 and T_4 may also be bound to albumin. Only about 0.1 per cent of the total plasma thyroid hormone circulates unbound as free thyroid hormone. It is the free hormone concentration which correlates best with the level of thyroid function. TBG may be increased on a genetic basis and by estrogens (birth control pills), hypothyroidism, and liver disease. TBG is decreased by genetic factors, adrenal steroids, acidosis, testosterone, liver disease, and chronic illnesses with protein wasting. Since the gene which controls TBG production is on the X chromosome, genetic disorders associated with TBG excess or deficiency are sex-linked. Salicylates and phenytoin may displace thyroid hormone from binding proteins by successfully competing for binding sites rather than by altering the concentration of TBG or TBPA per se.

FREE THYROXINE

Although most of the circulating thyroid hormone is bound to carrier proteins, a small fraction (approximately 0.1 per cent of the total) is not protein-bound but travels free in the plasma. Most of the investigations relative to free hormone have dealt with free T_4. Free T_4 concentrations do not always correlate with the thyroid functional status of the patient. For example, inappropriate elevations in free T_4 concentrations have been observed in patients with liver disease and other acute and chronic illness. It seems likely that until it becomes possible to assess the combined free T_4–free T_3 concentration, apparent inconsistencies must be expected in special situations.

DISTRIBUTION AND METABOLISM OF THYROID HORMONE IN MAN

Normally the half-life of T_4 in the plasma is about 6 days, whereas that for T_3 is only about 1 day. The difference may relate in part to the relative binding affinity of T_4 and T_3 to TBG.

Infusion of T_4 labeled by a radioactive tracer is rapidly followed by a high concentration of the tracer in the liver. The hepatic T_4 pool is largely reversible and seems to represent predominantly a storage depot rather than the site of extensive T_4 metabolism. There is also a substantial early concentration of T_4 in the kidneys, whereas accumulation in muscle is slower and lesser in magnitude. The rate of disappearance of T_4 from the plasma is increased in hyperthyroidism and decreased in hypothyroidism and liver disease. The prolonged plasma T_4 half-life in patients with liver disease primarily reflects reduced hepatic storage capacity and only secondarily a reduction in T_4 metabolism. The absolute T_4 disposal in cirrhosis is normal.

The initial step in the peripheral metabolism of the thyroid hormones is deiodination. More than half of the T_3 in the blood is derived from partial T_4 deiodination. The released iodide is then available for reutilization by the thyroid or for renal excretion. The protein component may undergo hepatic conjugation with glucuronide or sulfate and then be excreted by the biliary tract. Bacterial enzymes may break down these conjugates, permitting reabsorption. Ultimately, about 15 per cent of the total secreted hormone is excreted in the feces.

Recent data indicate that phenobarbital, long used for hyperthyroidism for its sedative effects, may increase both hepatocellular hormonal binding and deiodination.

PERIPHERAL ACTION OF THYROID HORMONE

How thyroid hormone affects cellular function is not yet entirely clear. Thyroid hormone appears to act upon intracellular energy transport systems in the mitochondria. Thyroid hormone increases oxygen consumption; heat production; metabolism of carbohydrates, proteins, and fats; cardiac output; and nervous irritability. It is essential for maximal growth and development.

PART II. MODERN LABORATORY METHODS

An ever increasing number of sensitive and highly specific testing methods vie for physician acceptance in the workup of thyroid patients. The sequential application of appropriately selected tests provides diagnostic precision in most instances. However, the efficient use of modern thyroid tests requires a thorough understanding of what each test is measuring and the potential methodologic pitfalls.

Thyroid tests may be classifed under two general headings: tests of thyroid functional integrity and tests of thyroid structural integrity.

TABLE 1-1. TESTS OF THYROID FUNCTIONAL INTEGRITY

A. Tests providing data on thyroid secretory activity
  1. Free T_4 index, FTI (NR, 1.5 to 4.2)
  2. Serum T_3 concentration, T_3(RIA) (NR, 60 to 190 ng per 100 ml)
  3. Serum TSH concentration, TSH(RIA) (N, < 8 μU/ml)
B. Tests providing data on thyroid iodide clearance
  The 24-hour radioactive iodine uptake test, RAI (NR 10 to 40 per cent)[a]
C. Tests providing data on suppressibility of thyroid function
  The T_3 suppression test (N, a fall in RAI value to less than 20 per cent and less than 50 per cent of the baseline value)
D. Tests providing data on thyroid functional reserve
  The TSH stimulation test (N, an increment of 10 per cent or greater over the baseline RAI)
E. Tests providing data on TRH-induced pituitary TSH release
  1. An augmented release of TSH occurs with hypothyroidism or impaired thyroid function. This may replace the TSH stimulation test.
  2. A blunted response occurs with hyperthyroidism or nonsuppressible thyroid function, or in a patient taking full doses of thyroid hormone. In patients not taking thyroid hormone, this response is similar in significance to a nonsupressible RAI. (Of course, a blunted response will occur in hypopituitarism.)

[a]Many factors other than thyroid function influence RAI values. The *number* without careful clinical correlation may be misleading. See Table 1-3.

NOTE: Obsolete tests such as the BMR, PBI, BEI, and others, with which most physicians are familiar, are not included because they are too crude to be of continuing clinical utility. They have been replaced by more sensitive, more specific, and more reliable methods.

A discussion of the modern methods employed to assess thyroid functional integrity follows.

A. TESTS OF THYROID SECRETORY ACTIVITY

Highlights

> THE T_4(D) OR TBG(S) VALUES ALONE MAY BE GROSSLY MISLEADING SINCE BOTH ARE DEPENDENT UPON CARRIER PROTEIN CONCENTRATIONS.

> THE FTI PROVIDES A VALUE WHICH IS INDEPENDENT OF CHANGES IN CARRIER PROTEIN CONCENTRATION AND IS THE PREFERRED SCREENING TEST FOR THYROID FUNCTION.

   1. The Free T_4 Index (FTI).   The FTI is a reflection of the serum concentration of metabolically active thyroid hormone. Most of the circulating thyroid hormone is bound to thyroxine-binding globulin (TBG). Less than 0.1 per cent circulates unbound, or "free." The concentration of TBG may be increased by estrogens (birth control medication), liver disease, and occasionally by hereditary factors. By contrast, TBG may be decreased by androgens, protein-wasting diseases (e.g., nephrotic syndrome), liver disease, and again by genetic factors. Also, phenytoin and salicylates (the latter in high doses) may displace thyroxine (T_4) from TBG by effectively competing for binding sites. The serum-bound T_4 concentration (essentially the total T_4) varies with the TBG concentration and thus may be either inappropriately high or inappropriately low. It is the unbound, or free, T_4 that determines the patient's functional status. One can measure the free T_4 by equilibrium dialysis, but this method is difficult and not readily available.
   The FTI is a mathematically derived value which correlates well with the free T_4 concentration. The free T_4 concentration is proportional to the numerical product of the serum total T_4 concentration and an index of TBG saturation.
   The serum total T_4 concentration has been measured by competitive protein-binding radioassay in most modern laboratories for the past ten years. The designation T_4(D) is employed to indicate that what is measured is radioactive T_4 displaced from TBG in proportion to the amount of T_4 (from patient serum) added to the assay tube.
   Recently there has been a trend favoring the radioimmunoassay of T_4 over the T_4(D) method because of improved specificity, accuracy, and simplicity. Also, using the T_4(RIA) method eliminates problems inherent in the T_4(D) assay, including the variable efficiency of alcoholic extraction and results that are falsely elevated because of an increase in nonesterified fatty acids. The normal range for the T_4(RIA) test at Northland Thyroid Laboratory is 5.5 to 11.5 μg per 100 ml.
   A simple method for measuring TBG saturation is the familiar T_3 resin uptake test, now referred to as the TBG(S) test.

   NOTE: The T_3 resin uptake does not measure serum T_3 concentration. Radioactive T_3 is used in this assay, which actually measures TBG saturation, hence the designation TBG(S). Labeled T_3 and a resin are added to the patient's serum (of course containing TBG, saturated to some unknown degree by thyroid hormone). The greater the saturation of TBG, the less TBG binds labeled T_3, and the greater the TBG(S) (see Fig. 1–2). The normal TBG(S) range at Northland Thyroid Laboratory is 25 to 35 per cent.
   When T_4(RIA) and TBG(S) values deviate from normal in the same direction (e.g., both are elevated or both are subnormal), this indicates either hyperthyroidism or hypothyroidism, respectively. However, when these values deviate from normal in

opposite directions, it means that there is an alteration in carrier protein (principally TBG) concentration. For example, an elevated T_4(RIA) value with a depressed TBG(S) value indicates a high TBG concentration, whereas a depressed T_4(RIA) value and an elevated TBG(S) value indicate a low TBG concentration. Figure 1–2 is a diagrammatic explanation of why an estrogen-mediated increase in TBG will increase the T_4(D) or T_4(RIA) values while simultaneously decreasing the TBG(S) value.

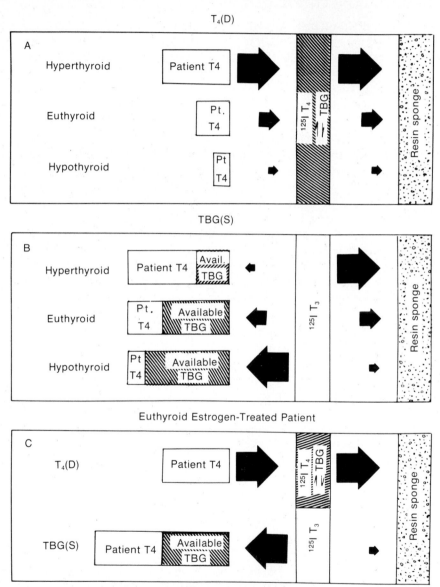

Figure 1–2. Correlation of methodology and results for T_4(D) and TBG(S). *T_4(D):* A large amount of T_4 is extracted from hyperthyroid serum, displacing more labeled T_4 from TBG; hence high sponge count. The reverse is true for hypothyroid serum, and euthyroid serum is intermediate.

TBG(S): Hyperthyroids have saturated TBG. Therefore, labeled T_3 is bound primarily by the resin sponge; hence high sponge count. The reverse is true for hypothyroids, and euthyroids are intermediate.

Euthyroid estrogen treated patient: Estrogen increases TBG, and therefore bound T_4; hence more T_4 is extracted from the serum, producing a high T_4(D) sponge count. However, since estrogen increases TBG, patient serum binds more labeled T_3; hence low TBG(S) sponge count.

By multiplying the T_4(RIA) value by the TBG(S) value, one obtains a new number which corrects for altered TBG concentration and may serve as an index of the serum free thyroxine, i.e., the FTI. The normal range for the FTI at Northland Thyroid Laboratory is 1.5 to 4.2. *Note: There are no units.* The FTI is simply an arbitrary numerical expression and not a direct measurement of anything. The following examples will show how the FTI corrects abnormal T_4(RIA) and TBG(S) values that are the result of abnormal serum TBG concentrations.

A normal T_4(RIA) might be 7 μg per 100 ml and a normal TBG(S) might be 30 per cent, giving an FTI of 2.1. The same patient on estrogens might have a T_4(RIA) of 12.0 μg per 100 ml, with a TBG(S) of 20 per cent, giving an FTI of 2.4. If the patient were taking androgens, the T_4(RIA) might be 4.0 μg per 100 ml with a TBG(S) of 50 per cent, but the FTI is 2.0. Thus, the FTI avoids the confusion which might arise from abnormal values for either the T_4(RIA) or TBG(S) alone.

Value of the Routine Use of the FTI

The importance of obtaining adequate data to calculate the FTI in all patients is evident from an evaluation of 300 consecutive patients studied at Northland Thyroid Laboratory. Sixty-six patients (22 per cent) had evidence for an alteration in carrier protein binding. The changes in T_4(D) and TBG(S) which resulted are summarized in Table 1–2.

In 24 of the 66 patients there was no history of any disease or ingestion of medication which would have accounted for the laboratory variations. More than 10 per cent of the patients in the study group acknowledged that they were taking estrogen-containing medications. Even if they had concealed this information, the studies would have exposed the abnormality in carrier protein, and the FTI would have eliminated concern for abnormal thyroid function.

Patients with unexplained abnormalities of these types should be informed of the findings to avoid confusion in the event of testing at some future time. I prefer to provide the patient with a copy of my report, which includes an explanation of the abnormal T_4(D) and TBG(S) values. This may avoid needless future anxiety, expense, and possibly mistreatment.

2. Radioimmunoassay (RIA). The low plasma concentration of many peptide hormones makes their assay by biological or chemical techniques impractical. They cannot be reliably distinguished from other plasma proteins which are present in concentrations 100 million times as great. The development of the radioimmunoassay (RIA) was a major breakthrough in diagnostic methodology. This technique

TABLE 1–2.   CHANGES IN T_4(D) AND TBG(S) VALUES RESULTING FROM CARRIER PROTEIN DISTURBANCES

CHANGES OBSERVED	NO. PATIENTS	EXPLANATION	NO. PATIENTS
Elevated T_4(D), depressed TBG(S)	55	Estrogens	39
		Unknown	14
		Pregnancy	2
Depressed T_4(D), elevated TBG(S)	9	Unknown	9
Normal T_4(D) although patient was hypothyroid, TBG(S) very low, and FTI subnormal	2	Estrogens	1
		Unknown	1
Total	66		66

permits an accurate assay of compounds that are present in very minute concentrations. RIA takes advantage of the high degree of specificity of an immunologic reaction between a peptide hormone as antigen and its biosynthesized antibody. The general principle of RIA can be viewed as a set of competing reactions. Unlabeled hormone, depending upon its quantity (extracted from patient serum), competes for specific antibody, displacing proportionate amounts of labeled hormone. Displaced labeled hormone is separated from antibody bound hormone, and is then assayed; it directly reflects the quantity of unlabeled hormone (from patient serum) introduced into the system.

A. THE T_3(RIA). This test is useful when a preferential increase in T_3 secretion might be anticipated, such as:

(1) In T_3 toxicosis—e.g., multinodular goiter, autonomously functioning thyroid adenomata, after thyroidectomy or ^{131}I therapy for hyperthyroidism, or an early stage in the development of Graves' disease.

(2) A compensatory mechanism in a failing thyroid—e.g., Hashimoto's disease, degenerating goiter, or after thyroidectomy or ^{131}I therapy.

The normal range (at Northland Thyroid Laboratory) is 60 to 190 ng per 100 ml.

CAUTION: Since an elevated T_3(RIA) value may mean either thyrotoxicosis or compensation by a functionally impaired thyroid gland, the intelligent use of this test requires careful clinical correlation.

B. THE TSH (RIA). In primary hypothyroidism TSH(RIA) levels rise as a consequence of negative feedback. The lack of an elevated TSH(RIA) in the presence of hypothyroidism suggests secondary hypothyroidism. Most assays will not distinguish between normal and hypopituitary levels of TSH. Relatively low values are obtained for both groups.

An elevated TSH(RIA) value may be an early indicator of a failing thyroid gland. Lack of suppression of an elevated TSH(RIA) value means that thyroid hormone dosage is inadequate. Conversely, a suppressed TSH(RIA) value indicates that a further increment in thyroid dosage will be needless and possibly hazardous.

Normal levels are less than 8 μU/ml. Values of between 8 and 12 μU/ml are of marginal significance. Most patients with clinically evident hypothyroidism have values in excess of 20 μU/ml, and many have values higher than 100 to 200 μU/ml. The magnitude of the elevation observed in the serum TSH concentration depends upon both the duration and the severity of the deficiency in thyroid function. Not all patients with elevated serum TSH concentrations have clinically evident hypothyroidism. Sometimes an elevated serum TSH concentration provides enough stimulus to a functionally impaired thyroid gland to produce an adequate hormonal output. Thus, the euthyroid state is preserved by virtue of the serum TSH elevation. This is seen in patients with Hashimoto's disease, simple thyroid enlargement from mild dyshormonogenesis, and occasionally after thyroidectomy or ^{131}I therapy. The magnitude of the elevation of serum TSH concentration is usually not great. Generally one will find values of 15 to 20 μU/ml.

NOTE: Those who have copies of my earlier books will observe changing numerical values for these tests. This is the inevitable result of the progressive shift to more reliable methods. The normal ranges are provided only to serve as a reference for the values in case reports, included elsewhere in this volume, of patients studied at Northland Thyroid Laboratory. These "normal ranges" give only a general idea of the values that might be recorded at other laboratories.

ANTITHYROID ANTIBODIES

These tests will be covered briefly at this point, even though they are not tests of thyroid secretory activity and do not fit anywhere in my outline of laboratory methods. The usefulness of antibody studies for the diagnosis of Hashimoto's disease is well established. Kits for the assay of antibodies to thyroglobulin and thyroid microsomes are available and are quite satisfactory. Elevated titers are more consistently found for the antimicrosomal antibody.

B. TESTS OF THYROID IODIDE CLEARANCE (THE RAI)

Highlights

THE RAI PROVIDES ONLY INDIRECT EVIDENCE OF THYROID FUNCTION, AND ITS VALUES MAY BE INCREASED OR DE-CREASED BY CORRESPONDING SHIFTS IN PLASMA INORGANIC IODIDE CONCENTRATIONS. THE RAI IS NO LONGER CONSID-ERED A USEFUL PRIMARY TEST OF THYROID FUNCTION. NEVER-THELESS, IN SPECIAL SITUATIONS IT IS HELPFUL. SUPPRESSION OR STIMULATION TESTS EXTEND THE USEFUL-NESS OF THE RAI.

The 24-hour radioactive iodine uptake (RAI) is a simple estimate of plasma clearance of iodide by the thyroid. Usual normal ranges are from 10 to 15 per cent to 35 to 40 per cent. However, low RAI values may not mean that hypothyroidism is present, since thyroid iodide clearance may not correlate with hormonal secretion. For example, a normal patient taking full doses of thyroid hormone is euthyroid; however, the RAI value will be low. If the RAI value were "normal," it would be *abnormal* and indicative of nonsuppressible function. Similarly, a patient with dyshormonogenesis may have an elevated RAI value, indicating increased iodide clearance. This indicates not hyperthyroidism but inefficient synthesis of thyroid hormone, possibly producing hypothyroidism. Table 1–3 outlines the more common situations in which RAI values may not directly relate to thyroid function.

Data on Changing Values in the RAI

Table 1–4 shows the changes observed in RAI values in euthyroid and hyperthyroid patients between 1962 and 1974.

Note that in both groups there seems to be a decreasing proportion of patients with higher values and an increasing proportion with lower values. It has been presumed that this change is the result of a higher iodide intake, in part related to the use of iodinated products in the baking of white bread. As already discussed, since so many things alter RAI values other than thyroid dysfunction, the RAI is not the best primary test for either hyperthyroidism or hypothyroidism. Nevertheless, the RAI continues to be a very useful diagnostic tool in clinical thyroidology. Table 1–5 outlines the current clinical applications for which the RAI has particular value.

Two confirmatory procedures have been employed to extend the usefulness of the RAI—i.e., the T_3 suppression test and the TSH stimulation test. The availability of the TRH test has rendered the older tests largely obsolete. The TRH test is much simpler, safer, and less expensive. Nevertheless, the earlier tests will be discussed, emphasizing situations in which they are still of value and indicating when TRH data may be of equivalent significance.

TABLE 1-3. CLINICAL SIGNIFICANCE OF RAI VALUES

I. Elevated RAI values may be seen in
  A. Hyperthyroidism
  B. Euthyroidism
    1. Rebound after withdrawal of thyroid hormone or antithyroid drugs
    2. Recovery from subacute thyroiditis
    3. Early phases of Hashimoto's disease
    4. Compensated dyshormonogenesis
  C. Hypothyroidism
    1. Decompensated dyshormonogenesis
    2. Hashimoto's disease
II. Normal RAI values may be seen in
  A. Hyperthyroidism
    1. When the patient is on antithyroid drugs
    2. When the patient has received iodides
    3. Toxic multinodular goiter or toxic autonomously functioning thyroid adenoma
  B. Euthyroidism
  C. Hypothyroidism
    1. Hashimoto's disease
    2. After treatment for hyperthyroidism (^{131}I or thyroidectomy)
    3. Decompensated dyshormonogenesis
    4. Recovering from subacute thyroiditis
III. Low RAI values may be seen in
  A. Hypothyroidism
  B. Euthyroidism
    1. When the patient has received iodides or thyroid hormone (less likely antithyroid drugs)
    2. Hashimoto's disease
    3. Subsiding subacute thyroiditis
  C. Hyperthyroidism
    1. When the patient has received iodides or antithyroid drugs
    2. During the hyperthyroid phase of subacute thyroiditis
    3. Iatrogenic or factitious hyperthyroidism
    4. Toxic struma ovarii

TABLE 1-4. CHANGING RAI VALUES IN EUTHYROID AND HYPERTHYROID PATIENTS

RAI VALUE (%)	1962–64	1965–67	1968–70	1971–72	1973–74
No. Euthyroid Patients					
16	3	6	5	6	6
16–30	24	30	25	43	37
30+	73	64	70	51	57
Total	100	100	100	100	100
No. (%) Hyperthyroid Patients					
20–45	25 (20)	32 (14)	63 (22)	67 (23)	80 (31)
46–70	72 (59)	139 (63)	165 (59)	180 (62)	145 (56)
70+	26 (21)	50 (23)	54 (19)	45 (15)	34 (13)
Total	123	221	282	292	259

TABLE 1-5. CURRENT CLINICAL APPLICATIONS OF THE RAI

A. DIAGNOSTIC
1. To exclude the hyperthyroid phase of subacute thyroiditis (SAT)
2. As part of the TSH stimulation test
    a. In the evaluation of the necessity for continued thyroid hormone administration to patients with prior diagnoses of hypothyroidism which are in doubt
    b. In the diagnosis of factitious hyperthyroidism
    c. In the diagnosis of SAT
    d. In the diagnosis of toxic struma ovarii (the RAI in the neck will be suppressed by the ovarian hormonal secretion but will respond to TSH stimulation)
    e. In the diagnosis of secondary hypothyroidism
3. As part of the T_3 suppression test
    a. In the diagnosis of mild hyperthyroidism (the TRH test is now preferred)
    b. In the evaluation of euthyroid patients with ophthalmopathy consistent with Graves' disease (the TRH test is now preferred)
    c. To confirm or exclude a diagnosis of hyperthyroidism in a patient taking antithyroid drugs for whom the original diagnosis of hyperthyroidism is questioned
4. To diagnose nonsuppressible function
B. THERAPEUTIC
1. To assure that the RAI is high enough for ^{131}I therapy in hyperthyroidism
2. To assess the potential usefulness of ^{131}I therapy in patients with inoperable thyroid cancer

C. THE T_3 SUPPRESSION TEST

An elevated RAI on a compensatory basis (e.g., for iodine deficiency, dyshormonogenesis, a rebound in recovering subacute thyroiditis) will fall sharply in response to T_3 administration, 75 to 100 μg daily for 4 to 7 days. The usual fall in RAI is to less than half the baseline value (e.g., if the baseline RAI is 40 per cent, the RAI on the T_3 test is less than 20 per cent). If there is hyperthyroidism, the RAI value is not suppressed.

CAUTION: The RAI may not be suppressed in the nonhyperthyroid situations listed in Table 1-6.

Thus, although all hyperthyroid patients have nonsuppressible RAI values, all those with nonsuppressible RAI values do not have hyperthyroidism, and some patients with suppressible RAI values may have the pathophysiologic potential for future hyperthyroidism.

TABLE 1-6. THYROID CONDITIONS WITH T_3 NONSUPPRESSIBLE RAI

A. Hyperthyroid
1. Toxic diffuse goiter (classic Graves' disease)
2. Toxic multinodular goiter (TMNG)
3. Toxic autonomously functioning thyroid adenoma (AFTA)
B. Nonhyperthyroid
1. Euthyroid Graves' disease
2. Multinodular goiter
3. Nontoxic AFTA
4. After treatment of hyperthyroidism (^{131}I or thyroidectomy)

Note that in the nonhyperthyroid situations listed in Table 1–6, in which nonsuppressible RAI values may be present, suppressible values may also be observed in some patients.

1. Euthyroid Graves' disease. These patients present with ophthalmopathy or goiter. Early in the course of the disease, the RAI may be suppressible; later it may become nonsuppressible.

2. Multinodular goiter (TMNG). Portions of these goiters may function autonomously. The RAI will be suppressed by more than 50 per cent until more than half the tissue functions autonomously.

3. Nontoxic AFTA. The greater the AFTA secretory activity, the more completely will the extranodular thyroid tissue (ENT) be suppressed. Since the baseline RAI reflects uptake by both the AFTA and ENT, the fall in RAI in response to T_3 will vary inversely with the suppression of ENT function produced by the AFTA. For instance, if the ENT is fully suppressed, uptake of the tracer will be confined to the AFTA; hence, T_3 will produce no significant suppression of the baseline RAI. In contrast, if the AFTA is small and produces no appreciable suppression of the ENT, then T_3 administration will produce a sharp fall in the baseline RAI because of the fall in ENT tracer uptake.

CAUTION: It should now be obvious that a suppressible RAI does not exclude autonomous function, either in the TMNG or in a solitary functional nodule.

4. After treatment of hyperthyroidism. The RAI may revert to suppressibility or may remain nonsuppressible. A suppressible RAI may again become nonsuppressible months to years after treatment. This has important therapeutic implications, as we shall see. The mechanism which underlies these shifts in suppressibility as well as the initiation of nonsuppressible function remains unknown.

CAUTION: The T_3 suppression test is contraindicated whenever a temporary increase in circulating thyroid hormone level might be hazardous, particularly in elderly patients with marginally compensated cardiovascular systems. The TRH test now makes the T_3 suppression test unnecessary for these patients.

D. THE TSH STIMULATION TEST

For this test I give 5 units of TSH, followed by 5 μCi of [131]I 8 to 12 hours later. An RAI value is obtained in 10 to 18 hours. Table 1–7 outlines the major uses for TSH testing. The TSH stimulation test may be helpful in the diagnosis of subacute thyroiditis by permitting the identification by imaging of uninvolved or lesser in-

TABLE 1-7. CLINICAL UTILITY OF THE TSH STIMULATION TEST

A. Positive response
   1. Normal patient on thyroid hormone
   2. Normal patient with marginal baseline RAI value (TRH testing is a more sensitive and simpler method for diagnosis of impaired thyroid function)
   3. Secondary hypothyroidism (a blunted response to TRH would be observed)
B. Negative response
   1. Primary hypothyroidism or impaired thyroid function
     a. Hashimoto's disease or SAT
     b. After administration of ^{131}I or operation for hyperthyroidism
     c. After radiation to the thyroid, incidental to treatment of other adjacent disease
   2. Euthyroid patient who has ingested iodide

volved tissue (Figure 6–5). The test also may be employed to determine whether patients taking thyroid hormone actually need the medication. A poor response— an RAI value after TSH stimulation of less than 8 per cent—supports the need for thyroid hormone, whereas an RAI value of greater than 8 per cent suggests that thyroid hormone is not necessary.

Classically, this study has been employed to differentiate primary from secondary hypothyroidism. In the primary form, a subnormal RAI does not respond to parenteral TSH. In secondary hypothyroidism the post-TSH value is at least 10 per cent greater than the baseline RAI (e.g., if the baseline RAI is 5 per cent, the post-TSH RAI is 15 per cent or more). Some patients with secondary hypothyroidism will require more than one dose of TSH (usually 5 units daily for 3 days) to produce a positive response. Hence, if secondary hypothyroidism is the question (rather uncommon), the single dose TSH stimulation test should not be employed. In secondary hypothyroidism TRH would produce no significant increment in the baseline TSH(RIA) value. This test is simpler, but false positive tests may be obtained if the patient is taking thyroid hormone (and, of course, in hyperthyroidism).

CAUTION: RAI values of between 7 and 10 per cent after TSH stimulation (or even lower in some instances) may indicate iodide interference; hence, a positive response to TSH stimulation is more valuable than a subnormal response.

E. THE TRH TEST

This test is an important advance in diagnostic methods. Although different TRH doses and timing of taking blood for TSH(RIA) values have been suggested, I have found that administration of 100 μg of TRH intravenously, with baseline and 20 minute TSH(RIA) values, is a simple and effective protocol for clinical purposes. Normal patients respond with a mean increment in TSH(RIA) of 9.3 μU/ml (range 4.4 to 13.7. μU/ml). Patients with hyperthyroidism have a blunted response with no greater increment than 0.5 μU/ml. Patients with mild hypothyroidism (including those taking inadequate doses of thyroid hormone) had increased or augmented responses with increases of 20 μU/ml or greater. Note that overtly hypothyroid patients have greatly elevated baseline TSH(RIA) values and do not require TRH testing for diagnosis. It is for those with lesser impairments of thyroid function that the test is so helpful. Here the baseline TSH(RIA) level may be only slightly elevated or at the upper level of normal. This is often the case in patients with goiter (Hashimoto's disease) or those who have been treated for hyperthyroidism with ^{131}I or surgery. In these patients FTI values are also often within normal limits, although usually they are at the lower limits of normal. An augmented response to TRH may indicate that annoying but not severe complaints may be caused by subnormal thyroid function and may respond to thyroid hormone.

CAUTION: Some patients whom I have advised to discontinue thyroid hormone (taken for doubtful indications) and reevaluated 2 months later had normal FTI values and normal baseline TSH(RIA) values but augmented responses to TRH. This abnormality may be only temporary and should not be considered proof of hypothyroidism. A similar situation may occur after treatment of hyperthyroidism or in the recovery phase of SAT.

TABLE 1-8. CLINICAL UTILITY OF THE TRH TEST

A. Possible indications with a blunted response (i.e., no increment in TSH(RIA) level greater than 1 μU/ml). This result has the same significance as nonsuppressibility of the RAI in response to T_3.
  1. Hyperthyroidism
  2. Euthyroid patient
    a. with Graves' disease
    b. with AFTA
    c. with multinodular goiter
    d. after treatment of hyperthyroidism
    e. taking full doses of thyroid hormone
B. Possible indications with an augmented response (i.e., an increase of 20 μU/ml or more over the baseline TSH(RIA) value)
  1. Hypothyroidism
    a. untreated
    b. on inadequate replacement therapy
  2. Impaired thyroid function
    a. Hashimoto's disease
    b. simple goiter
    c. after thyroidectomy or ^{131}I therapy
  3. After withdrawal from thyroid hormone. (An augmented TRH response may persist for 3 to 6 months, even though the patient has normal thyroid function.)

The TRH test has in large measure replaced the T_3 suppression test and the TSH stimulation test because of the following advantages:

  1. The risks of administering T_3 are avoided.
  2. The test can be done in a single brief visit.
  3. No TSH (a foreign protein) is given.

The same nonhyperthyroid situations in which the RAI is nonsuppressible (Table 1-7) will have blunted TRH responses. Blunted responses also are seen in patients taking full doses of thyroid hormone. For these patients an unsuppressed RAI value is of more help in the diagnosis of hyperthyroidism than a blunted TRH response.

Spurious Alterations in Thyroid Test Values Produced by Medications

Table 1-9 summarizes the alterations in test values produced by medication. Routine use of the FTI obviates concern for variations in TBG. FTI values may be affected by thyroid hormone (depending upon dosage), the type of thyroid, and whether the patient's own thyroid function is normally suppressible. The normal circulating thyroid hormone is a mixture of T_4 and T_3. Since the T_3 component is about four times as potent as T_4 and thus is present in much smaller amounts, T_3 concentrations are not reflected by the FTI value. The patient treated with a pure T_3-containing compound will have low FTI values even if toxic doses are given.

CAUTION: We see two or three patients yearly who have been given toxic amounts of T_3 in a vain attempt to elevate the results of blood tests to normal. If the patient initially had low normal values, the physicians were often surprised to find that as the dose of T_3 was increased, these values fell rather than rose (because of progressively increasing suppression of endogenous T_4 output with replacement by T_3).

Treatment with a proper dose of a pure T_4 preparation produces an FTI value

TABLE 1-9. SPURIOUS ALTERATIONS IN THYROID FUNCTION
TEST VALUES PRODUCED BY MEDICATIONS

| | | MEDICATIONS | | | | | |
| | | *Thyroid Hormone*[a] | | | | *Drugs Affecting TBG Concentrations*[b] | |
TEST	WHAT IS MEASURED	*Iodide*	T_3	T_4	T_3-T_4	↑ *TBG*	↓ *TBG*
T_4(D) or T_4(RIA)	Serum total T_4 concentration	0	↓	0	0	↑[c]	↓
TBG(S)	TBG saturation	0	↓	0	0	↓	↑
FTI	Index of serum free T_4 concentration	0	↓	0	0, ↓	0	0
T_3(RIA)	Serum total T_3 concentration	0	↑	0	[d]	↑	↓
TSH(RIA)	Serum TSH concentration	0	↓	↓	↓	0	0
RAI	Plasma iodide clearance	↓	↓	↓	↓	0	0

[a]Assuming full replacement doses. Lesser doses produce less marked alteration or none.

[b]TBG concentrations may also be altered by disease or heredity. Phenytoin or high doses of salicylates may simulate decreased TBG concentration.

[c]Euthyroid jaundiced patients may have increased T_4(D) values. Bilirubin increases TBG binding of T_4. The FTI will be normal.

[d]The result depends upon the time lapse between the administration of the hormone and drawing the blood for the test.

Key: ↓ = decrease, ↑ = increase, 0 = no change.

within normal limits. Serum T_3 concentrations will also be normal, the T_3 being derived from T_4 by deiodination. In the past it was thought that one had to administer enough T_4 to produce a slightly elevated FTI for adequate treatment of hypothyroidism. Recent studies correlating FTI and TSH(RIA) values indicate that these doses were probably excessive, and that most hypothyroid patients can be treated adequately with 0.1 to 0.2 mg daily of levothyroxine.

The primary impetus to the introduction of the newer mixtures of T_3 and T_4 was avoidance of the high FTI values observed when pure T_4 products were given in what is now appreciated as excessive doses. It was also thought that, since the thyroid gland produces both T_3 and T_4, a mixture of the two hormones might more nearly reproduce "normal" physiology.

It has since been shown that most of the T_3 utilized at the tissue level results from T_4 deiodination rather than from thyroidal secretion. Thus, the rationale for T_3–T_4 mixtures is not valid. Furthermore, the T_3 component of these mixtures produces spiking rather than sustained serum T_3 levels. This is at least theoretically undesirable. Also these products are more costly. Hence, I do not use them. Most patients who are taking them seem to have a lower FTI than would have been expected. The T_3(RIA) varies depending upon the time lapse between the last dose of the medication and the drawing of the blood sample.

For desiccated thyroid preparations the ratio of T_3 to T_4, and indeed the hormonal content itself, are uncertain and inconsistent; hence, test values are unpredictable. An inappropriately high T_3(RIA) level with a relatively lower T_4(RIA) level is very common.

CAUTION: If patients are treated with desiccated thyroid preparations (a practice which I emphatically discourage), the PBI test (now obsolete) should definitely not be used for follow-up. This study measures iodinated protein, whether hormonally active or not. I recall a hyperthyroid girl treated with a combination of antithyroid drugs and 180 mg of desiccated thyroid daily. Her complaints of rather severe hypothyroidism were dismissed by a pediatric endocrinologist because the PBI was "normal." On further testing, the T_4(D) was exceedingly low and the TSH(RIA) greatly elevated.

Medications containing either thyroid hormone or iodide may reduce RAI values. The duration of the suppression depends upon the patient's intrinsic thyroidal function and the dosage and duration of the medication administered. For example, although thyroid hormone administration suppresses the RAI of normal patients, it will not suppress the RAI in hyperthyroid patients. This is the basis of the suppression test. By contrast, hypothyroid patients (except those with dyshormonogenesis) have low RAI values, whether they are taking thyroid hormone or not. Therefore, for the patient taking thyroid hormone, the question of how long to wait before RAI testing after discontinuing the medication is irrelevant. If hyperthyroidism is suspected, an immediate suppressed RAI excludes the diagnosis, whereas a nonsuppressed high value is strong evidence in favor of hyperthyroidism. If hypothyroidism is considered, there is little point in waiting. An RAI value which remains subnormal in spite of TSH administration is good evidence for impaired thyroid function, whereas a normal value suggests that the thyroid gland is capable of normal function (or, rarely, secondary hypothyroidism).

Iodides (Quadrinal, SSKI, Lugol's solution, Combid, Ornade, Vioform, Floraquin, Itrumil, kelp from "health food" stores, and many others) will not affect the FTI. If hyperthyroidism is suspected, an elevated RAI should be observed if the iodides are withheld for 2 to 3 weeks. An occasional patient with toxic multinodular goiter (TMNG) may have a more prolonged suppression of RAI. Patients with TMNG often have normal RAI values even when iodide has not been given. Of course, hypothyroid patients (except those with dyshormonogenesis) have low RAI values regardless of iodides.

Selected Current References

1. Vagenakis AG, Braverman LE, Azizi F, et al: Recovery of pituitary thyrotropic function after withdrawal of prolonged thyroid-suppression therapy. *New Eng J Med* 293:681–684, 1975

   This article emphasizes the necessity for waiting 2 months after withdrawal of thyroid hormone before reevaluating the patient's pituitary thyroid axis. Short of this, one may find subnormal serum thyroid hormone concentrations which are only temporary.

2. Molitch ME, Spare SV, Arnold GL, et al: Pituitary-thyroid function after cessation of prolonged thyroid suppression. *New Eng J Med* 295:231, 1976

   Wouldn't you know it, just when everything was so nicely settled, we have to have the exception — i.e., a patient who was euthyroid 2 months after withdrawal of thyroid hormone, but who became hypothyroid 2 months later. This must be a rare event, but the cautious physician might be well advised to follow patients withdrawn from thyroid hormone until the outcome is certain. How long is that? Incidentally, this patient's serum T_4 concentration was 5 µg per 100 ml (NR 5.0 to 13 µg per 100 ml) at the 2-month point; hence, the authors should have been suspicious.

TABLE 1-10. TESTS OF THYROID STRUCTURAL INTEGRITY

A. Thyroid imaging
    1. Radioactive iodine image (^{123}I preferred). This image reflects the distribution of iodide *currently* being incorporated into thyroglobulin.
    2. Technetium-99m image. This image reflects the distribution of active trapping of the tracer throughout the thyroid.
    3. Fluorescent image. This image reflects the iodide which *had previously* been incorporated into thyroglobulin.
B. Ultrasound evaluation
    This study permits the differentiation of cystic from solid nodular thyroid lesions.

A. THYROID IMAGING

Thyroid imaging provides a visual display of the thyroid anatomy. Thyroid imaging has become somewhat more complex than it was in the early days when ^{131}I was the only tracer, and the only imaging device was the rectilinear scanner. Since different methods and tracers provide information that may be substantially different in some circumstances, it is necessary to discuss both the differences between imaging devices and the tracers that may be used for imaging.

Imaging Devices

1. The Rectilinear Scanner. This was the first practical instrument for producing an image of the thyroid. The patient is given a tracer substance; after a suitable interval, during which the tracer is concentrated by the thyroid, the image can be produced by the scanner. The detector in this instrument moves back and forth over the thyroid, indexing in the vertical direction after each horizontal passage, so that in time the entire thyroid gland is surveyed. The radioactivity detected by the scanner is translated as a printout in which the concentration of darkness in each area is in proportion to the intensity of activity in that area of the gland. Because the instrument "scans" the organ it is called a scanner, and the image produced is called a scan.

2. The Gamma Camera. This newer instrument is capable of viewing the entire thyroid gland from a single position. Since the detector does not move, it is not a scanner, and the image produced is not properly called a scan. The term "image" is applicable regardless of the instrument employed. I will continue to refer to images produced by the rectilinear scanner as scans, but pictorial representations of the thyroid in general or those produced by the gamma camera I shall call images.

The gamma camera utilizes a pinhole collimator and produces high resolution images of a quality superior to those obtainable with a rectilinear scanner. Relatively small defects that may not be readily visible on scans often can easily be seen on gamma camera images. However, there are disadvantages:

a. The gamma camera is about five times as expensive as a rectilinear scanner.

b. The image bears no specific relationship to the actual size of the organ imaged.

c. Serial studies must be performed with the thyroid gland at the same distance from the face of the collimator if one hopes to draw any inferences as to the relative size of images obtained at different times.

d. Localization of nodules is more cumbersome with the gamma camera.

Tracers Used in Thyroid Imaging

There are two classes of tracer that are employed for thyroid imaging, and there is another method of imaging which does not involve the administration of a tracer. Since the resultant information may be quite different, physicians must have some understanding of this aspect of the imaging procedure.

1. Radioactive Iodine. The availability of radioactive iodine in the form of ^{131}I made thyroid imaging possible. The tracer is given orally, and after an appropriate period of time (usually but not necessarily 24 hours), the imaging proceeds. When radioactive iodine is used the image that results represents the distribution of iodide that has been not only trapped by the thyroid but also incorporated into the thyroglobulin.

Other isotopes of iodine have been used more recently, including ^{125}I and ^{123}I. I shall discuss the relative merits of these isotopes later.

2. Technetium-99m (Tc). This tracer is also trapped by the thyroid but is not incorporated into thyroglobulin. It may be given orally (imaging proceeds 30 to 45 minutes later) or intravenously (imaging proceeds 20 minutes later).

Since there are thyroid diseases in which trapping may be preserved or enhanced, even though the later steps which result in the incorporation of iodide into thyroglobulin are defective, it should be clear that images obtained after administration of Tc may be quite different from those after administration of ^{131}I. These differences may have clinical relevance in two important situations:

a. Hashimoto's disease and those forms of dyshormonogenesis which trap but only poorly organify iodide may be confusing. In these disorders the output of thyroid hormone is often subnormal, giving rise to increased TSH stimulation and enhanced trapping. A Tc image will reveal a uniform intense concentration of tracer. This image will closely resemble that obtained in patients with toxic diffuse goiter. Of course, serum FTI and TSH(RIA) levels will easily differentiate these two conditions. However, a radioactive iodine image will reveal a patchy irregular tracer uptake. Later in the course of Hashimoto's disease, when there has been extensive fibrotic replacement of functioning tissue that produces patchy areas in which neither trapping nor organification can proceed, radioactive iodine and Tc images may be similar. Therefore, we must have additional clinical information before attempting to draw functional and pathophysiologic inferences from Tc images.

b. A generation of experience with radioactive iodine scans has established the principle that neoplastic nodules (excluding AFTA) are hypofunctional (cool or cold). They incorporate iodide into thyroglobulin poorly in comparison with the surrounding thyroid tissue. Unfortunately, some neoplasms, occasionally malignant ones, may trap Tc as well as the normal thyroid tissue, so that they appear functional. If a suspected thyroid neoplasm appears hypofunctional on a Tc image, it will also be hypofunctional on a radioactive iodine study. However, if the neoplasm appears to be functional with Tc, another study using radioactive iodine should be done unless autonomous function can be demonstrated by either a post-TSH stimulation image or a suppression image. Obviously, if the lesion is an AFTA, it will be functional whether studied with Tc or radioactive iodine.

At this point it may be appropriate to ask how to know whether to do suppression imaging or a post-TSH stimulation image when a functional nodule is seen on a baseline Tc study. It is easy but also essential to select the proper test.

(1) If the nodule concentrates all or essentially all of the tracer, repeat the image after TSH stimulation, looking for a shift in relative activity away from the nodule to the extranodular tissue.

(2) If there is considerable tracer concentration by the extranodular tissue, repeat the image after 3 weeks of treatment with levothyroxine, 0.15 or 0.2 mg daily. Look for preferential suppression of tracer concentration by extranodular tissue.

Failure to follow these guidelines will lead to inconclusive data.

3. The Fluorescent Image. This is a new method of thyroid imaging in which no tracer is given to the patient. The machine contains a number of sealed sources of americium-241 which irradiate the thyroid, causing the iodide stores to become transiently radioactive. As the activity is induced it is detected and recorded in rectilinear fashion. The information obtained by this instrument may differ from that obtained from either radioactive iodine or Tc images.

a. The fluorescent image reflects what the thyroid gland *has done in the past* by way of iodide incorporation into thyroglobulin, whereas the radioactive iodine image is dependent upon *current* iodide organification. Two examples illustrate how this difference may have clinical relevance:

(1) The thyroid gland of a patient taking SSKI for asthma will be loaded with iodide, but current radioactive iodine uptake will be very low.

(2) A patient taking full doses of thyroid hormone for several months for an erroneous diagnosis of hypothyroidism will have suppressed pituitary TSH release. Therefore, radioactive iodine uptake will be suppressed. However, since TSH is suppressed, iodide stores within the thyroid will remain intact, and a fluorescent image will be normal.

b. The fluorescent image will differ from the Tc image because the latter requires only trapping of the tracer, whereas a satisfactory fluorescent study depends upon trapping *and* organification of iodide.

There is yet another aspect of thyroid imaging which requires consideration — i.e., radiation safety. Table 1–11 provides data on the amount of radiation delivered to the thyroid gland with various imaging methods.

It is obvious that different sources deliver vastly different amounts of radiation to the thyroid gland. Although ^{131}I has been the standard tracer employed for over 40 years, its continued use has been challenged on the grounds of radiation safety. Recent reports on thyroid cancer as a late sequela of radiation therapy to the thymus, tonsils, and other parts of the upper body indicate that cancers have occurred after as little as 50–100 rads exposure to the thyroid gland. The probability that cancer would develop increased as the exposure increased up to 700–1000 rads. The risk is greatest in children and young adults. The following guidelines are now gaining broad acceptance:

1. Neither ^{131}I nor ^{125}I should be given for thyroid imaging with the following exceptions, in which ^{131}I is still preferred: (a) the study of substernal thyroid masses, and (b) the search for metastatic thyroid cancer.

TABLE 1–11. THYROID RADIATION FROM VARIOUS IMAGING METHODS

SOURCE AND DOSE OF RADIATION	RADIATION DELIVERED TO THE THYROID PER IMAGE (RADS)
^{131}I (100 μCi)	100–300
^{125}I (100 μCi)	90–250
^{123}I (300 μCi)	5–10
Tc (10 mCi)	2–3
^{241}Am (fluorescent image)	0.1

TABLE 1-12. INDICATIONS FOR THYROID IMAGING

1. To provide an objective evaluation of thyroid size and shape
   a. Before and after ^{131}I therapy
   b. Before and after thyroidectomy
2. To establish the thyroid origin of neck masses
3. To locate ectopic foci of thyroid tissue in
   a. Substernal goiter
   b. Benign ectopic thyroid tissue
   c. Metastatic thyroid cancer
4. To demonstrate nonuniform thyroid function in
   a. Inflammatory disease
   b. Degenerated goiter
5. To evaluate the functional activity of thyroid nodules

2. Either ^{123}I or Tc is the tracer of choice from the standpoint of radiation safety; either permits the production of excellent images.

3. When imaging is necessary in children, the fluorescent image is particularly advantageous since there is low radiation dose to the thyroid and no radiation to the rest of the body.

At times a combination of imaging procedures will be of value in elucidating the pathophysiology. For example, an excellent Tc image and a very poor fluorescent image will be seen whenever trapping is active but organification of iodide is defective. This is most commonly seen in Hashimoto's disease but also occurs in certain types of dyshormonogenesis. Discordant images of this type will be illustrated later.

Thyroid imaging provides valuable information, but it has distinct limitations which must be appreciated.

One cannot make a diagnosis of hyperthyroidism from a thyroid image because the same pattern of a diffuse goiter, multinodular goiter, or solitary autonomously functioning thyroid adenoma may be seen in euthyroid patients. As already noted, Tc images in patients with Hashimoto's disease or dyshormonogenesis may be indistinguishable from images in patients with TDG.

Although the literature is replete with reports indicating that one technique or another is superior for the imaging of thyroid nodules, the reader should be wary. A thyroid nodule is a mass which is detected by physical examination. Some nodules produce defects on thyroid images and some do not. The presence or absence of defects on thyroid images depends upon a number of factors such as:

1. The functional activity of the nodule.

2. The tracer employed — e.g., some nodules which appear hypofunctional with radioactive iodine will be functional with Tc for reasons already discussed.

3. The size of the nodule. The smaller the nodule, the more often it will fail to produce a defect that is visible on the image.

4. The location of the nodule. A small functionless nodule in the thickest

TABLE 1-13. THYROID IMAGING WILL *NOT*

1. Make a diagnosis of hyperthyroidism
2. Make a diagnosis of a thyroid nodule (nodules)
3. Make a diagnosis of a thyroid cancer

portion of the lobe may be obscured by overlying or underlying normal thyroid tissue.

Furthermore, some non-nodular pathologic processes produce defects on images which are indistinguishable from the defects produced by nodules. Therefore, it is essential to correlate the physical findings with any defect observed on the image if one is to be certain that a palpable nodule actually coincides with a recognizable defect. Failure to do this can lead to gross misinterpretation of thyroid images.

In the absence of a palpable nodule the significance of any defect on a thyroid image remains in doubt. It could represent an impalpable nodule or it could be an area of fibrosis or inflammatory involvement. The more experienced the examiner, the less often will nodules that produce visible defects on imaging be impalpable.

By this point, it should be obvious that a thyroid image alone is not sufficient for a diagnosis of cancer. Thyroid cancers are uniformly hypofunctional, and, when they reach an adequate size for their location, they produce hypofunctional defects. However, nonmalignant nodules and nonmalignant non-nodular pathologic processes can produce identical defects. In fact, at least two thirds of hypofunctional nodules, even when firm and discrete, turn out to be benign.

The diagnosis of thyroid cancer is a clinical exercise in which the image plays primarily a negative role. Evidence of nodular function as good as or better than that within the rest of the thyroid is strong evidence *against* thyroid cancer. However, do not forget to repeat Tc images with radioactive iodine when necessary.

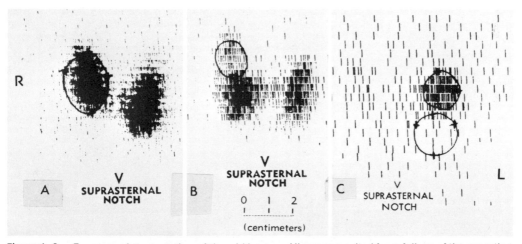

Figure 1–3. *Erroneous interpretation of thyroid images.* All errors resulted from failure of the reporting physician to examine the thyroid gland. *A,* The phantom cold nodule. This patient was referred for a scan because of the discovery of a nodule in the right thyroid lobe. A cold nodule was initially reported because of the asymmetry and absence of activity below the higher lying right lobe. On the scan shown the nodularity is outlined and includes the entire right lobe. *B,* The phantom hot nodule. A hot nodule in the lower pole of the right lobe was initially reported. On the scan shown the actual nodule was located in the upper pole and was hypofunctional. It was a carcinoma. *C,* A patient with a visible nodule reported as hot on the basis of imaging. Actually, the patient had two nodules—the larger visible nodule was hypofunctional, and the hot nodule was not visible but was easily palpable.

B. ULTRASOUND EVALUATION

Diagnostic ultrasound is a simple method by which one can differentiate a cystic from a solid thyroid nodule. Since ultrasound findings are not always reliable, and since we now employ diagnostic needling as part of our routine evaluation of thyroid nodules, we no longer use ultrasound. If the nodule is cystic it will contain fluid that may be aspirated. If it does not contain fluid, obviously it is solid, and we then obtain material for cytologic and histologic evaluation. Needling is more reliable and provides more information.

Imaging and ultrasound studies will now be illustrated.

Selected Current References

1. Vagenakis AG and Braverman LE: Thyroid function tests — which one? *Ann Intern Med* 84:607–608, 1976
2. Pilch BZ, Kahn CR, Ketcham AS, et al: Thyroid cancer after radioactive iodine diagnostic procedures in childhood. *Pediatrics* 51:898–902, 1973
3. Silverman C and Hoffman DA: Thyroid tumor risk from radiation during childhood. *Prev Med* 4:100–105, 1975
4. Foster RS, Jr: Thyroid irradiation and carcinogenesis. *Am J Surg* 130:608–611, 1975
5. Steinberg M, Cavalieri RR and Choy SH: Uptake of technetium 99-pertechnetate in a primary thyroid carcinoma: need for caution in evaluating nodules. *J Clin Endocrinol* 31:81–84, 1970
6. Alderson PO, Sumner HW and Siegel BA: The single palpable thyroid nodule. Evaluation by ^{99m}Tc-pertechnetate imaging. *Cancer* 37:258–265, 1976

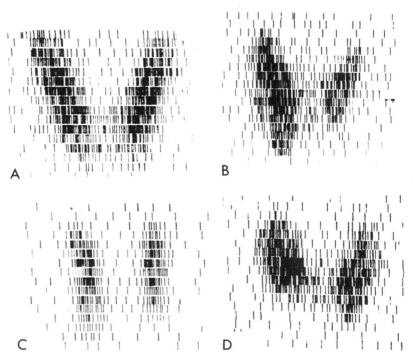

Figure 1–4. *Four thyroid scans from normal patients demonstrating varying shapes and degrees of asymmetry. A,* The usual normal scan. *B,* A longer right lobe. *C,* Poor representation of the isthmus. *D,* A longer left lobe.

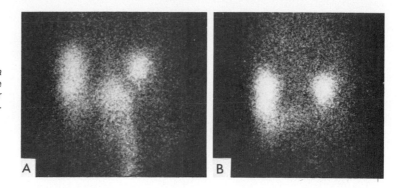

Figure 1-5 *Saliva artifact on gamma camera image. A,* The initial image shows a peculiar midline smear caused by the tracer. *B,* A repeat image after a drink of water.

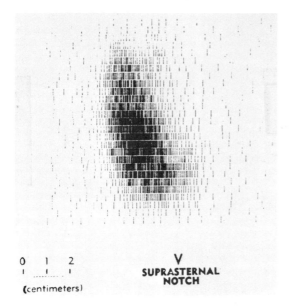

0 1 2
(centimeters)

V
SUPRASTERNAL
NOTCH

Figure 1-6. *Thyroidal hemiagenesis.*

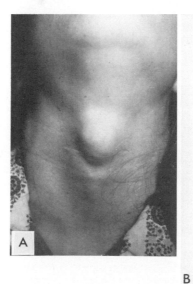

Figure 1-7. *Submental ectopic thyroid. A,* Anterior view. *B,* The fluorescent scan.

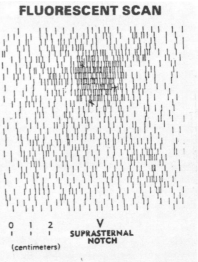

FLUORESCENT SCAN

0 1 2
(centimeters)

V
SUPRASTERNAL
NOTCH

B

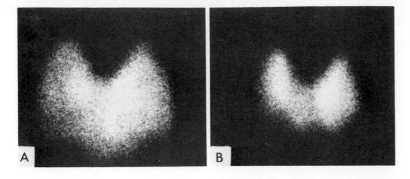

Figure 1-8. *Toxic diffuse goiter before and after therapy. A,* The initial image. *B,* The image after ^{131}I therapy.

Figure 1-9. *Toxic multinodular goiter before and after therapy. A,* The initial image. *B,* The image after ^{131}I therapy.

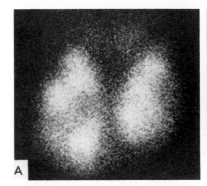
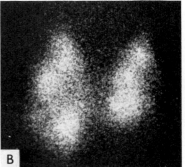

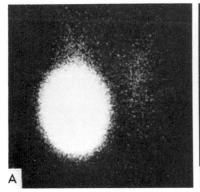
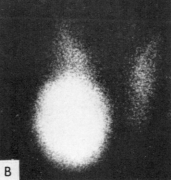

Figure 1-10. *Autonomously functioning thyroid adenoma. A,* The initial image. *B,* A repeat image after TSH stimulation.

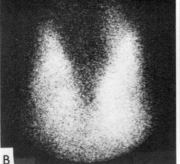
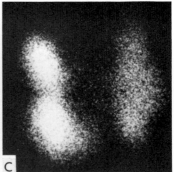

Figure 1-11. *Hashimoto's disease. A,* The fluorescent scan. *B,* the Tc image shows excellent trapping. *C,* A later stage in the disease shows irregular trapping resulting from patchy fibrosis.

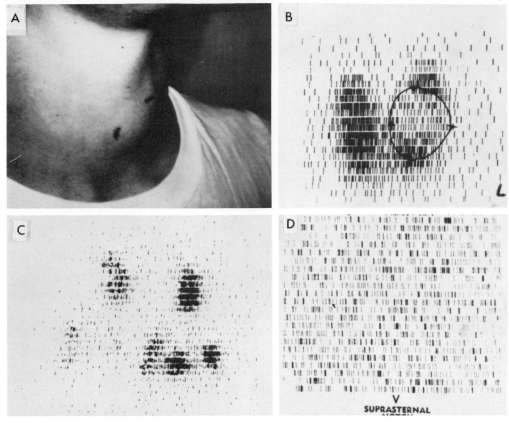

Figure 1–12. *A differentiated thyroid cancer. A,* The visible nodule. *B,* Nodule is hypofunctional on scanning. *C,* Residual ^{131}I concentrating in tissue after surgery. *D,* After ^{131}I therapy.

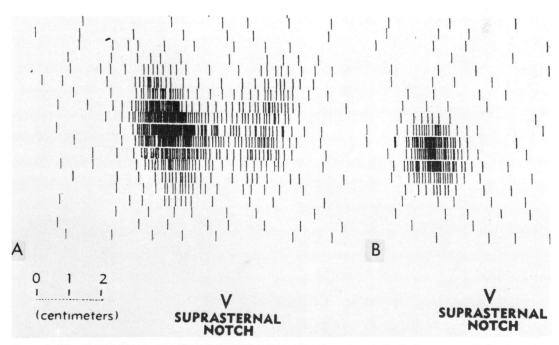

Figure 1–13. *Suppression scan demonstrating autonomous function. A,* Preliminary scan. *B,* Suppression scan reveals right lobe autonomously functioning thyroid adenoma.

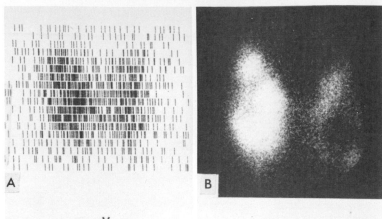

SUPRASTERNAL
NOTCH

Figure 1-14 *Superior resolution of gamma camera image compared to rectilinear scan. A*, The scan. *B*, The gamma camera image.

Figure 1-15. *The solid hypofunctional nodule. A*, The gamma camera image reveals an indentation of the lateral aspect of the left lobe, the site of the nodule. *B*, The ultrasound study reveals a solid pattern.

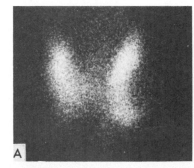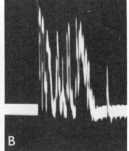

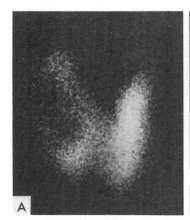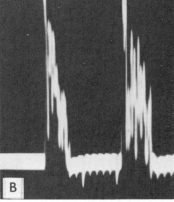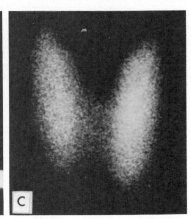

Figure 1-16. *A large cyst. A*, The gamma camera image. *B*, The ultrasound study. *C*, A repeat gamma camera image 3 months later, after regression of hemorrhage.

Figure 1-17. *A partially cystic nodule. A*, The gamma camera image reveals a defect in the left upper pole. *B*, The ultrasound study shows a gap in the echoes through about half the thickness of the nodule.

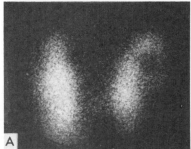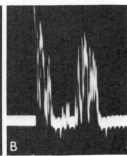

PART III. SELF-ASSESSMENT

These are difficult cases. Remember that the purpose of the exercise is the analysis of the problems. Do not be concerned about the "right" answer. More than one choice may have merit. If you work through these and all subsequent self-assessment sections, you should find that you have expanded your grasp of how to deal with thyroid patients.

CASE 1–1. HYPERTHYROIDISM WITH A LOW RAI

A 43 year old, divorced, delivery-room nurse reported a weight loss of 30 pounds in the past 3 to 4 months, increasing nervousness, tremor, heat intolerance, and palpitation. The heart rate was 130, the BP was 140/60, the reflexes were hyperactive, there was a marked hand tremor, and the thyroid gland was impalpable.

The FTI was 6.8, the T_3(RIA) 350 ng per 100 ml, and the RAI less than 1 per cent. A repeat RAI after TSH stimulation was 19 per cent. The thyroid image was normal.

With which of the following statements do you agree?

a. She is taking a large dose of either desiccated thyroid or a T_3–T_4 mixture but not a pure LT_4-containing product.

b. She may be taking a large dose of a pure LT_4-containing product.

c. One should check for uptake of radioactive iodine in the ovaries at 24 hours.

d. It would be better to check for uptake of radioactive iodine in the ovaries at 48 hours.

e. After administration of an oral tracer dose, a 48-hour urine assay for radioactive iodine might be helpful.

f. A TRH test should be done. A blunted response will make the diagnosis.

g. An ESR is important to rule out SAT.

h. The diffuse activity on the gamma camera image suggests that the patient has TDG. The RAI was blocked by iodide absorbed through the skin when the patient helped in preparing her delivery-room patients.

Comment—Case 1–1

a. This is not correct. She might be taking an overdose of a pure LT_4 product and still have a high T_3(RIA) value. Most of the T_3 measured in the serum is derived from T_4 by deiodination.

b. This could be correct.

c, d. A toxic struma ovarii is possible, and it would be better to check for ovarian tracer uptake at 48 hours when the bladder will be less likely to contain urine with radioactive iodine. It is important to ask the patient to urinate before counting, even at 48 hours.

e. If there is no uptake of radioactive iodine in the neck one would expect nearly all of the tracer to be excreted in the urine (i.e., 85 per cent or more). If this is not the case, one must consider the possibility of an ectopic location for thyroid tissue.

f. The TRH test is useless. The response will always be blunted when the FTI is elevated, regardless of the source of the excess thyroid hormone.

g. This patient does not have SAT. The response of the RAI to TSH stimulation is too vigorous for SAT in the hyperthyroid phase of the disease; the impalpable thyroid gland is inconsistent with SAT.

h. If you selected this one you get an A for imagination.

This patient did have factitious hyperthyroidism. She was presented to me as a diagnostic problem when I was a visiting professor in South Bend, Indiana.

CASE 1–2. A LOW FTI VALUE WITHOUT AN ELEVATED TSH(RIA) VALUE IN A PATIENT TAKING THYROID HORMONE

A 35 year old woman was referred for evaluation. She had been given a full replacement dose of thyroid hormone 3 months earlier but still complained of fatigue, lethargy, cold intolerance, and constipation. The FTI was 1.4, but the TSH(RIA) was 3 μU/ml.

With which of the following statements do you agree?

a. She is not taking her medication regularly.

b. Increase her dose of thyroid hormone — the TSH(RIA) value is wrong.

c. If TRH produces an augmented release of TSH, then the dose of thyroid should be increased. If the TSH response is blunted, the present dose is adequate, assuming the patient does not have secondary hypothyroidism.

d. She may be taking T_3.

e. She could only be taking desiccated thyroid; and if she is, the T_3-(RIA) level may be toward the upper level of normal.

f. She may be taking desiccated thyroid or a T_3–T_4 combination.

g. She is taking a pure LT_4 preparation.

h. The T_3 (RIA) value will be normal.

i. A fluorescent scan or a TSH stimulation test may provide useful information.

j. Her symptoms are probably unrelated to thyroid disease.

Comment — Case 1–2

a. This is possible if she had been given a pure T_3 preparation, did not need thyroid hormone, and was taking her medication only sporadically — i.e., often enough to partially suppress endogenous T_4 output.

b. This conclusion is not justified. There are too many alternate possibilities. Increasing her dose of medication may produce iatrogenic thyrotoxicosis.

c. The second part of this statement is correct. I am not sure about the first part and will not be until I have some TRH to work with. Wouldn't it be interesting if an accentuated response to TRH proves to be a more sensitive index of inadequate replacement (or early hypothyroidism) than a spontaneous elevation in the serum TSH concentration?

d, e, f, g, h. She could be taking either desiccated thyroid or a T_3–T_4 combination product. With either of these preparations it is common to find a slightly lowered FTI value, a TSH(RIA) value that is not elevated, and a T_3(RIA) value that is normal (occasionally elevated), indicating a disproportionate T_3 component in the serum hormonal pool. These laboratory data are not consistent with administration of a full dose of pure T_3 because the FTL in that case would be much lower. The FTI would be higher if pure LT_4 had been given. She was in fact taking desiccated thyroid, and the T_3(RIA) value was 145 ng per 100 ml.

i. A normal fluorescent scan or a normal response to TSH stimulation would suggest that she might not require thyroid hormone at all. Her fluorescent scan was normal (Fig. 1–18). Thyroid hormone was discontinued, and 2 months later her thyroid function studies were normal.

j. This is a reasonable conclusion. After all, without an elevated serum TSH concen-

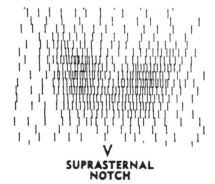

Figure 1-18. Normal fluorescent scan.

tration, it is safe to conclude that her symptoms are out of proportion to any possible minimal hormonal deficit that might be exposed by TRH testing, unless of course she had secondary hypothyroidism. Forget about tertiary.

CASE 1-3. GRAVES' DISEASE?

A 24 year old woman had been told she had Graves' disease after a thyroid scan 1 year earlier. No treatment was given. She had now been referred for a second opinion. In the previous 3 months she had gained 22 pounds and now weighed 152 pounds. Her height was 62 inches. She complained of tremor, nervousness, and difficulty climbing stairs. There was no palpitation, loose bowels, or heat intolerance, and the skin and reflexes were normal. The heart rate was 62. There was a moderate hand tremor. The thyroid gland was one and a half times normal size, but there were no nodules. The gamma camera image is shown in Figure 1–19B. The upper lids were at the limbus, and the sclera was exposed above the edge of the lower lids (Fig. 1–19A). The exophthalmometric measurements were 18 mm right and 17 mm left (upper limit of normal).

The FTI was 3.5, the T_3(RIA) was 195 ng per 100 ml, and the RAI was 37 per cent. A repeat RAI after 1 week of T_3, 50 μg twice a day, was 40 per cent.

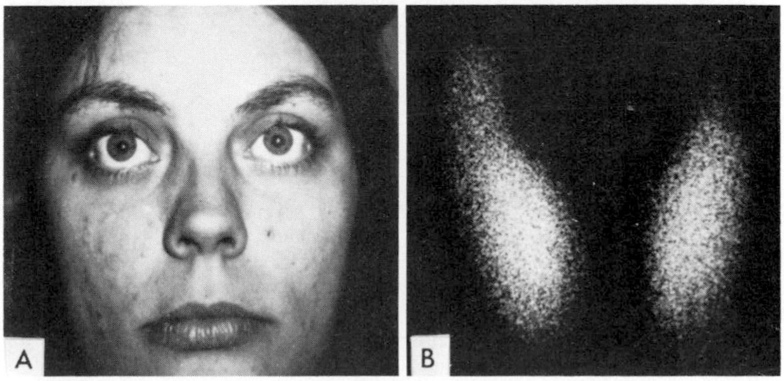

Figure 1-19. *A,* The patient. *B,* The gamma camera image.

With which of the following statements do you agree?

    a. The patient has Graves' disease.
    b. The patient has hyperthyroidism.
    c. If the TSH response to TRH is blunted, she has hyperthyroidism.
    d. Treatment is indicated.
    e. Observation is all that is required.

f. Her weight gain is incompatible with hyperthyroidism.

g. She has T_3 toxicosis.

Comment—Case 1–3

a. A diffuse goiter with a nonsuppressible RAI is diagnostic of Graves' disease.

b, c, d, e, and g. A diagnosis of hyperthyroidism requires clinical features of hyperthyroidism and elevated serum levels of thyroid hormone. This patient's clinical features are not impressive. The FTI is not elevated, and the T_3(RIA) of 195 ng per 100 ml does not move me. The TRH response should be blunted but tells us nothing more than the T_3 suppression test. These data are compatible with, but not diagnostic of, hyperthyroidism. Since a diagnosis of hyperthyroidism is not certain, treatment is not mandatory. This patient has been observed for 6 months without any significant change in her status.

f. Her obesity and weight gain do not exclude hyperthyroidism. In a series of 400 consecutive hyperthyroid patients I found that 58 were more than 21 per cent overweight. Five of 17 obese hyperthyroid patients had gained weight prior to treatment for their hyperthyroidism. Three gained more after treatment, and two lost weight after treatment.

CASE 1–4. NECK PAIN, SAT?

A 44 year old business executive's wife was referred for evaluation of neck pain of 2 months' duration. The patient complained of low grade fever and malaise. Ten years earlier she had been given x-ray therapy for SAT. She thought she was experiencing a recurrence of the disease. There had been no weight loss or palpitations. The heart rate was 118, and the temperature was 99° F. There was no tremor. The thyroid gland was tender, firm, and about twice the normal size.

The FTI was 4.8, the T_3(RIA) 210 ng per 100 ml, the RAI 1 per cent, and the ESR 48 mm/hour. A 48-hour urine collection contained 84 per cent of the tracer. The RAI after TSH stimulation was 9 per cent. The gamma camera image is shown in Figure 1–20.

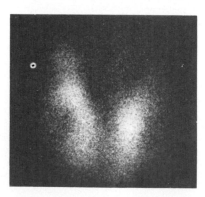

Figure 1–20. The gamma camera image obtained after TSH stimulation.

With which of the following statements do you agree?

a. The response to TSH stimulation and the nearly normal gamma camera image are incompatible with SAT.

b. The patient has TDG and has received iodide. The pain is a red herring.

c. A repeat gamma camera image in 3 months will look different.

d. The abnormality on the gamma camera image may only reflect the previous x-ray therapy.

e. The patient is neurotic and has factitious thyrotoxicosis. A substantial proportion of factitious thyrotoxic patients come from the families of executives.

f. She may have a toxic struma ovarii.

g. Recovery of only 84 per cent of the tracer in a 48-hour urine test suggests that she may have a toxic ovarian struma.

Comment—Case 1–4

a. This is a response to TSH which is commonly seen in SAT, a definite but slightly subnormal response. The irregular moth-eaten appearance of the right lobe is suggestive of the patchy involvement common in SAT.

b. What about the high ESR and the moth-eaten appearance of the right lobe?

c. The repeat image was entirely normal (Fig. 1–21). Of course, it might not have been even though the patient had SAT. Most, but not all, SAT patients recover within 3 months. Some have persistent goiter, and others have evidence of continuing activity of the inflammatory process when imaging is repeated.

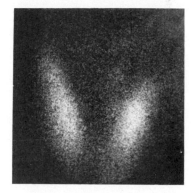

Figure 1–21. The repeat gamma camera image 3 months later after recovery from SAT.

d. I suppose this was possible.

e. Worth considering, but the high ESR, the slightly subnormal response to TSH, and the initial gamma camera image point away from factitious hyperthyroidism. Spontaneous complete recovery, of course, proves that the diagnosis of SAT was correct. Nevertheless, a proper attitude of skepticism is useful, so do not downgrade yourself too much for this choice.

f. Important to remember, but a real long shot with all the data pointing to SAT.

g. An 84 per cent recovery is about as complete a recovery as one will get with no significant retention in any location in the body. Some of the tracer is lost in the stool, and some is excreted through the respiratory tract. A much larger discrepancy would be expected if the patient had a toxic ovarian struma.

CASE 1–5. HYPERTHYROIDISM WITH A LOW RAI

A 49 year old woman was referred for treatment of hyperthyroidism. She had been hospitalized for an acute episode of cholecystitis with pancreatitis 1 month earlier, and 3 weeks earlier she had had a cholecystogram. While in the hospital, FTI values were 6.7 and 5.9 on two separate evaluations. These values were obtained 3 and 5 days after the cholecystogram. No RAI was done because of the cholecystogram. She was given propranolol, 40 mg four times a day, to control her tachycardia and was still taking the medication when first seen. She was also taking long-acting capsules of Combid twice daily. Her complaints included palpitation, tremor, loose bowels, and difficulty climbing stairs, but there had been no weight loss.

The skin was fine textured, the heart rate 64, the reflexes normal. The exophthalmometric measurements were 18 mm right and 18.5 mm left. Her appearance is shown in Figure 1–22. She weighed 148 pounds and was 61 inches tall. The thyroid gland was twice normal size, smooth, normal in consistency, and not tender.

The FTI was 3.7, the RAI 11 per cent, and the gamma camera image revealed a uniform tracer uptake in a small diffuse goiter.

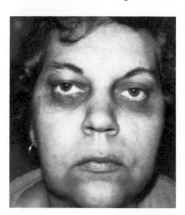

Figure 1–22. The patient.

With which of the following statements do you agree?

a. The patient had jodbasedow's disease, which is now subsiding spontaneously.

b. The patient had tachycardia from the pancreatitis, and the elevated FTI values were caused by the cholecystogram. She does not have hyperthyroidism.

c. She has hyperthyroidism, but the hyperthyroidism was suppressed by the iodide in the gallbladder contrast medium in conjunction with that in the Combid.

d. A TRH test might be of value.

e. A T_3 suppression test would be definitive, assuming all iodide-containing drugs are discontinued.

f. Discontinue propranolol and Combid.

g. Discontinue Combid, and repeat the FTI and RAI in 6 weeks.

h. Discontinue Combid, and repeat the FTI and RAI in 2 weeks.

i. This patient's weight, lack of weight loss, and facial appearance suggest that she is not hyperthyroid.

j. She might have had SAT while in the hospital and is now recovering.

Comment—Case 1–5

a. The absence of a nodular goiter makes this choice less appealing. Nevertheless, there have been cases reported of jodbasedow's phenomenon precipitated by the relatively small amount of iodine in radiographic contrast media.

b. The tachycardia might have been caused by the pancreatitis, but the FTI is not influenced by iodide in any form. She was hyperthyroid all right.

c. A distinct possibility and one that seems to have been true. Two weeks later the FTI rebounded to 6.2, and the RAI was 50 per cent. The heart rate increased to 80, even though propranolol had been continued.

d. The TRH response should have been blunted; if not, it would have suggested that the previous hyperthyroidism was temporary and is now clearing.

e.   A T_3 suppression test could have been performed, looking for a rising RAI value—e.g., 11 per cent baseline and 40 to 50 per cent while on T_3. However, I elected simply to wait 2 weeks.

f, g, h.   While waiting, continuing propranolol was a good idea to minimize the tachycardia which might have occurred without this protection if the hyperthyroidism had rebounded vigorously. There is no need to wait more than 2 weeks. Almost every month I receive a call from a physician who has been told by the director of his hospital nuclear medicine laboratory that he must wait 6 weeks after iodide exposure for a valid RAI. When one is looking for hyperthyroidism this is bad advice. The hyperthyroid patient with TDG will almost always have an elevated RAI value within 2 weeks. (This may not be the case with TMNG or toxic AFTA.) If not, the patient is not very hyperthyroid. In fact, the rapidity with which the RAI rebounds is a good test for hyperthyroidism. As already noted, this patient's RAI increased from 11 to 50 per cent in 2 weeks. I have seen it rise from 8 to 70 per cent in 1 week.

i.   Her hyperthyroidism was temporarily suppressed by iodide. However, these clinical features are not definitive.

j.   A reasonable thought, but not borne out by subsequent events.

CASE 1–6.   HASHIMOTO'S DISEASE

June, 1975.   A 24 year old woman was referred for evaluation of a goiter discovered on a routine examination. She had noted some hoarseness and loss of pep but no other symptoms of thyroid dysfunction. The skin and reflexes were normal. The thyroid gland was diffusely enlarged to twice the normal size and was quite firm. The heart rate was 70. The FTI was 0.2, the TSH(RIA) 80 μU/ml, the antimicrosomal antibody titer positive at 1 to 100,000. The gamma camera image revealed a diffuse goiter with relatively uniform trapping of the tracer (Fig. 1–23).

Treatment was begun with LT_4, 0.15 mg daily, and the patient was asked to return in 2 months.

August, 1975.   The patient reported a definite increase in pep and energy. Her hoarseness had cleared. The heart rate was 80. The thyroid gland was unchanged in size. The FTI was 4.2, and the TSH(RIA) was 1.5 μU/ml. She was advised to continue LT_4, 0.15 mg daily, and return in 1 year.

January, 1976.   The patient returned prematurely because of extreme nervousness, a 5 pound weight loss, and disturbing palpitation. The heart rate was 120, and there was a marked hand tremor. The thyroid gland was unchanged in size. The FTI was 5.6, and the T_3(RIA) was 220 ng per 100 ml.

With which of the following statements do you agree?

a.   She is taking more thyroid hormone than ordered.

b.   She has TDG; the previous diagnosis of hypothyroidism was based

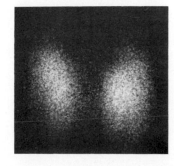

Figure 1–23.   The gamma camera image.

upon erroneous laboratory data which were inconsistent with the lack of clinical features of hypothyroidism.

    c.   She has Hashitoxicosis.

    d.   An immediate RAI would be helpful.

    e.   Discontinue thyroid hormone and recheck in 6 weeks.

    f.   A blunted response on TRH testing will be of great value.

    g.   The excellent trapping demonstrated on the initial gamma camera image was inconsistent with the diagnosis of hypothyroidism.

OF THE FOLLOWING THREE OPTIONS, SELECT THE ONE WHICH IS MOST LIKELY

    h.   An RAI at this point will be less than 5 per cent.

    i.   An RAI at this point will be no more than 25 per cent.

    j.   An RAI at this point might be more than 50 per cent.

Comment — Case 1–6

    a.   This is possible, but she wasn't taking an excess dose of thyroid hormone.

    b.   She did have Graves' disease, and her previous laboratory data were not erroneous. To expect that the FTI and TSH were both wrong and that the very high antibody titer was coincidental is not reasonable.

    c, d.   The RAI was 21 per cent. This test immediately exposes the underlying pathophysiology—i.e., diffuse nonsuppressible function (the gamma camera image was unchanged)—and makes the diagnosis of Graves' disease. The previous data were diagnostic of Hashimoto's disease. Put the two together and you have Hashitoxicosis—i.e., Graves' disease in which the expression of the hyperthyroidism is limited by the concurrent Hashimoto's disease. The development of hyperthyroid features was precipitated by the administration of thyroid hormone. Why there was a change from practically no thyroid hormone output initially to an output adequate (when combined with the exogenous hormone) to produce thyrotoxicosis is unclear. This is a very unusual sequence of events.

    e.   Thyroid hormone should be discontinued, but not until after the RAI value is obtained. Otherwise, the diagnosis of a nonsuppressible RAI will be missed.

    f.   The TRH test would be useless. The response is always blunted in hyperthyroidism regardless of the mechanism. This tells us nothing we do not already know.

    g.   Excellent trapping with impaired organification of iodide is the characteristic finding in early Hashimoto's disease.

    h, i, j.   One would expect that the RAI would be unsuppressed, but would still not be very high; otherwise, the patient would have had higher FTI and T_3(RIA) values. After all, these values measure the summation of endogenous secretion and exogenous hormone. The values are only modestly elevated. Furthermore, in the face of known Hashimoto's disease, one might anticipate some limitation in the endogenous functional capacity. Therefore, the best guess is *i*.

    Incidentally, after discontinuation of thyroid hormone for 2 months, the patient was mildly hypothyroid. She has done well on LT_4, 0.05 mg daily. This is likely to be an unstable situation and will be followed carefully.

Selected Current References

1. Rapoport B and Ingbar SH: Production of triiodothyronine in normal human subjects and in patients with hyperthyroidism. *Am J Med* 56:586–591, 1974
2. Blum M, Kranjac T, Park CM, et al: Thyroid storm after cardiac angiography with iodinated contrast medium. *JAMA* 235:2324–2325, 1976
3. Editorial: Iodide-induced thyrotoxicosis. *Lancet* 2:1072–1073, 1972
4. Bremner WJ and Griep RJ: Graves' thyrotoxicosis following primary thyroid failure. *JAMA* 235:1361, 1976
5. Stewart JC and Vidor GI: Thyrotoxicosis induced by iodine contamination of food — a common unrecognised condition? *Brit Med J* 1:372–375, 1976

CHAPTER 2

HYPERTHYROIDISM

PART I. PATHOPHYSIOLOGY

Hyperthyroidism is a complex clinical syndrome resulting from an excess of thyroid hormone. Since thyroid hormone affects every organ system, the clinical features of hyperthyroidism are usually multiple and diffuse. The intensity of the signs and symptoms depends not only upon the duration and severity of the disease but also upon the general health status of the patient.

Table 2–1 is a list of the various types of hyperthyroidism as encountered in the medical literature. Each type will be described briefly in terms of pathophysiology. The entities included in this list are not necessarily pathophysiologically distinct. The intention of this table is to provide a very inclusive listing of variations on the general theme of hyperthyroidism. For rare cases or those with which I have limited or no experience, literature citations will be provided.

TOXIC DIFFUSE GOITER (TDG, GRAVES' DISEASE)

This is by far the most common form of hyperthyroidism. The thyroid gland is diffusely involved, and all of the functioning tissue is hyperactive. The driving

TABLE 2–1. TYPES OF HYPERTHYROIDISM

1. Toxic diffuse goiter (Graves' disease)
2. Toxic multinodular goiter
3. Toxic autonomously functioning thyroid adenoma (AFTA)
4. Transient hyperthyroidism of subacute thyroiditis (SAT)
5. Iatrogenic hyperthyroidism
6. Factitious hyperthyroidism
7. T_3 toxicosis
8. Apathetic hyperthyroidism
9. Hyperthyroidism resulting from abnormal ectopic thyroid stimulators
10. Toxic struma ovarii
11. Hyperthyroidism resulting from functioning metastatic thyroid cancer
12. Jodbasedow's disease
13. Neonatal hyperthyroidism
14. Thyroid storm (crisis)
15. Hyperthyroidism resulting from excessive pituitary TSH secretion

mechanism is as yet unknown. LATS or some variant thereof, although a common accompaniment of the disease, seems to me unlikely to be the cause. For the present, I prefer the view that LATS is simply another manifestation of Graves' disease.

Hyperthyroidism is only one part of the syndrome of Graves' disease. The other elements include ophthalmopathy, dermopathy, and acropachy — features which may precede, accompany, or follow the expression of the hyperthyroidism itself. Restoration of the euthyroid state seems to have no regular influence on the course of these phenomena.

TOXIC MULTINODULAR GOITER (TMNG)

This is another disorder characterized by hypersecretion of thyroid hormone. In this case the hypersecretion seems to have been grafted upon a pre-existing goiter of long-standing duration. The goiter of TMNG is characteristically present for 10 or more years before the hyperthyroidism begins. In contrast, the goiter of TDG usually develops concurrently with the hyperthyroidism and seldom precedes the hyperthyroidism by more than a few months. The abnormal physiology appears to be a development of widespread functional autonomy. The nodular portions of the goiter may participate in the hypersecretory process or may be functionless by virtue of prior degeneration. Patients with TMNG are usually older than those with TDG — most of them are over 50 years old. There are none of the associated phenomena of Graves' disease with TMNG. Bilateral upper lid retraction may lead to the erroneous conclusion that Graves' ophthalmopathy is present. However, the regression of this finding after restoration of the euthyroid state will clarify this issue.

Of course, it is possible to have Graves' disease in conjunction with a multinodular goiter, but this is uncommon. One must take care to differentiate an irregular or lobulated goiter of Graves' disease from a multinodular goiter. In practice, this is not difficult. The goiter of TMNG is always large and bulky, the patient is older, the hyperthyroidism is milder, and the absence of the associated findings of Graves' disease makes the distinction between these two forms of hyperthyroidism rather clear. TDG is about 20 times as common as TMNG in my laboratory.

TOXIC AUTONOMOUSLY FUNCTIONING THYROID ADENOMA (AFTA)

In this case we have an autonomous hypersecreting nodule in an otherwise normal (at least macroscopically) thyroid gland. The hypersecretion of the AFTA produces suppression of pituitary TSH release, which in turn suppresses function of the extranodular thyroid tissue. Toxic AFTA are distinctly unusual lesions in the United States. In my laboratory, TDG is about 40 times as common. Nontoxic AFTA are present about seven times as often as the toxic variety. Toxic AFTA resemble TMNG in that, with rare exceptions, they occur in older patients. Also, these patients do not have the associated phenomena of Graves' disease.

Since the hypersecretion arises from the AFTA, ablation of this lesion, either with ^{131}I or surgically, is all that is necessary for a cure.

Miller has shown that patients with AFTA often have microscopic lesions elsewhere in the thyroid gland that seem to have functional characteristics identical to those of macroscopic AFTA. In association with a large AFTA, smaller AFTA are occasionally present somewhere else in the gland. These are most often recognized on a suppression image. With about equal infrequency one may see two or three macroscopic AFTA of similar size in the same thyroid gland. However, toxicity is almost always associated with a single lesion. Toxic AFTA are generally 3 cm or larger in diameter.

I know of only one reported case in which removal of one toxic AFTA was followed by the development of a recurrent toxic AFTA. This was reported in a Dutch paper. It should be noted that in Europe toxic AFTA account for up to one-third of the cases of hyperthyroidism, compared to less than 5 per cent in the United States. The basis for this geographic difference is unknown.

References

1. Hamburger JI: Solitary autonomously functioning lesions. *Am J Med* 58:740–748, 1975
2. Wiener JD: A systemic approach to the diagnosis of Plummer's disease (autonomous goitre) with a review of 224 cases. *Neth J Med* 18:218–233, 1975

TRANSIENT HYPERTHYROIDISM OF SUBACUTE THYROIDITIS (SAT)

In the phase of this disease in which the inflammatory process is active there is characteristically a discharge of preformed thyroid hormone into the circulation. Most of the time this is not associated with many of the features of hyperthyroidism. Occasionally there is tachycardia, tremor, or loose bowels. The process is usually mild, always self-limited, and generally rather brief (a matter of only a few weeks). As the inflammatory reaction regresses, hormonal stores are depleted, since new synthesis of hormone is temporarily suspended. The hyperthyroidism then spontaneously subsides and is often followed by a brief period of hypothyroidism until normal hormonal synthesis and secretion recover.

IATROGENIC HYPERTHYROIDISM

This is a rather common problem. There are two mechanisms that can give rise to this disease. The first and most frequent is simply the administration of too large a dose of thyroid hormone to a patient who has either no significant endogenous secretory capacity or a normally suppressible thyroid gland. There are a number of reasons why too large a dose may be ordered:

1. The physician is treating the patient's symptoms — symptoms which are not related to hypothyroidism (e.g., fatigue) — and fails to monitor the serum hormone concentrations or to appreciate the clinical features of hyperthyroidism.

2. The physician orders Cytomel, a pure T_3-containing product, and is misled by persistently low serum T_4 values into thinking that even higher doses are needed. One should not use this drug for maintenance therapy. It is more costly than T_4, provides spiking rather than sustained serum levels, and exposes the patient to the risk of misinterpreted laboratory values. If the physician insists upon using T_3, he should not exceed the dose needed to suppress the elevated TSH(RIA) level (which presumably would have been obtained to establish the diagnosis of hypothyroidism prior to institution of treatment).

3. A similar problem can occur if one orders $T_3 - T_4$ combinations and monitors treatment with a serum T_4 or FTI. Since the T_3 component is not measured, the patient may be overtreated when the FTI is beyond the midnormal level. These products are more costly than T_4 and are best avoided. Incidentally, desiccated thyroid products also commonly have an inappropriate excess T_3 component, which is another reason for avoiding them.

There is a second mechanism which may lead to iatrogenic hyperthyroidism, even when only physiologic doses of thyroid hormone are given. This occurs when the patient's thyroid gland is not normally suppressible. Hyperthyroidism then results from the combination of the exogenous hormone and the continued secretion of endogenous hormone. Again, there is more than one situation in which one should anticipate this problem:

1. The euthyroid patient with a diffuse goiter may be in the euthyroid stage of TDG. Thyroid function is nonsuppressible but not hypersecretory. The addition of exogenous thyroid hormone causes hyperthyroidism. Therefore, whenever one administers thyroid hormone to a patient with a diffuse goiter, it is prudent to check the suppressibility of the RAI before pursuing the treatment too long, particularly if the goiter fails to regress. Also, one should remember that the demonstration of suppressible function at one time does not preclude the subsequent development of nonsuppressible function. Hence, all goiter patients treated with thyroid hormone should be observed annually.

2. Similarly, patients with multinodular goiters or single functional nodules may prove to have autonomous function and thus be intolerant of exogenous thyroid hormone. Some degree of autonomous function should be assumed to be present in all long-standing goiters in elderly patients.

3. After ^{131}I therapy or thyroidectomy for hyperthyroidism the thyroid remnant may be nonsuppressible or may recover nonsuppressible function years, even many years, later. In the interim, thyroid hormone may be not only well tolerated but even needed to correct temporary hypothyroidism. The recovery of nonsuppressible function may necessitate discontinuation of the previously tolerated exogenous thyroid hormone.

A variant on this theme is the patient who has a thyroid remnant which is incapable of sustaining the euthyroid state but is nevertheless nonsuppressible. Such a patient must be given a supplemental dose of thyroid hormone. Unfortunately, after a satisfactory balance is achieved, there is no guarantee that the function of the remaining thyroid tissue will be stable. It may either increase or decrease.

FACTITIOUS HYPERTHYROIDISM

In this situation, the patient covertly takes large doses of thyroid hormone to satisfy some neurotic tendency. Paramedical personnel, nurses, pharmacists, medical students, and their spouses should be particularly suspect. The diagnosis is established when the hyperthyroid patient has elevated serum concentrations of thyroid hormone and a suppressed RAI which responds to TSH stimulation, after which one can demonstrate a normal thyroid gland with an imaging procedure. A toxic struma ovarii would give the same findings and must be considered when the patient is female.

If the patient happens to take T_3, the serum T_4 and FTI levels will be low. A T_3-(RAI) value would be required to clarify the situation.

Reference

1. Gorman CA, Wahner HW and Tauxe WN: Metabolic malingerers: Patients who deliberately induce or perpetuate a hypermetabolic or hypometabolic state. *Am J Med* 48:708–714, 1970

T_3 TOXICOSIS

T_3 toxicosis is hyperthyroidism resulting from the secretion of excessive quantities of T_3 without a simultaneous excess output of T_4. Criteria for the diagnosis of T_3 toxicosis include:

1. An elevated T_3(RIA) value which is not the result of increased TBG concentration.
2. A normal FTI value.
3. Clinical hyperthyroidism.
4. A normal or increased RAI value which is nonsuppressible.
5. A blunted TSH response to TRH.

T_3 toxicosis should be anticipated in the following clinical settings:
1. Toxic AFTA.
2. Toxic multinodular goiter.
3. Recurrent thyrotoxicosis after thyroidectomy or ^{131}I therapy.
4. Early in the development of toxic diffuse goiter.

The concept of T_3 toxicosis carries the implication that without a T_3(RIA) value the diagnosis will be missed. For more than 2 years I have been obtaining T_3(RIA) values in all suspected hyperthyroid patients. More than 1000 patients have been tested, and about half had hyperthyroidism. There were three patients in whom the criteria for T_3 toxicosis were met, and in all three the diagnosis was obvious from the clinical evaluation. FTI values, although not elevated, were at or near the upper limit of normal. In none of these patients was the diagnosis of such urgency that immediate treatment was essential to the patient's welfare.

Nevertheless, there are rare cases of this type, and one should be on the alert in the special circumstances just listed. The problem is most important in the elderly patient with long-standing multinodular goiter and a compromised cardiovascular system. These patients tolerate even mild hyperthyroidism poorly, and have a tendency to develop either atrial fibrillation, congestive heart failure, or both. When it is finally available, the TRH test will be of value in supporting the diagnosis, for it is obvious that such a patient should not be subjected to T_3 suppression testing. Since these patients should be prepared with antithyroid drugs prior to ^{131}I therapy, the clinical response to administration of these drugs, correlated with falling T_3(RIA) values, is also of diagnostic value.

Reference

1. Ivy HK, Wahner HW and Gorman CA: Triiodothyronine (T_3) toxicosis: Its role in Graves' disease. *Arch Intern Med* 128:529–534, 1971

APATHETIC HYPERTHYROIDISM (MASKED HYPERTHYROIDISM)

My teacher used to say (and maybe still does) that the mask of masked hyperthyroidism is over the eyes of the physician. I prefer the term apathetic, for by now every physician should think of hyperthyroidism as a possible explanation for weight loss and tachycardia in the elderly patient with goiter. A flattened affect and the absence of nervous hyperactivity are principal features of this form of hyperthyroidism. These patients may have anorexia, and if they do, the weight loss may be startling. The presenting event may be atrial fibrillation with congestive heart failure. There is no special pathophysiologic feature that distinguishes these patients from other patients with hyperthyroidism.

HYPERTHYROIDISM RESULTING FROM ECTOPIC THYROID STIMULATORS

Certain tumors including choriocarcinoma, embryonal carcinoma of the testis, and hydatidiform mole are capable of producing humoral substances with thyroid-stimulating properties which have caused hyperthyroidism. They are rare. I have never seen a case. The hyperthyroidism could be treated with ^{131}I if the tumor could not be ablated.

References

1. Karp PJ, Hershman JM, Richmond S, Goldstein DP and Selenkow HA: Thyrotoxicosis from molar thyrotropin. *Arch Intern Med* 132:432–436, 1973
2. Cohen JD and Utiger RD: Metastatic choriocarcinoma associated with hyperthyroidism. *J Clin Endocrinol* 30:423–429, 1970
3. Steigbigel NH, Oppenheim JJ, Fishman LM and Carbone PP: Metastatic embryonal carcinoma of the testis associated with elevated plasma TSH-like activity and hyperthyroidism. *New Eng J Med* 271:345–349, 1964

TOXIC STRUMA OVARII

This is another rare condition which I have yet to see. Since this condition causes an elevated FTI and a suppressed RAI value (in the neck), it must be included in the differential diagnosis along with the hyperthyroidism of SAT and factitious hyperthyroidism. Valuable differential points that favor toxic struma ovarii include a normal response to TSH stimulation, no goiter, no elevation of ESR, and, of course, the pathognomonic finding of a mass concentrating radioactive iodine in the area of the ovary.

Reference

1. Kempers RD, Dockerty MB, Hoffman DL and Bartholomew LG: Struma ovarii — ascitic, hyperthyroid, and asymptomatic syndromes. *Ann Intern Med* 72:883–893, 1970

HYPERTHYROIDISM RESULTING FROM FUNCTIONING METASTATIC THYROID CANCER

This rare entity crops up in the literature every few years. Once again, I have never seen it. One should not infer that the cancer tissue is hyperfunctional — it is not. Function per unit mass is less than that of normal thyroid tissue. However, if the mass of the tumor is great enough, by its very bulk it may produce enough thyroid hormone to cause toxicity. These cancers may also produce humoral substances with thyroid-stimulating properties which presumably would compound the problem.

Reference

1. Ghose MK, Genuth SM, Abellera RM, Friedman S and Lidsky I: Functioning primary thyroid carcinoma and metastases producing hyperthyroidism. *J Clin Endocrinol* 33:639–646, 1971

JODBASEDOW'S DISEASE

The induction of hyperthyroidism by the administration of iodide has received renewed attention in Boston in the past few years. This is most likely to happen if iodide is given to a patient with a multinodular goiter. These goiters may have the potential to produce hyperthyroidism, but under ordinary circumstances they are prevented from expressing this potential because of both inefficient utilization of iodide and the limited amount of iodide ordinarily available. When large quantities of iodide are administered, the secretory activity may increase to the degree necessary for the development of hyperthyroidism. In my experience, this condition is seen most often in asthmatic patients who have been treated with iodides for mucolytic purposes. However, it has been reported in such unusual situations as after the administration of iodinated contrast media.

References

1. Vagenakis AG, Wang C, Burger A, Maloof F, Braverman LE and Ingbar SH: Iodide-induced thyrotoxicosis in Boston. *New Eng J Med* 287:523–527, 1972
2. Blum M, Kranjac T, Park CM and Englemen RM: Thyroid storm after cardiac angiography with iodinated contrast medium. *JAMA* 235:2324–2325, 1976

NEONATAL HYPERTHYROIDISM (SEE ALSO P. 275)

Neonatal hyperthyroidism has been thought to result either from transplacental transfer of LATS to the fetus in utero from a mother who has or has had Graves' disease or from an inherited, genetically conditioned disease. The former lasts only a few weeks until the infant has metabolized the LATS. The latter may be more prolonged. Both are very uncommon.

References

1. Riopel DA and Mullins CE: Congenital thyrotoxicosis with paroxysmal atrial tachycardia. *Pediatrics* 50:140–144, July, 1972
2. Hollingsworth DR, Mabry CC and Eckerd JM: Hereditary aspects of Graves' disease in infancy and childhood. *Pediatrics* 81:446–459, 1972

THYROID STORM (CRISIS)

Thyroid storm is defined as an exacerbation (usually acute) of all of the features of hyperthyroidism. Prominent manifestations are tachycardia, with heart rates of 160 or more per minute, and fever, occasionally of alarming degree. Thyroid storm is almost exclusively associated with TDG. It is seen most often when an unprepared patient is subjected to the added stress of major surgery. Storm also may be precipitated by an infection in a patient with severe long-standing TDG. Iodine-131 therapy has been incriminated as a cause of thyroid storm on rare occasions. I have never experienced this problem, probably because I prepare severely toxic patients with antithyroid drugs before giving [131]I.

My personal experience with thyroid storm is very limited because I deal exclusively with outpatients. Nevertheless, I do offer telephone advice to anxious physicians who have had to face this problem unexpectedly. After outlining my usual regimen, I offer to come to the hospital to see the patient if there is insufficient improvement in 24 hours. So far, I have not had to make good on this offer.

Reference

1. Shafer, RB and Nuttall FQ: Thyroid crisis induced by radioactive iodine. *J Nucl Med* 12:262–264, 1970

HYPERTHYROIDISM RESULTING FROM EXCESSIVE PITUITARY TSH SECRETION

A few children with TSH-secreting pituitary tumors have been described. When I see one, I will publish the case.

Reference

1. Hamilton CR, Jr, Adams LC and Maloof F: Hyperthyroidism due to thyrotropin-producing pituitary chromophobe adenoma. *New Eng J Med* 283:1077–1079, 1970

Miscellaneous Current References

1. Green WL: Humoral and genetic factors in thyrotoxic Graves' disease and neonatal thyrotoxicosis. *JAMA* 235:1449–1450, 1976
2. Cave WT, Jr, and Dunn JT: Choriocarcinoma with hyperthyroidism: Probable identity of the thyrotropin with human chorionic gonadotropin. *Ann Intern Med* 85:60–63, 1976

PART II.   CLINICAL DIAGNOSIS OF HYPERTHYROIDISM

The cardinal clinical features that suggest a working diagnosis of hyperthyroidism include:

1. Ophthalmopathy.
2. Goiter.
3. Tremor.
4. Tachycardia.
5. Weight loss.

These easily documented findings indicate the need to search for further corroboration by obtaining a history and performing a physical examination of each of the systems likely to be involved.

A.   THE EYES

History.   The patient may report changes in appearance, resulting from protrusion of the globes, retraction of the upper eyelids, periorbital edema, chemosis, extraoculomotor muscle imbalance, or varying combinations of these abnormalities. The principal complaints other than changes in appearance include lacrimation, photophobia, foreign body sensation, retro-orbital pain, diplopia, and, rarely, diminished visual acuity or constricted visual fields when there is severe involvement.

Physical Findings.   The ophthalmic features of Graves' disease are generally classified in two categories, noninfiltrative and infiltrative.

1. NONINFILTRATIVE OPHTHALMOPATHY, i.e., changes relating to an elevation in the level of thyroid hormone in the circulation regardless of cause. As a result there is a retraction of the upper eyelids. This finding probably results from excessive activity of the sympathetic nervous system, producing spasm of Müller's muscle, an integral part of the retractile mechanism of the upper eyelid.

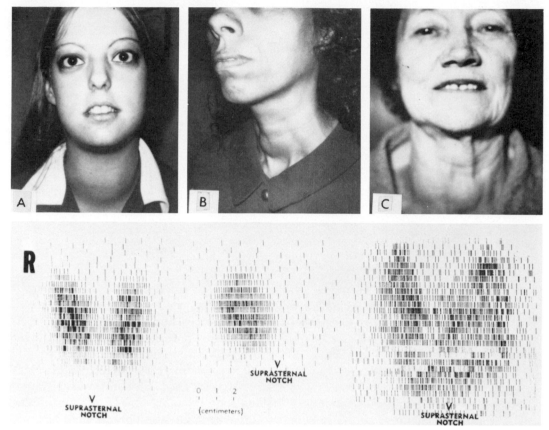

Figure 2–1. *The faces of hyperthyroidism. A,* Toxic diffuse goiter. *B,* Toxic autonomously functioning thyroid adenoma. *C,* Toxic multinodular goiter.

Similar retraction can be caused by fright. Since the underlying mechanism is an excess of thyroid hormone, this change may be seen with not only toxic diffuse goiter but also toxic multinodular goiter, toxic AFTA, and every other form of hyperthyroidism.

The key to the diagnosis is awareness of the normal lid positions. Normally the upper lid covers one-half or more of the distance from the limbus to the pupil (Fig. 2–2 *A*). With minimal lid retraction the edge of the lid may lie at the limbus

Figure 2–2. *Graves' ophthalmopathy— diagrammatic. A,* Normal. *B,* Upper lid retraction. *C,* Marked upper lid retraction. *D,* Abnormal upper and lower lid positions— proptosis.

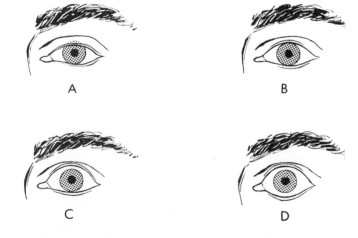

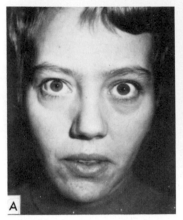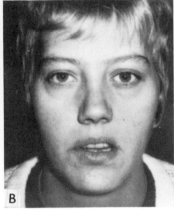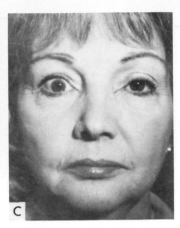

Figure 2–3. *A*, Upper lid retraction (noninfiltrative ophthalmopathy). *B*, Improvement after treatment of hyperthyroidism. *C*, Unilateral upper lid retraction.

(Fig. 2–2 *B*). This is abnormal. It is not necessary for the sclera to be exposed (Fig. 2–2 *C*) for one to conclude that lid retraction has occurred. By contrast, note that the normal position of the edge of the lower lid is at the limbus (Fig. 2–2 *A–C*). This lid position is not altered in noninfiltrative ophthalmopathy, for the retractile mechanism of the lower lid is much less effective than that of the upper. Thus, exposure of sclera between the edge of the lower lid and the limbus usually signifies that there is actual proptosis of the globe and that infiltrative involvement is present (Fig. 2–2 *D*). Retraction of the upper lid may be seen in noninfiltrative ophthalmopathy alone or in conjunction with infiltrative ophthalmopathy. However, failure of the lower lid to cover the sclera usually indicates proptosis, i.e., infiltrative ophthalmopathy.

Since upper lid retraction usually is a simple consequence of hyperthyroidism per se, it is regularly reversible with restoration of the euthyroid state (Fig. 2–3 *A* and *B*). However, upper lid retraction due to fibrous shortening of the levator palpebrae superioris is also possible as part of the infiltrative form of the disease. These changes are not reversible. A possible clue as to whether lid retraction is the result of infiltrative or noninfiltrative ophthalmopathy is the symmetry of the change. Whenever the lid retraction is asymmetrical, one should

TABLE 2–2. MANIFESTATIONS OF INFILTRATIVE OPHTHALMOPATHY

I. Complications Resulting from Increased Intraorbital Pressure
  A. Proptosis
    1. Exposure keratitis
    2. Corneal ulceration
    3. Optic nerve injury from traction or compression at the optic foramen
  B. Interference with venous drainage of the orbit
    1. Periorbital edema
    2. Chemosis
    3. Orbital pain
    4. Glaucoma
II. Complications Resulting from Extraoculomotor Muscle Involvement
  A. Muscular paresis or paralysis
  B. Muscular fibrosis and shortening; strabismus
  C. Lagophthalmos

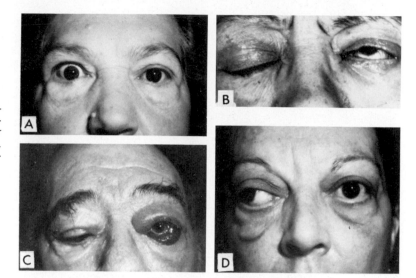

Figure 2–4. *Features of infiltrative ophthalmopathy. A,* Periorbital edema and unilateral upper lid retraction. *B,* Severe chemosis. *C,* Lagophthalmos. *D,* Lateral rectus contraction.

be suspicious that the infiltrative form of the disease is involved and should guard against offering a favorable prognosis (Fig. 2–3 *C*). Of course, when there are features of infiltrative ophthalmopathy in addition to lid retraction one should be particularly hesitant to predict the future course.

2. INFILTRATIVE OPHTHALMOPATHY. This finding is considered pathognomonic of Graves' disease. The various elements of this process may be attributed to the effects of an infiltration of the retrobulbar space and the extraoculomotor muscles by an acid mucopolysaccharide substance, fat, edema fluid, and various inflammatory cells. As a result, several types of phenomena may be seen.

One of the most common features of infiltrative ophthalmopathy is periorbital edema (Fig. 2–4 *A*). Injection and edema of the conjunctiva (chemosis) may become so severe that there is prolapse of the conjunctiva over the lid (Fig. 2–4 *C*). The usual complaints derived from chemosis include excessive lacrimation, photophobia, and foreign body sensation.

Lagophthalmos — i.e., inability of the upper lid to cover the globe — results from both shortening of the levator, which limits the downward movement of the lid, and proptosis, which makes it more difficult for the upper lid to cover the globe (Fig. 2–4 *B*). The inferior rectus muscle is the most commonly involved

Figure 2–5. *Use of the Hertel exophthalmometer.* Relatively minor deviations from normal may be masked if the lids accommodate and cover the globes reasonably well. However, an occasional patient has truly dramatic proptosis for which only orbital decompression can provide a satisfactory cosmetic solution (Fig. 2–6).

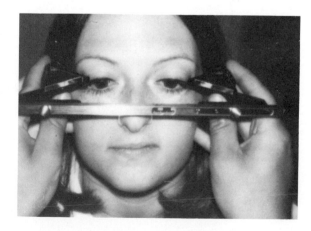

muscle affecting movement of the globe; as the fibrotic process progresses, the eye will be pulled inferiorly. Next most commonly involved is the lateral rectus muscle, which causes lateral deviation of the globe (Fig. 2–4 *D*).

The Hertel exophthalmometer (Fig. 2–5) permits accurate measurement of the distance between the anterior surface of the globe and the lateral orbital rim. Normal measurements are 18 to 20 mm or less. Proptosis is usually a slowly progressive process, and protrusion seldom exceeds more than 1 to 4 mm.

Relatively minor deviations from normal may be masked if the lids accommodate and cover the globes reasonably well. However, an occasional patient has truly dramatic proptosis for which only orbital decompression can provide a satisfactory cosmetic solution (Fig. 2–6).

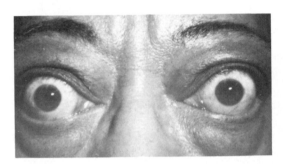

Figure 2–6. *Severe proptosis.* In addition to the cosmetic problems caused by proptosis, there may be more serious complications which may lead to loss of vision. This may result either from the consequences of exposure of the globe, leading to corneal ulceration and panophthalmitis, or from traction upon or compression of the optic nerve.

In addition to the cosmetic problems caused by proptosis, there may be more serious complications that may lead to loss of vision. This may result either from the consequences of exposure of the globe, leading to corneal ulceration and panophthalmitis, or from traction upon or compression of the optic nerve.

Reference

1. Hamburger JI and Sugar HS: What the internist should know about the ophthalmopathy of Graves' disease. *Arch Int Med* 129:131–139, 1972

B. THE THYROID GLAND

History. The patient may know of the existence of a goiter for months or years prior to the development of toxicity. Multinodular goiters (TMNG) and toxic autonomously functioning thyroid adenomas (AFTA) characteristically are present for 5 to 10 years and sometimes longer before toxicity becomes evident. One of my patients with TMNG had a visible enlargement of the thyroid for 73 years (between ages 13 and 86) before developing hyperthyroidism. By contrast, the goiter of TDG usually precedes the onset of hyperthyroidism by only a few months, if at all. There are exceptions to this generalization: I have seen patients with diffuse goiters which were detected 1 or 2 years before the onset of hyperthyroidism, but this is not the ordinary course of events.

Physical Findings. Examination will readily differentiate between the diffuse and often firm goiter of Graves' disease and the toxic multinodular goiter or the solitary toxic autonomously functioning thyroid adenoma. Remember, most

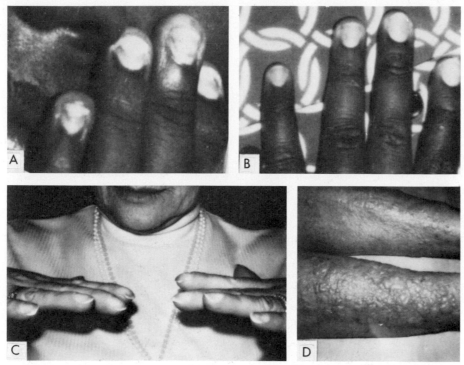

Figure 2–7. *Acral findings of Graves' disease. A,* Onycholysis. *B,* Improvement after treatment of hyperthyroidism. *C,* Acropachy. *D,* Pretibial myxedema.

toxic AFTA are large lesions, usually over 3 cm in diameter. Thus, in the absence of a readily palpable nodule the probability of a toxic AFTA is much reduced. While palpating the thyroid gland one can usually note vigorous pulsations of the carotid arteries in hyperthyroid patients. Bruits may be heard, particularly over the vascular goiters of Graves' disease.

C. THE CUTANEOUS SYSTEM

History.   Excessive sweating, hair loss, and pruritus are the most common complaints. Hair loss is also associated with hypothyroidism, but it is more consistently present in hyperthyroidism. Hair loss is a diffuse thinning. Alopecia areata or alopecia totalis is not a feature of thyroid disease.

Physical Findings.   Fine textured, velvety, soft, warm, moist skin is most characteristic. Vitiligo may be seen with hyperthyroidism and Hashimoto's disease (euthyroid or hypothyroid). Peripheral edema may be found occasionally in the absence of any other cause. Pretibial myxedema is seen in less than 5 per cent of patients with Graves' disease. The lesions are raised, firm plaques, usually on the lateral aspect of the leg. The overlying skin has an orange peel or pigskin appearance and is generally darker in color than adjacent normal tissue. The application of topical adrenal steroids followed by occlusive wrapping is helpful if the condition is mild. For more severe disease there is no effective treatment. Attempts at excision or even biopsy may be followed by a failure to heal. Onycholysis (separation of the nail from the nail bed), most commonly involving the nails of the fourth or fifth fingers, will be found in some degree surprisingly often if regularly sought. Recovery is spontaneous after the hyperthyroidism has been eliminated.

D. THE CARDIOVASCULAR SYSTEM

History. The tachycardia may be described as palpitation, pounding, or simply the onset of an awareness of the heart beat. Complaints referable to congestive heart failure may be reported, particularly if hyperthyroidism is engrafted upon a pre-existing organic heart disease. The characteristic heat intolerance may also be described.

Physical Findings. Sinus tachycardia or atrial fibrillation, high pulse pressure, friction rub in the pulmonic area (Means-Lerman scratch), and evidence of congestive heart failure may be found. In most hyperthyroid patients auscultation over the femoral arteries will reveal the pistol shot sounds indicative of the high pulse pressure. Peripheral edema and even anasarca may be seen without evidence of another form of organic heart disease.

E. THE NERVOUS SYSTEM

History. Increased nervousness, irritability, and irresponsible behavior are common complaints. Probably the best example of efficient but irresponsible behavior I can recall is that of a middle-aged woman who had diagnostic studies performed on Wednesday and Thursday and was scheduled for ^{131}I therapy on Friday. When she failed to appear for the treatment, we called her home and found that her husband was standing in a bare apartment. Between Thursday evening and Friday morning the patient had withdrawn all funds from the joint checking and savings accounts, emptied the safety deposit box, hired movers to pick up the furniture and personal belongings, and left for Tennessee. Hyperthyroid patients frequently cry during the evaluation. The change in personality in conjunction with the physical changes is a source of severe anxiety. Many patients are convinced that they have a malignant disease.

Physical Findings. The tremor of hyperthyroidism is of low amplitude and high frequency, about 6 per second. Deep tendon reflexes are brisk in both the initial and return phases.

F. THE GASTROINTESTINAL SYSTEM

History. Increased frequency of bowel movements, the usual finding, may progress to frank diarrhea associated with nausea and vomiting as the disease reaches the crisis level. Although weight loss in spite of an increased appetite is the usual history, elderly apathetic patients may present with marked anorexia, which greatly exacerbates the weight loss.

G. THE MUSCULOSKELETAL SYSTEM

History. Weakness of the proximal girdle muscles may be pronounced. This is often recognized in activities such as stair climbing and rising from a chair. Muscular involvement improves after correction of the hyperthyroidism. It may take up to 6 months before strength returns to normal. Patients with myasthenia gravis have an increased incidence of hyperthyroidism. However, hyperthyroid patients only rarely have myasthenia gravis. I have seen only two such patients. The effect produced on the myasthenia by controlling the hyperthyroidism is unpredictable. Hypokalemic periodic paralysis is a rare syndrome seen primarily in Orientals with hyperthyroidism. Control of hyperthyroidism leads to relief. Nausea, vomiting, constipation, and polyuria may signify symptomatic thyrotoxic hypercalcemia, a condition that results from excessive mobilization of calcium from the bones.

Physical Findings. Muscular atrophy is often readily visible in the suprascapular area (Fig. 2–8). Clubbing of the fingers (acropachy) is seen in only about 1 per cent of hyperthyroid patients. Although there has been one report of a remission in acropachy, as a rule the changes are permanent. Findings similar to acropachy may be seen with other illnesses.

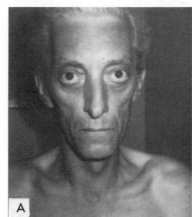
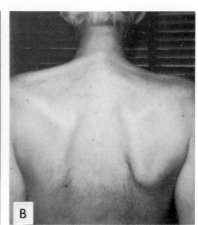

Figure 2–8. *Muscular atrophy in severe hyperthyroidism. A,* Pectoralis muscle atrophy. *B,* Atrophy of shoulder girdle musculature.

H. THE REPRODUCTIVE SYSTEM

History. Loss of libido, scanty menses, amenorrhea, infertility, and an increased frequency of spontaneous abortion are all common in hyperthyroidism. The cessation of menses soon after treatment has begun may signify that infertility is no longer a problem.

Physical Findings. Temporary gynecomastia has been reported in males with hyperthyroidism.

Assuming that this more complete survey of the history and physical findings supports the working diagnosis of hyperthyroidism, one may proceed with laboratory confirmation as indicated in Part III.

References

1. Meier DA, Arnstein AR and Hamburger JI: Symptomatic thyrotoxic hypercalcemia. *Mich Med* 73:19–24, 1974
2. McAnulty JH and Sisson JC: Thyroid acropachy: Improvement with time. *Univ Mich Med Center J* 38:154–156, 1972
3. Siegler M and Refetoff S: Pretibial myxedema—a reversible cause of foot drop due to entrapment of the peroneal nerve. *New Eng J Med* 294:1383–1384, 1976

PART III.   LABORATORY CONFIRMATION OF A DIAGNOSIS OF HYPERTHYROIDISM

The selection of appropriate laboratory studies for confirmation of a clinical diagnosis of hyperthyroidism may be simple or complicated, depending upon the circumstances. The flowsheet provides an approach to the solution of the more common problem situations, but deserves amplification.

A.   UNTREATED NEW PATIENTS NOT TAKING INTERFERING MEDICATION

1. The FTI Is Clearly Elevated. In these patients an elevated FTI confirms the diagnosis of hyperthyroidism. However, that is not the end of the problem. To be sure that the hyperthyroidism is not caused by SAT, toxic struma ovarii, or factitious administration of thyroid hormone, the RAI is important. In most cases, it will be greater than 30 per cent, usually in the 50 to 70 per cent range. A value between 5 and 30 per cent, in the presence of a distinctly elevated FTI and clinical features of hyperthyroidism, is most frequently an indication of iodide interference. Patients with the hyperthyroidism of SAT, toxic struma ovarii, or factitious hyperthyroidism will have RAI values of less than 5 per cent. The only exceptions will be the unusual situation in which the patient happens also to have nonsuppressible function. These patients will have goiter, either diffuse or multinodular. If the RAI is between 10 and 20 per cent and the patient recently received iodide (e.g., radiographic contrast medium, SSKI, or Lugol's solution), and if ^{131}I therapy is planned, it would be preferable to have a higher RAI value. The simple expedient of waiting a week or two is often effective. If the patient is so sick that prompt action seems called for, one could administer antithyroid drugs for a few weeks, taking advantage of the rebound elevation of the RAI which will occur when the ATD are withdrawn.

When the RAI is less than 5 per cent, do not make the mistake of assuming that iodide is the cause. If no history of iodide ingestion is obtained, the patient probably has painless or occult SAT or, rarely, either toxic struma ovarii or factitious hyperthyroidism. An elevated ESR supports the diagnosis of SAT. A TSH stimulation test is an additional essential procedure. A normal response suggests either toxic struma or factitious hyperthyroidism. The former diagnosis should have been made before the TSH stimulation test by counting over the ovaries. This should be a routine procedure for every patient with an elevated FTI and a suppressed RAI (unless another explanation is obvious). However, if you forgot to do it, you can still do it after the TSH stimulation test. TSH will not produce uptake of radioactive iodine by normal ovaries. Hence, substantial activity would be diagnostic.

CAUTION: Do not mistake scatter from the bladder for ovarian uptake. If high counts are obtained over the bladder, have the patient void. A toxic struma will always produce higher activity over the ovaries than over the bladder, especially after voiding. An imaging procedure will be diagnostic.

FLOWSHEET FOR CONFIRMATION OF WORKING DIAGNOSIS OF HYPERTHYROIDISM

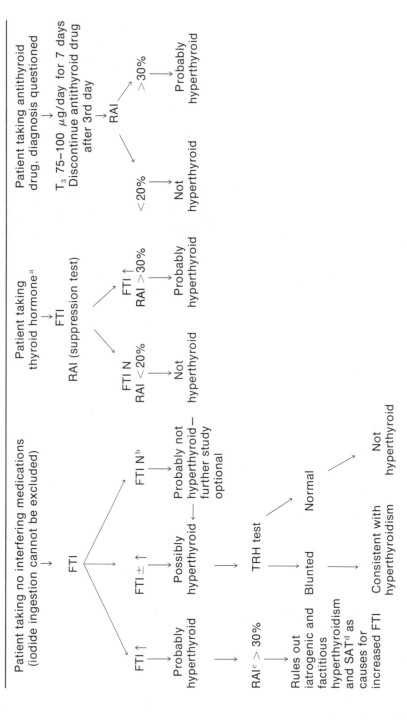

[a]If also taking iodides, wait 2 weeks with no further administration before obtaining RAI
[b]N = Normal
[c]In case of recent iodide ingestion, wait 2 weeks with no further iodide administration before obtaining RAI.
[d]SAT = Subacute thyroiditis

CAUTION: The suppressed RAI of SAT usually does not respond to TSH stimulation. When it does, the response is marginal, and imaging will reveal either unilateral or patchy tracer concentration in areas of lesser involvement. Therefore, a response to TSH stimulation in the absence of an ovarian struma, although suggestive of factitious hyperthyroidism, may not be diagnostic unless occult SAT can be excluded.

2. The FTI Is Only Slightly Elevated or at the Upper Level of Normal. This may indicate early TDG, TMNG, or toxic AFTA. An elevated T_3-(RIA) would provide support for the diagnosis of hyperthyroidism, but do not expect to find this very often. When the FTI is at the upper level of normal, the T_3(RIA) will usually be either normal or also at the upper level of normal. If the RAI is compatible with hyperthyroidism, a TRH test will be very helpful. A blunted response does not make the diagnosis of hyperthyroidism but does confirm the presence of an abnormal state of thyroid function consistent with that diagnosis.

How one would proceed from that point would depend upon the severity of the clinical findings and the risk to the patient of hyperthyroidism. Older patients with marginal cardiovascular reserve or patients with other diseases that may become unstable when complicated by hyperthyroidism (e.g., diabetes mellitus) might best be treated promptly and definitively. Younger patients who are otherwise in good health may be observed for further developments or treated with ATD or possibly iodide.

Older patients with long-standing multinodular goiter, cardiac decompensation, or atrial fibrillation may have either marginal elevations of FTI and T_3-(RIA) values or values at the upper level of normal. RAI values are often not very high, usually within the 20 to 30 per cent range. Again, TRH testing should be helpful. After all, if the patient has hyperthyroidism or even nonsuppressible function, the response to TRH should be blunted. Nevertheless, this is one situation in which a therapeutic trial has both diagnostic and therapeutic value, assuming that there are objective clinical abnormalities which can be assessed to judge the response. Most important would be tachycardia and weight loss. If a trial of ATD produces improvement in these indices with a concomitant fall in FTI and T_3(RIA) values, this would be strong support for the conclusion that hyperthyroidism is a material factor in the patient's disability. Under these circumstances, one could be more confident that ablative therapy would be not only indicated but likely to be of value.

A therapeutic trial of ATD should employ enough medication so that a judgment on the response can be made within a reasonable period of time — e.g., 4 to 6 weeks. I never give less than 300 mg of propylthiouracil four times a day. TMNG are generally more resistant to ATD than TDG. If the patient is so sick that the correct diagnosis is immediately important, then it makes no sense to give smaller ATD doses. They may either prove inadequate or take so long to produce their effect that the patient will suffer irreparable harm from the debilitating effects of the disease.

B. THE PATIENT IS TAKING THYROID HORMONE

Hardly a month goes by when I do not receive a call from a worried physician who has a patient with hyperthyroidism who happens to be taking thyroid hormone. He reports that his request for a tracer study to confirm the diagnosis has been rejected by the radiology department of his hospital because

TABLE 2-3. THYROID CONDITIONS WITH NONSUPPRESSIBLE RAI VALUES

I. Hyperthyroid conditions
   A. TDG (classical Graves' disease)
   B. TMNG
   C. Toxic AFTA
II. Nonhyperthyroid conditions
   A. Euthyroid Graves' disease
   B. Multinodular goiter
   C. Nontoxic AFTA
   D. After treatment of hyperthyroidism (^{131}I or thyroidectomy)

the patient must be off thyroid hormone for 6 weeks to obtain a "valid reading." Often the patient seems so sick that the attending physician is not sure that she will survive for 6 weeks if something is not done. This is the epitome of bureaucratic bungling. The hospital was practicing medicine by the book but reading the wrong page.

Obviously a patient taking thyroid hormone is an ideal candidate for an immediate RAI if hyperthyroidism is suspected. If the diagnosis is correct, a high value will be obtained, and a high value under these circumstances is even more valuable than a spontaneous high value. This is in essence a suppression test. Although it is possible that the high FTI was the result of an overdose of thyroid hormone, the RAI in an otherwise euthyroid or even hypothyroid patient would be suppressed. Also, the high RAI that results from any nonhyperthyroid process (e.g., dyshormonogenesis or rebound after SAT) will always suppress in response to a dose of thyroid hormone large enough to elevate the FTI. Hence, an elevated RAI (i.e., greater than 30 per cent) is virtually pathognomonic of hyperthyroidism if enough thyroid hormone has been taken to elevate the FTI.

Nonsuppressible function of lesser degree (i.e., an RAI of greater than 5 per cent but less than 30 per cent) is abnormal but need not be associated with hyperthyroidism. Table 2–3 lists the hyperthyroid and nonhyperthyroid conditions which may have nonsuppressible RAI values.

C. THE PATIENT IS TAKING ANTITHYROID DRUGS FOR A QUESTIONABLE DIAGNOSIS OF HYPERTHYROIDISM

This problem comes up ten or twelve times each year. There are three possibilities:
   1. The patient had hyperthyroidism and still has it.
   2. The patient had hyperthyroidism and is now in remission.
   3. The patient never had hyperthyroidism.

A simple solution is available through the T_3 suppression test. The antithyroid drug may be continued for the first few days of T_3 administration to shorten the block-free period and thus reduce the risk of recurrent manifestations of toxicity should hyperthyroidism still be active. The RAI either will be suppressed (often to less than 10 per cent) or will remain at a level compatible with hyperthyroidism. An intermediate value is uncommon but possible if the patient happens to have one of the nonhyperthyroid conditions associated with nonsuppressible RAI (Table 2–3).

PART IV.   TREATMENT OF HYPERTHYROIDISM

As already noted, hyperthyroidism is a term that includes a broad spectrum of disorders that have in common an excess of thyroid hormone. Treatment must be individualized and should be based upon an assessment of a number of factors, including:

1. The age of the patient.
2. The type of goiter.
3. The source of the hormone.
4. The severity of the disease.
5. The presence of other illnesses which complicate or are complicated by hyperthyroidism.
6. The response to previous treatment, if there was any.
7. The ability and willingness of the patient to cooperate with the treatment.
8. The facilities available to the patient.
9. The experience of the patient's physician.
10. Patient and physician prejudices.

The multiplicity of therapeutic methods that may be applied to correct hyperthyroidism makes it both practical and necessary to tailor the treatment to specific and individual features of the disease and the patient. Therefore, I shall discuss the following important therapeutic modalities in terms of indications, advantages, and disadvantages and then comment on the methods that I follow in applying these treatments: (1) antithyroid drugs (ATD), (2) thyroidectomy, (3) stable iodide, (4) propranolol, (5) radioactive iodine (^{131}I).

A. ANTITHYROID DRUGS (ATD)

The ATD propylthiouracil (PTU) and methimazole (Tapazole) became available almost simultaneously with ^{131}I in the 1940's. ATD produce their effects by blocking the synthesis of thyroid hormone. PTU also seems to interfere with the peripheral conversion of T_4 to T_3. ATD do not halt the secretion of preformed stored thyroid hormone. Table 2–4 lists the indications, advantages, and disadvantages of ATD.

The principal disadvantages of ATD are the high rate of failure in inducing a remission, even after 1 or 2 years of treatment, and the possibility of a relapse even when a remission does occur. A 50 per cent remission rate has been claimed for ATD therapy. However, this high rate will not be achieved unless patients are very carefully selected, including principally those less than 20 years old who have minimal thyroid enlargement and mild hyperthyroidism. Children who do not fulfill these criteria may still be given ATD with the objective of controlling the hyperthyroidism until they are old enough to be given ^{131}I.

Another drawback to ATD is their toxicity. Toxic reactions occur in about 10 per cent of patients. These reactions may be quite alarming in their explosive onset and severity. However, with rare exceptions they subside promptly upon

TABLE 2-4. INDICATIONS, ADVANTAGES, AND DISADVANTAGES FOR THE TREATMENT OF HYPERTHYROIDISM WITH ANTITHYROID DRUGS

INDICATIONS
1. Preparation for thyroidectomy or ^{131}I therapy
2. Long-term treatment for children, or for young adults with mild hyperthyroidism and small goiters
3. Hyperthyroidism in pregnancy
4. Thyroid storm

ADVANTAGES
1. No hospitalization
2. No destruction of thyroid tissue—hence, no increased likelihood of hypothyroidism

DISADVANTAGES
1. Inadequate or delayed response
2. Failure to induce permanent remission
3. Toxicity
   a. hematologic: granulocytopenia, agranulocytosis, anemia, thrombocytopenia, hypoprothrombinemia
   b. cutaneous: pruritus, angioedema, urticaria, maculopapular eruption
   c. rheumatologic: lupus-like syndrome, rheumatoid arthritis-like syndrome, serum sickness-like syndrome
   d. hepatocellular
   e. oversuppression causing goiter enlargement and hypothyroidism
   f. in pregnant hyperthyroid patients: fetal hypothyroidism and goiter, prematurity, abortion, and possible physical and mental maldevelopment if safe levels of exposure are exceeded at critical periods of gestation

discontinuation of the drug. Cutaneous reactions are the most common. Agranulocytosis is rare but potentially serious. My first experience with this complication involved a medical technologist who performed her own blood counts periodically. One day she presented me with a blood smear upon which she could find no neutrophils. Neither could I. Fortunately, discontinuation of ATD was followed by prompt recovery. Most toxic reactions occur within the first 2 months of treatment, but occasional instances of gradually declining neutrophil counts have been reported. An initial white blood cell count and differential is important, since hyperthyroidism per se is associated with a relative reduction in neutrophil count. Therefore, the assessment of any further reduction requires a baseline. Although periodic blood counts are no guarantee against an explosive decline, they may indicate a progressive decline.

Other toxic reactions are listed in Table 2–4. It is sound medical practice to inform the patient (or parent) of the possible reactions and what to do in case one occurs. I use a handout which I ask the patient to post near his or her phone. I also request the pharmacist to label the medication with the following warning: "In case of fever, sore throat, or skin eruption, stop this medication and contact your physician." I emphasize to the family that if in doubt it is never wrong to stop the medicine. The patient should also be checked by a physician as soon as practical, both to verify that a toxic reaction has occurred and to rule out the more serious hematologic problems.

References

1. Arnheim JA, Kenny FM and Ross D: Granulocytopenia, lupus-like syndrome, and other complications of propylthiouracil therapy. *Pediatrics* 76:54–63, 1970

2. Wartofsky L: Low remission after therapy for Graves' disease. *JAMA* 226:1083–1088, 1973
3. Wise PH, Marion M and Pain RW: Single-dose, "block-replace" drug therapy in hyperthyroidism. *Brit Med J* 4:143–145, 1973

Specific Applications of ATD

Preparation for Thyroidectomy or [131]I Therapy

The primary goal of preparation is to restore the patient to the euthyroid state as quickly as possible. A second objective is to reduce the vascularity of the goiter so that technical problems related to the thyroidectomy will be minimized. In addition, attention should be paid to controlling or correcting any associated abnormalities that might increase the surgical risk (e.g., congestive heart failure, hypertension, obesity, anemia, hypercalcemia).

The Usual Regimen. ATD are the backbone of the preparation. The initial dose depends upon the severity of the hyperthyroidism, but usually I begin with PTU, 200 mg four times a day. If the patient is more severely hyperthyroid, I increase the dose to 300 mg four times a day. With these doses the patient can be rendered euthyroid in 4 to 6 weeks in most instances. Lesser doses will prolong the preparation for no useful purpose. Every year I treat with ^{131}I one or two patients for whom operation was initially planned, but the preparation became so drawn out that either the patient or the physician became disgusted with the procedure. I might add that the initial decision for thyroidectomy in these cases was at best arguable. Nevertheless, if thyroidectomy is indicated, expeditious preparation is proper.

I recheck the patient at 2-week intervals, noting the weight, blood pressure, and pulse, and also looking for signs of regression in the other clinical features of hyperthyroidism. The FTI and T_3(RIA) are helpful guidelines of progress. When the patient is euthyroid I add Lugol's solution, 5 drops three times a day for 10 days, and the operation is usually uneventful.

NOTE: I do not discontinue the ATD when I begin Lugol's solution. For reasons which are obscure to me, this is a common practice. Since the ATD block iodide uptake by the thyroid and permit release of preformed stored hormone, an iodide-starved gland is produced. If iodide is given and the ATD block removed, a rapid recrudescence in the hyperthyroidism may occur.

Preparation for Thyroidectomy When ATD Cannot Be Used. Occasionally I am called upon to assist in the preparation of a patient who has developed a toxic reaction to ATD. Usually it is better to administer ^{131}I to these patients, but in the following circumstances ^{131}I may be contraindicated or thyroidectomy might be considered preferable:

1. The pregnant hyperthyroid patient. The reason for the contraindication to ^{131}I in pregnancy is obvious.

2. The prepubertal child. Although some physicians administer ^{131}I to hyperthyroid patients at all ages, most prefer to avoid giving this treatment to growing children. Experience indicates that radiation therapy to the thymus, tonsils, and adenoids, for acne or other minor conditions during childhood can predispose the child to the development of thyroid cancer years later. In my opinion this justifies continued caution in the use of ^{131}I in the individual who has not achieved full growth and development. At this time I consider ^{131}I therapy in children still investigational, and it will require many years before the potential risks can be quantified accurately. Nevertheless, the principal alternative therapy, thyroidectomy, also has risks, and under special circum-

stances the risks of ^{131}I may be considered less. With this qualification I accept the prepubertal state as a partial contraindication to ^{131}I therapy.

Whenever ATD cannot be used, preparation for operation will be less than ideal. Nevertheless, I have had success with the following regimen: (1) Lugol's solution, 5 drops three times a day for 2 weeks; (2) propranolol in a dose adequate to slow the resting heart rate to less than 90. The usual dose will be 20 to 40 mg four times a day. Propranolol should be given at bedtime the night before the operation and 1 hour before the operation; it should be given orally with just a sip of water. If needed, propranolol can be given intravenously during the operation; however, this is usually unnecessary. After the operation the patient can be weaned from the drug over 3 to 4 days. (3) A routine adrenal corticosteroid preparation is helpful. I give cortisone acetate, 100 mg intramuscularly the night before, the morning of the operation, and that afternoon. Additional cortisone is seldom needed. If there is more than minimal elevation in heart rate during the operation, supplemental cortisol may be given intravenously.

Long-Term Treatment of Hyperthyroidism with ATD

1. The Initial Evaluation. This includes an adequate clinical and laboratory investigation to confirm the diagnosis, permit recording of vital signs, and describe the clinical features which will be checked on subsequent visits. Exophthalmometer measurements are taken, and I photograph the face as well. A baseline complete blood count is obtained.

2. The Initial Dose. I begin treatment with PTU, 100 to 300 mg four times a day, depending upon the severity of the disease. If the disease is unusually mild, a smaller initial dose may be employed.

3. Followup. The first followup visit is at 1 month. This examination is performed primarily to evaluate the accuracy of the initial estimate of the patient's sensitivity to ATD. If there has been slight or no improvement the dose is increased. If the patient is already showing signs of hypothyroidism, or if values for the FTI are at the lower level of normal, the dose may be reduced. If an adjustment in the dose is made, it is best to recheck in 1 month. If a suitable dose was selected, the patient should be euthyroid or nearly so. The initial dose may then be continued and the patient rechecked at 3-month intervals. One should attempt to reduce the ATD dose as soon as possible. If the treatment is favorable, it will be possible to decrease the daily PTU dose progressively by 50 mg at 3-month intervals without a recurrence of hyperthyroidism. The dose may be decreased at times as soon as 3 to 6 months after treatment is instituted. If reductions are not possible without a recurrence of the hyperthyroidism, the prognosis is less favorable. If the maintenance dose is less than 200 mg per day, a single daily dose may be employed. This simplifies the program and improves the chances for maintaining patient cooperation over the long treatment period.

4. Termination of Treatment. One should seldom expect to terminate ATD treatment in less than 1 year, and more often the treatment must be maintained for 2 years or more. If actual withdrawal of the drug is not followed by a relapse, a remission has been realized.

5. Postremission Followup. A remission is no guarantee that there will be no recurrence of hyperthyroidism. Further followup is needed. I suggest that the patient be seen 1 month after discontinuing the PTU (to exclude the occasional rapid relapse), then at 6 months if all is well, and then annually thereafter. Of course, the patient is advised that if the disease seems to be recurring prior to the projected return visit, prompt reevaluation is necessary.

NOTE: I do not advise either of the following measures, which have been enthusiastically advocated by others.

1. Supplemental Thyroid Hormone (ST$_4$). It is common practice to give a full blocking dose of ATD and then add a full dose of ST$_4$ (e.g., LT$_4$, 0.2 mg daily). This approach is touted as simpler. No ATD dosage adjustments are needed, and there need be no concern about overtreatment, since the ST$_4$ will protect the patient from hypothyroidism. My objections are (1) it is simpler to assure faithful self-administration of one medication than two; (2) ATD in combination with ST$_4$ negates the most useful sign suggesting that the patient is heading for a remission — i.e., the failure of the FTI to rise in spite of a progressive reduction in ATD dosage.

2. Suppression Testing as a Prognostic Aid. It has been suggested that a return to suppressibility of the RAI in response to thyroid hormone (the T$_3$ suppression test) is an indication that a remission has been achieved, whereas persistent nonsuppressible function carries the opposite implication. However, one cannot rely upon the proposed significance for either response. The only reliable prognostic index is the clinical response of the patient on repeated followup examination. If the patient is doing well clinically and if the FTI and T$_3$(RIA) values are favorable, I pursue progressive ATD dose reduction whether the RAI is suppressible or not. Granted that if the patient is not doing well, the RAI will remain nonsuppressible, but this may be inferred from the usual clinical and laboratory data without suppression testing.

EXPERIENCE WITH LONG-TERM ATD THERAPY

One hundred and five patients less than 40 years old were given a trial of ATD to control hyperthyroidism in the hope that a spontaneous remission would be realized. For most of the patients older than 25 ATD therapy was advised by the attending physician, although we had suggested [131]I. Toxicity to ATD in 16 patients led to discontinuation of the drugs. In addition, ATD were discontinued in three pregnant patients because of toxic reactions. The toxic reactions were cutaneous in 13 patients, rheumatologic in two patients, and hematologic in two patients. The final two patients developed severe throat infections with only marginal reductions in white blood cell counts; but it was thought safer to discontinue the ATD. Thus, excluding the pregnant patients (for whom ATD were planned only as a temporary measure) and the two patients with questionable reactions, there were 14 instances of toxicity in 105 patients, for a rather high incidence of 13.3 per cent.

In 11 patients ATD were discontinued after less than 1 year for the following reasons: the attending physician reconsidered and advised ^{131}I for five patients; the goiter became unsightly in four patients; one patient failed to take the medication regularly; and one patient heard of ^{131}I from a friend and requested this treatment.

In 78 patients treatment was pursued for 1 year or longer unless a remission was obtained. Table 2–5 summarizes the results of treatment by age group for different sizes of goiters.

Forty-one of the 79 patients obtained a remission, but 14 of the 41 suffered a relapse within 4 years. In patients 20 years of age or older, there were sustained remissions in only 12 of 47 patients (26 per cent), and these occurred exclusively in patients with the smallest goiters. No remission occurred in any patient with a goiter larger than three times the size of a normal thyroid gland. The highest incidence of sustained remissions (7 out of 9 patients, or 78 per cent) occurred in

TABLE 2-5. CORRELATION OF GOITER SIZE AND AGE WITH THE FREQUENCY OF REMISSION AND SUBSEQUENT RELAPSE IN ATD-TREATED PATIENTS

	AGE (YEARS)								
	< 20			20–29			30–39		
GOITER SIZE	No. Patients	No. Remissions	No. Relapses	No. Patients	No. Remissions	No. Relapses	No. Patients	No. Remissions	No. Relapses
2 × Nᵃ or less	9	8	1	12	10	5	12	8	1
2–3 × N	19	10	2	8	2	2	8	3	3
>3 × N	4	0	0	4	0	0	3	0	0
Total	32	18	3	24	12	7	23	11	4

ᵃNormal (estimated weight, 20 grams)

patients less than 20 years of age with goiters no larger than twice the size of a normal thyroid gland.

From this experience I have concluded that long-term ATD therapy is a poor choice for most patients over 20 years of age, unless the goiter is quite small; and ATD therapy is not likely to be successful at any age if the goiter is large. For practical purposes, ATD therapy is suitable only for children and the occasional adult with a small goiter who also has mild hyperthyroidism.

Note that the percentages of success, as unimpressive as they are, would look even worse if we had not excluded patients for whom ATD were discontinued because of toxic reactions or various other reasons before an adequate trial had been given. A similarly disappointing experience elsewhere has been reported recently.

ATD Therapy for Children with Hyperthyroidism. We have included patients who are less than 20 years of age in this category. The younger the age at which one draws the line, the rarer the disease. The youngest patient in my series was 5 years old; and through 1974 I had seen a total of only 11 patients 10 years old or younger. The principal treatment for those less than 20 years of age is ATD. These patients will have the best results with long-term ATD treatment. Nevertheless, there are some problems which, if they occur, necessitate an alternate form of treatment. These include:

1. TOXIC REACTIONS. Toxic reactions to ATD occur in about 10 to 15 per cent of patients. A toxic reaction to one drug is not always followed by a reaction to the other, but this may happen. Therefore, unless there is some compelling reason to pursue long-term treatment with ATD, I usually advise an alternate method of treatment after a toxic reaction. After all, one cannot be certain that the second toxic reaction will be as benign as the first.

2. THE UNCOOPERATIVE PATIENT. This is a frequent problem with children, particularly teenagers. One must include under this heading the uncooperative parent, for the net result is the same — i.e., the ATD are not taken regularly and the patient does not return for the necessary evaluations to assure safe and effective management.

3. THE LARGE UNSIGHTLY GOITER. I have had a few patients who either could not tolerate the teasing of other children or were depressed by the unsightliness of a large goiter and requested that something be done to solve the problem promptly.

For the three foregoing indications, I recommend an operation for the prepubertal child and offer ^{131}I treatment or thyroidectomy to the older child after an explanation of the advantages and disadvantages of both methods.

4. POSSIBLE COINCIDENTAL THYROID CANCER. An occasional patient has coincidentally a nodule that is suspicious for cancer, and for these patients thyroidectomy eliminates both problems.

For other children, long-term ATD therapy may be undertaken either with the hope that a remission will be experienced within 1 to 3 years or to control the hyperthyroidism until the patient reaches the age at which ^{131}I therapy may be comfortably administered.

It is probably incorrect to think that ATD induce or cause a remission in hyperthyroidism. It seems more likely that they act as a kind of holding action, permitting time to elapse during which a spontaneous remission may occur. The following clinical features are useful indicators predicting that a remission will take place: (1) a relatively small goiter—i.e., no more than twice the size of a normal thyroid gland; (2) relatively mild hyperthyroidism; (3) age less than 20 years; and (4) control of hyperthyroidism achieved by a small dose of ATD.

On the contrary, patients with very large goiters almost never experience a remission.

Table 2–6 gives the age and sex distribution of 113 children with hyperthyroidism seen at Northland Thyroid Laboratory.

The female to male ratio was only 2.32 to 1, less than the ratio of 4.77 to 1 for patients with toxic diffuse goiter over 20 years of age, but the difference is not statistically significant.

Two patients had iatrogenic thyrotoxicosis and were cured by the simple expedient of discontinuing the unnecessary thyroid hormone. Of the remaining 111 patients, two had such mild hyperthyroidism that no treatment was given. They are simply being observed at 6 month intervals. Fifteen others were treated by their own physicians without followup at Northland Thyroid Laboratory.

Twenty patients were treated with ^{131}I in spite of their age. Fifteen of these were either 18 or 19 years old. The remaining five patients were 17 years old (2), 16 years old (1), 15 years old (1), and 9 years old (1). The last patient had Down's syndrome. The principal indication for ^{131}I was large goiter and, for those younger than 18 years, refusal of operation.

Nine patients were treated with thyroidectomy without a trial of antithyroid drugs. Three of the nine developed toxic recurrent goiter and were subsequently treated with [131]I. One patient later developed iatrogenic thyrotoxicosis. She had been given thyroid hormone for hypothyroidism postoperatively, and later her residual thyroid tissue became nonsuppressible.

The 65 remaining patients were given a trial of ATD therapy. Five have been lost to followup. The experience with the remaining 60 is summarized in Table 2–7.

TABLE 2–6. AGE AND SEX DISTRIBUTION OF HYPERTHYROID CHILDREN

AGE (YEARS)	MALE	FEMALE
5–10	2	9
11–15	11	29
16–19	21	41
Total	34	79

TABLE 2-7. RESULTS OF ATD THERAPY FOR 60 PATIENTS WITH CHILDHOOD HYPERTHYROIDISM

ATD discontinued without remission		28
Treated with [131]I	24	
Treated surgically	3	
Treated with Lugol's solution	1	
Still on ATD with hyperthyroidism controlled		14
Remission induced		18
Subsequent relapse	4	
ATD resumed	3	
[131]I therapy	1	
Total		60

The reasons for terminating ATD treatment in 28 children are shown in Table 2-8.

TABLE 2-8. REASONS FOR ABANDONING ATD IN 28 CHILDREN

Large goiter	8
No remission after 2 to 6 years	8
Toxic reactions	4
Poor patient cooperation	4
Attending physician dissatisfied	4

Treatment of the Pregnant Hyperthyroid Patient

Hyperthyroidism is a rare complication of pregnancy, occurring in less than 1 per cent of pregnant women. The mainstay of treatment for the pregnant hyperthyroid woman is ATD. Thyroidectomy is reserved for patients who experience resistance or toxic reactions to ATD or are uncooperative. The decline in popularity of surgical treatment for the pregnant patient is based upon the same objections to operation as exist for the nonpregnant patient, plus the additional concern for the fetus. A combined series of surgically treated patients experienced a fetal loss of 9.9 per cent, about what might be expected with uncomplicated pregnancies. Nevertheless, medical management is at least equally effective.

The major drawback to the use of ATD during pregnancy is the ease with which these drugs cross the placenta. An excessive exposure of the fetus to ATD may cause hypothyroidism or goiter, and may contribute to abortion, prematurity, fetal death, and possibly intellectual retardation. Therefore, it is important to minimize fetal exposure to the drug. Obviously, fetal exposure will be minimal when the maternal dose is as low as possible.

It has been claimed that the use of ATD in conjunction with full replacement doses of supplemental thyroid hormone (ST_4) prevents maternal hypothyroidism and also fetal hypothyroidism and goiter. This method is subject to criticism on the basis of both concept and experience.

CONCEPTUAL OBJECTIONS TO COMBINED ST_4-ATD THERAPY

1. In pregnant patients whose hyperthyroidism is not in remission, ST_4 will be additive to the maternal secretion unless maternal secretory activity is fully blocked by ATD. It requires a larger dose of ATD to block fully the maternal

secretion than would be necessary if no ST_4 were given and the maternal thyroid were permitted to provide the hormone needed to maintain the euthyroid state. Therefore, in pregnant patients whose hyperthyroidism is not in remission, ST_4 necessitates a larger dose of ATD, and increases fetal ATD exposure.

2. Hyperthyroidism tends to improve as pregnancy advances and frequently remits during the last trimester, permitting the discontinuation of ATD, a highly desirable situation. The best indication that a remission may be in the offing is a reduced requirement for ATD, signalled by a falling FTI value. If ST_4 is given, the FTI will not fall; thus the possibility of reducing or even discontinuing ATD will be obscured.

3. Although ST_4 will prevent maternal hypothyroidism, experimental data indicate that the placenta presents a relative barrier to the flow of the thyroid hormone from mother to fetus. Ample clinical experience indicates that a normal maternal plasma concentration of thyroid hormone does not protect the fetus from either hypothyroidism (e.g., the athyreotic cretin) or ATD-induced goitrous hypothyroidism.

OBJECTIONS TO COMBINED ST_4–ATD MANAGEMENT BASED UPON EXPERIENCE

1. Publications from clinics where ST_4 is not given reveal results as good as or superior to results from clinics which advocate ST_4.

2. Identification of remissions and discontinuation of ATD in advanced stages of pregnancy are reported only by those who do not administer ST_4. Therefore, ST_4 is inconsistent with the goal of administering the smallest possible ATD dosage to the pregnant hyperthyroid patient.

PRINCIPLES UNDERLYING MANAGEMENT OF THE PREGNANT HYPERTHYROID PATIENT

1. ATD cross the placenta readily, thyroid hormone far less well.

2. Hyperthyroidism tends to improve as pregnancy advances.

3. Mother and fetus tolerate mild hyperthyroidism better than any degree of hypothyroidism.

4. Minimal fetal ATD exposure will be assured if the ATD dosage is adjusted to maintain the FTI at the upper level of normal.

5. Dosage adjustment should be made in anticipatory fashion, assuming that as the hyperthyroidism improves the FTI will decline during the interval between one visit and the next.

6. Optimal control requires evaluation at 3- to 4-week intervals throughout the pregnancy.

PROTOCOL FOR MANAGEMENT OF THE PREGNANT HYPERTHYROID PATIENT

1. **The Initial ATD Dose.** Assuming the patient is first seen when already pregnant, the initial ATD dose depends upon one's estimate of the severity of the hyperthyroidism. Since severely hyperthyroid women seldom become pregnant, it can be anticipated that the patient will have mild to moderate hyperthyroidism. Hence, I usually begin with PTU, 100 mg four times a day, and almost never give more than 200 mg four times a day.

2. Followup Evaluations:

a. The patient is rechecked in 3 weeks. If there has been some clinical improvement, even if the FTI is still substantially elevated, the same dose may be continued for another 3 weeks. An increased dose should be given if there has been no improvement. If the FTI has fallen to the upper level of normal or lower, I reduce the dose by 25 to 50 per cent and continue to make anticipatory reductions as long as the FTI does not rise to an undesirably high level.

b. By the third trimester most patients can be maintained on a total daily PTU dose of 200 mg or less, and for some, ATD may be discontinued.

c. If the patient requires in excess of 400 mg PTU per day, there may be an increased risk of fetal goiter, and consideration should be given to elective thyroidectomy. This is the prevailing opinion. This opinion is based upon an analysis of cases in which fetal goiter resulted from an excessive dose of ATD which might have been because of poor management rather than the absolute magnitude of the dose itself. I suspect that ATD in any dose actually required (barring unusual resistance) will be less risky than thyroidectomy. My experience is too limited to prove the point, however. Therefore, I recommend adherence to the prevailing opinion.

3. Postnatal Evaluations. After termination of the pregnancy, the problem is not over. If the mother is in remission, a relapse should be anticipated within 3 months. If this fails to occur, annual reevaluation is in order. Persistent hyperthyroidism or relapse deserves definitive therapy with [131]I. I can find no justification for allowing women who intend to have more children to remain hyperthyroid under control with ATD. One episode of hyperthyroidism complicating pregnancy is enough for any patient.

The question of hyperthyroidism in pregnancy leads to a related problem which is much more common. What advice should one give the young woman who is about to be married or is already married and contemplates starting a family within a year or two and also happens to have hyperthyroidism? I consider this situation a contraindication to long-term ATD therapy, even if ATD otherwise would be suitable (e.g., relatively small goiter and mild hyperthyroidism). ATD treatment simply constitutes an invitation to the problem of hyperthyroidism during pregnancy. In my opinion, these women should be treated with [131]I. An operation would be preferable to ATD, but it is the therapy of second choice.

I should add that I still see patients who have been told that ^{131}I can cause sterility. There is absolutely no basis for this statement. It is clear that the radiation delivered to the ovaries incidental to the treatment of hyperthyroidism with ^{131}I is roughly equivalent to that of a gastrointestinal x-ray series. Many thousands of patients have been treated with ^{131}I in the childbearing age group, and no increase in either infertility or fetal abnormalities has been reported beyond that which occurs in the population at large. Much larger doses of radiation directed to the ovaries specifically have not led to sterility. Finally, doses of ^{131}I are commonly given to children and young adults for treatment of cancer, and these may exceed 50 times the magnitude of the ^{131}I doses employed for hyperthyroidism. Even these doses have not caused either sterility or fetal abnormalities. In fact, among the risks to the future progeny of a young woman treated for hyperthyroidism, by far the greatest risk is the possibility of not surviving a thyroidectomy. As small as this risk is, it is a factual, quantifiable actuality and should be considered far more serious than risks from ^{131}I, which exist so far only as unsubstantiated speculations.

EXPERIENCE WITH TREATMENT OF HYPERTHYROIDISM DURING PREGNANCY

Table 2–9 summarizes my experience with hyperthyroidism in 32 pregnant patients.

For 30 of the 32 patients ATD was the initial treatment advised.

Two patients failed to receive any treatment for the reasons indicated. In both instances the hyperthyroidism was mild. One of the patients previously had been treated with [131]I. Her baby was normal. The other patient also had scleroderma, refused treatment, and was lost to followup.

One patient had an abortion in the first trimester because of persistent bleeding. She had received PTU for only 3 weeks. A second patient spontaneously aborted in the first trimester. Four patients developed toxicity to ATD. Two were treated with Lugol's solution, 3 drops daily for the balance of the pregnancy. These mothers and babies did well. At that time, I was unaware of the risks of fetal goiter from iodides. Although reports of infants with this complication reveal that much larger iodide dosage was given than I employed, I elected nevertheless not to take this risk in the two patients seen more recently. They were prepared for operation with iodides, propranolol, and cortisone. Thyroidectomy was uneventful. The subsequent deliveries were uncomplicated, and the infants were normal.

For two patients elective thyroidectomy was performed in the second trimester at the insistence of the attending physician. One mother subsequently delivered a premature but otherwise normal infant. The other delivery was full term, and the infant was normal.

Twenty-one patients were treated satisfactorily with ATD; for seven of these ATD were discontinued in the third trimester of pregnancy. All babies were normal.

The final patient received Lugol's solution for mild hyperthyroidism during pregnancy, having experienced an incomplete remission of hyperthyroidism after ^{131}I therapy administered several months before she conceived.

Following delivery, 13 mothers were treated with ^{131}I because of persistent or recurrent hyperthyroidism. Six patients maintained remissions (three of whom

TABLE 2–9.   TREATMENT OF HYPERTHYROIDISM DURING PREGNANCY

ATD		23
[131]I therapy given after delivery	13	
Remission after delivery	6	
Lost to followup after delivery	2	
Pregnancy aborted in first trimester owing to persistent bleeding	2	
ATD INITIALLY, ABANDONED FOR THYROIDECTOMY OWING TO		4
Toxicity from ATD	2	
Preference of attending physician	2	
LUGOL'S SOLUTION GIVEN		3
After ATD toxicity	2	
After ^{131}I therapy prior to pregnancy	1	
NO TREATMENT GIVEN		2
Patient refused ATD	1	
Attending physician failed to order ATD	1	
Total	32	32

TABLE 2-10. CLINICAL AND LABORATORY DATA ON A PATIENT WHO EXPERIENCED A REMISSION IN HYPERTHYROIDISM WHILE PREGNANT[a]

DATE OF EXAM	WT (lb)	HEART RATE	GOITER SIZE	FTI[c]	PTU DOSE (mg/day)
9/28/70	120	120	3 × N[b]	3.9	400
11/03/70	125	120	3 × N	2.9	300
12/11/70	132	90	3 × N	1.8	200
1/28/71	140	88	3 × N	1.5	100
2/08/71	143	84	3½ × N	1.4	0
3/04/71	144	86	3½ × N	1.3	0
4/10/71	Delivery, normal infant				

[a]Patient was a 31 year old female, 62½ inches in height, pregnant 3 months.
[b]N = normal weight (estimated to be 20 grams).
[c]NR = 1.1 to 3.4.

had received ^{131}I prior to conception but had incomplete remission in the hyperthyroidism).

Table 2–10 summarizes the data for a patient who experienced a remission in hyperthyroidism while pregnant. Soon after delivery, there was a relapse for which ^{131}I was given.

From this experience it is concluded that ATD without ST_4 is satisfactory for control of hyperthyroidism during pregnancy. Anticipatory dosage reductions will insure minimal fetal exposure to ATD and permit discontinuation of ATD if a remission occurs.

References

1. Goluboff LG, Sisson JC and Hamburger JI: Hyperthyroidism associated with pregnancy. *Obstet Gynecol* 44:107–116, 1974
2. Ayromlooi J, Zervoudakis IA and Sadaghat A: Thyrotoxicosis in pregnancy. *Am J Obstet Gynecol* 117:818–823, 1973
3. Stoffer SS and Hamburger JI: Inadvertent ^{131}I therapy for hyperthyroidism in the first trimester of pregnancy. *J Nucl Med* 17:146–149, 1976
4. Bullock JL, Harris RE and Young R: Treatment of thyrotoxicosis during pregnancy with propranolol. *Am J Obstet Gynecol* 121:242–245, 1975
5. Worley RJ and Crosby WM: Hyperthyroidism during pregnancy. *Am J Obstet Gynecol* 119:150–155, 1974
6. Talbert LH, Thomas CG, Jr, Holt WA, et al: Hyperthyroidism during pregnancy. *Obstet Gynecol* 36:779–785, 1970

Thyroid Storm (Crisis)

Thyroid storm may be defined as the end stage of thyrotoxicosis in terms of severity. The heart rate is more than 150 per minute, and there is fever, nausea, vomiting, diarrhea progressing to dehydration, congestive heart failure, shock, renal shut-down, and death. Therapeutic intercession will halt this progression, often producing a dramatic reversal of the condition in a matter of hours.

Thyroid storm or crisis (like myxedema coma) is a disease of neglect. One does not develop spontaneous thyroid storm overnight. It is the result of long-standing untreated hyperthyroidism. Either the patient fails to seek medical consultation (often fearing to learn that the diagnosis is cancer) or to cooperate with the treatment advised, or the diagnosis is overlooked. While writing this section, I saw a young girl for a followup examination for whom a diagnosis of hyperthyroidism had been missed by five physicians over many months. The last physician advised a psychiatrist, and it was the psychiatrist who suggested that she have her thyroid checked. When I finally saw her she was in imminent danger of going into thyroid storm, although she had not yet crossed the imaginary border.

Thyroid storm after thyroidectomy is almost unheard of these days. Proper preparation reduces the likelihood of storm to nil. Nevertheless, I can recall one example of this complication twice in the same patient as a result of really trying. This was a 50 year old woman with a large toxic goiter who was prepared for thyroidectomy for 6 months with inadequate doses of ATD and never restored to the euthyroid state. She was also more than 100 pounds overweight and hypertensive. On two separate occasions, she was given anesthesia for thyroidectomy, only to have sudden severe acceleration of the heart rate. After the second episode she was advised that her condition was incurable. Needless to say, ^{131}I following ATD preparation effectively eliminated the problem.

The principles for management of thyroid storm may be outlined as follows:

1. Look for a precipitating factor. Thyroidectomy is obvious. When storm appears to be spontaneous, suspect infection, particularly urinary, pulmonary, or gynecologic.
2. Treat the peripheral effects of excess thyroid hormone.
   a. Propranolol, 40 mg four times daily.
   b. Fluid therapy for dehydration.
   c. Sedation.
   d. High caloric food supplements.
3. Give adrenal steroids to counter the possibility of adrenal exhaustion.
   a. Immediate intravenous administration of cortisol, 200 mg.
   b. Cortisone acetate, 100 mg intramuscularly immediately and every 6 hours until there is clear-cut improvement — then taper off over 3 to 4 days.
4. Stop the synthesis and secretion of thyroid hormone.
   a. PTU, 300 mg every 4 to 6 hours.
   b. Sodium iodide, 1 gram intravenously every 12 hours for 48 hours. Further iodide will probably not be necessary.

Case Report

As this book was in the final stages of publication, I received a call from a very concerned surgeon who had been up most of the previous evening repairing extensive bowel lacerations in a 41 year old woman who had been in an automobile accident. She had been treated for hyperthyroidism with [131]I 1 week earlier. Four hours after the operation a rapidly increasing tachycardia developed with a heart rate of between 160 and 170. The temperature climbed to 102° F. The surgeon assured me that the blood volume had been restored. It seemed clear that she was in thyroid crisis. One gram of sodium iodide had been given intravenously. Since the patient was on continuous gastric suction, the problem was how to administer the propranolol and PTU which were clearly indicated. Propranolol may be given intravenously but requires close monitoring. No parenteral preparation of PTU is available. This type of problem comes up every 2 to 3 years, and it is useful to recall that almost anything that can be given orally can also be given rectally.

PTU, 300 mg, and propranolol, 40 mg, were crushed and placed in a gelatin capsule and inserted into the rectum. In 45 minutes the heart rate had slowed to 120 and in 2 hours it was down to 100. The elevated temperature fell to about

100° F over the next 24 hours. This combination of medications was continued rectally at 6-hour intervals until the patient was able to take oral medication, and there were no further problems from the hyperthyroidism for the duration of her hospitalization. Adrenal steroids were held in reserve and would have been given if the response had been less satisfactory.

Reference

1. Mackin JF, et al: Thyroid storm and its management. *New Eng J Med* 291:1396–1398, 1974

B. THYROIDECTOMY

Thyroidectomy was the first effective definitive treatment for hyperthyroidism, and it still retains a useful, if somewhat curtailed, role in the management of this disease (Table 2–11).

The major drawbacks to thyroidectomy are the unavoidable risks, of which by far the most serious is the unexpected death of the patient. Mortality rates have fallen in all the major centers, so that it is possible to read of 500 or 1000 consecutive operations without a death. However, it should not be concluded that these outstanding safety records are representative of the results realized in the usual community hospital. On the contrary, a number of surgical reports on 100 to 200 patients include one or more deaths. To be sure, these deaths can often be explained on the basis of some totally unpredictable catastrophic event, perhaps related to the anesthesia. In other cases, including two of my own patients, the cause of death was never satisfactorily explained. If death were a complication confined to elderly infirm patients, perhaps one could more easily accept it as

TABLE 2–11. INDICATIONS, ADVANTAGES, AND DISADVANTAGES OF THYROIDECTOMY IN THE TREATMENT OF HYPERTHYROIDISM

INDICATIONS
1. Pregnant patients or children who experience toxic reactions to ATD
2. Children with large unsightly goiters
3. Patients who refuse medical management
4. Young patients with toxic AFTA
5. Patients with coexistent nodules suggesting cancer

ADVANTAGES
1. On occasion the only suitable treatment
2. Relatively rapid elimination of goiter and hyperthyroidism

DISADVANTAGES
1. Mortality rate, 0.1 to 1.0 per cent
2. Permanent hypoparathyroidism, 2 to 5 per cent
3. Permanent impairment of voice, 1 to 2 per cent
4. Wound complications: keloid, hemorrhage, infection
5. Permanent tracheostomy, rare
6. Thyroid storm, rare with proper preparation
7. Permanent hypothyroidism, up to 50 per cent
8. Recurrent hyperthyroidism, up to 15 per cent
9. Unwarranted lay and professional fear of thyroidectomy
10. Possibility of legal action against surgeon for lack of informed consent

inevitable. However, death from thyroidectomy may occur at any age (one of my patients was in her 20's, the other in his 40's) and thus is a very difficult complication to justify, particularly with the availability of nonlethal alternative forms of therapy.

The necessity for hospitalization is another important drawback to thyroidectomy. When other methods of treatment can be employed, the unnecessary use of scarce and expensive hospitals beds is unwarranted.

The disadvantages of thyroidectomy and the availability of suitable alternatives have led to a dramatic reduction in the frequency of thyroidectomy for hyperthyroidism in most leading institutions. For example, at the Mayo Clinic, where it had been common for thousands of patients annually to undergo thyroidectomy for hyperthyroidism, in 1968 only 12 patients had operations for toxic diffuse goiter.

A new problem faces the surgeon who remains unimpressed by the advantages of alternative methods of treatment for hyperthyroidism. He must now consider the legal implications of the doctrine of informed consent. The patient has the legal right to full disclosure not only of the risks of the proposed treatment but also of the other available methods. Since thyroidectomy per se involves unavoidable expense and pain beyond that of medical management, the surgeon takes the risk of legal action if fully informed consent is not obtained, even if the patient survives thyroidectomy without a major complication. Any complication peculiar to surgery will, of course, increase this risk.

Nevertheless, in the special situations listed in Table 2–11, thyroidectomy remains an important treatment for hyperthyroid patients. As the number of patients who require operation falls, it seems prudent to suggest that those who must have it be directed to surgeons with extensive experience.

Experience with Thyroidectomy for Hyperthyroidism

For 34 patients the primary treatment was thyroidectomy. An additional 10 patients had thyroidectomy after a trial of antithyroid drugs which were abandoned for reasons that shall be cited. Of the 44 surgically treated patients, 38 were female and 6 were male. The majority of patients were young, less than 40 years of age. Thirty-nine of these surgically treated patients had TDG. An operation was advised for three patients with toxic AFTA because they were less than 40 years

TABLE 2–12. INDICATIONS FOR THYROIDECTOMY IN 39 TDG PATIENTS

Adult patients with TDG			30
Preference of attending physician		26	
Attending physician a surgeon	16		
Attending physician not a surgeon	10		
Pregnant with toxicity to ATD		2	
Possible coexistent cancer		1	
Preference of patient over [131]I		1	
Children with TDG			9
Prepubertal and no success with ATD		4	
Disfiguring goiter		3	
Possible coexistent cancer		1	
Preference of patient over [131]I		1	
Total			39

TABLE 2-13. INTERVAL BETWEEN OPERATION AND RECURRENCE OF HYPERTHYROIDISM

INTERVAL (YEARS)	NO. PATIENTS
< 2	3
2– 5	9
5–10	7
10–20	8
20–44	8
No data	11
Total	46

old. A fourth patient was advised to have a thyroidectomy for a large obstructing toxic AFTA. One patient with TMNG was treated surgically for obstruction.

Two patients given a choice of ^{131}I or thyroidectomy chose the latter. For 26 patients for whom ^{131}I might have been employed, the decision favoring an operation was made by the attending physician. Most surgically treated patients were not available for reevaluation; hence, no systematic assessment of surgical complications can be made. However, three of these patients were referred back to Northland Thyroid Laboratory for treatment of recurrent thyrotoxicosis, and one additional patient has permanent hypoparathyroidism.

Toxic Recurrent Goiter (TRG)

Forty-six patients have been seen for recurrent hyperthyroidism following previous thyroidectomy. There are no data upon which to determine the incidence of this complication in the metropolitan Detroit area.

Almost half the patients were over 50 years of age when they developed recurrent hyperthyroidism.

The earliest recurrence was perhaps not a recurrence at all but an outright failure of thyroidectomy to control the hyperthyroidism in a 47 year old man. The patient was treated with ^{131}I during the same hospital stay. It is of interest to note how many patients had recurrences of hyperthyroidism many years after an apparently successful operation. Thus, one must consider not only the possibility of a late onset of hypothyroidism but also late recurrence of hyperthyroidism in a surgically treated population.

References

1. Memery HN: Anesthesia mortality in private practice. A ten-year study. *JAMA* 194:1185–1188, 1965
2. Sanfelippo PM, Beahrs OH, McConahey WM and Thorvaldsson SE: Indications for thyroidectomy. *Mayo Clin Proc* 48:269–272, 1973.
3. Hamburger JI: Recurrent hyperthyroidism after thyroidectomy. *Arch Surg* 111:91–92, 1976

C. STABLE IODIDE SOLUTION (LUGOL'S SOLUTION)

Lugol's solution, containing about 8 mg of iodide per drop, will suppress not only hormonal synthesis but also thyroglobulin degradation. This reduces the secretion of preformed thyroid hormone. That is why Lugol's solution improves hyperthyroidism more rapidly than ATD. Saturated solution of potassium iodide (SSKI), containing about 50 mg of iodide per drop, also may be used. Since the usual adult requirement for iodide is only about 200 μg daily, one drop of either solution can be considered a pharmacologic quantity.

Stable iodide became more widely used after Henry Plummer in the 1920's reported its effectiveness in the preparation of patients with toxic diffuse goiter for thyroidectomy. This remains the principal use of Lugol's Solution. The usual dose of 5 drops three times a day is arbitrary and probably more than necessary. However, there is no compelling reason for greater precision in dosage. Iodides given for the last 10 days of ATD preparation for operation will reduce the size and firm up the goiter and decrease its vascularity. Lugol's solution should be given concomitantly with ATD; otherwise, the delivery of iodide to an iodide-depleted goiter (the result of prior ATD therapy) may precipitate a relapse in the toxicity.

Concern for escape from the suppressant effects of iodide, a common occurrence after a few weeks to a few months of treatment, has given rise to the opinion that stable iodide alone is not useful for the suppression of hyperthyroidism. Although this principle has general validity, patients with very mild disease, especially those with minimal thyroid enlargement, may be exceptions. I have been successful in treating an occasional patient in this simple, inexpensive, and relatively complication-free fashion, and I believe it is worthy of consideration for patients with very mild hyperthyroidism.

Lugol's solution may also be given after ^{131}I therapy if only partial correction of the hyperthyroidism has been achieved. The previously irradiated toxic thyroid gland seems to be more sensitive to the suppressant effects of iodide, and this treatment may obviate the need for repeat ^{131}I therapy. Earlier, it had been thought that smaller ^{131}I doses, followed by iodide to control any residual hyperthyroidism until thyroid function gradually fell to the euthyroid range, might be a means of curtailing the high incidence of hypothyroidism that is observed after ^{131}I therapy. Further experience with this method indicates that it is necessary

TABLE 2-14. INDICATIONS, ADVANTAGES, AND DISADVANTAGES OF STABLE IODIDE IN THE TREATMENT OF HYPERTHYROIDISM

INDICATIONS
1. Supplemental to ATD in preparation for thyroidectomy
2. Supplemental to ^{131}I therapy
   a. Short-term use to hasten resolution of hyperthyroidism
   b. Long-term suppression after low ^{131}I doses
3. Thyroid storm
4. Occasionally for suppressive treatment of mild hyperthyroidism
5. Neonatal hyperthyroidism

ADVANTAGES
1. Simple and inexpensive
2. Almost free of toxicity
3. No destruction of thyroid tissue; hence, less likelihood of eventual hypothyroidism

DISADVANTAGES
1. Escape from suppression of hyperthyroidism
2. Recurrence of hyperthyroidism if ATD are inadvertently discontinued in the course of preparation for thyroidectomy
3. Relapse after discontinuation of treatment
4. Iodism (fever, skin eruption, salivary gland swelling) — seen only with unnecessarily excessive doses

ultimately to re-treat many of these patients and that the others still develop hypothyroidism quite frequently, although somewhat later than might have been the case with larger ^{131}I doses. The morbidity of the disease obviously is increased by this method of treatment. I use supplemental Lugol's solution only if the patient has rather mild hyperthyroidism that persits after an initial ^{131}I dose. If the hyperthyroidism is then not much improved, I prefer to administer a second ^{131}I dose 3 months after the initial unsuccessful therapy.

For long-term treatment of hyperthyroidism, either primary therapy or supplemental to ^{131}I, I prescribe 3 drops of Lugol's solution daily. One drop may be enough, but the extra drops provide insurance against incomplete self-administration. The iodide solution is taken with fruit juice to mask the taste. Treatment may be continued for 6 months, more or less, when given after ^{131}I, or for 1 to 2 years if it is the primary therapy. If escape occurs or if the proposed course of treatment is not followed by a sustained remission, I then resort to ^{131}I.

Of 25 patients with hyperthyroidism who were given Lugol's solution as the primary treatment, 21 were females and 4 were males. They ranged in age from 18 to 62 years. All these patients had mild hyperthyroidism and goiter that was no larger than twice the normal size. No followup data are available for five patients. Of the remaining 20, four failed to respond satisfactorily, one experienced an escape after several months of good control, and two had relapses after successful control for over 1 year. Thus, seven patients (35 per cent) had a poor response to treatment. In another seven patients (35 per cent) a remission was induced and sustained for 1 or more years after withdrawal of Lugol's solution. One of these patients was successfully treated with Lugol's solution after several trials with ATD over a 4-year period failed to lead to a remission. In six patients (30 per cent) the disease has been controlled by the medication.

From this experience it is concluded that Lugol's solution is a reasonable method of treatment in selected patients in the hope of avoiding therapy that is destructive to the thyroid. Only about 1 to 2 per cent of hyperthyroid patients are suitable for this simple treatment.

NEONATAL HYPERTHYROIDISM

I have no personal experience with this rare form of hyperthyroidism. It usually lasts only a few weeks but occasionally may be prolonged. Sometimes it is severe enough to precipitate congestive heart failure. Treatment is simply accomplished by the addition of Lugol's solution to the infant's formula. Three drops daily should be adequate. Propranolol, 2 mg/kg, and PTU, 5 mg/kg, also may be helpful.

Reference

1. Friend DG: Iodide therapy and the importance of quantitating the dose. *New Eng J Med* 263:1358–1360, 1960

D. PROPRANOLOL (INDERAL)

In my opinion, propranolol is the most important single advance in the management of hyperthyroidism since ^{131}I (i.e., in the last 30 years). I say this even though this drug is not used as a primary treatment for hyperthyroidism but

TABLE 2–15. INDICATIONS, ADVANTAGES, AND DISADVANTAGES OF PROPRANOLOL IN THE TREATMENT OF HYPERTHYROIDISM

INDICATIONS
1. Preparation of patients for thyroidectomy (in conjunction with stable iodide and possibly adrenal cortical steroids) when ATD cannot be given
2. Thyroid storm
3. Relief of tachycardia and tremor while awaiting the response to definitive therapy

ADVANTAGES
1. The response is dramatic and appreciated within hours.
2. Does not interfere with other therapeutic modalities
3. Does not affect thyroid function tests

DISADVANTAGES
1. Contraindicated in asthmatics, in whom it may induce status asthmaticus
2. May aggravate congestive heart failure. The risk of this complication in hyperthyroid patients has not been well studied but is probably less than in euthyroid patients
3. May mask hypoglycemic manifestations of insulin overdosage in patients with coexistent diabetes mellitus
4. Occasional cutaneous, hematologic, gastrointestinal, and other miscellaneous reactions as with all drugs

only as a supplemental agent. Nevertheless, the usefulness of propranolol in controlling tachycardia and tremor while awaiting the results of definitive therapy is so outstanding that it has virtually revolutionized our methods of management. For example, it is almost never necessary to hospitalize patients with hyperthyroidism, no matter how severe. The onset of action of propranolol is so prompt that within a few hours there is significant clinical improvement. I keep a supply of the medication on hand and often administer it on the initial visit, indicating to the patient that by the time she is home she will be feeling better, and she is.

CAUTION: If given to asthmatics, propranolol may precipitate status asthmaticus. Also, it may aggravate congestive heart failure.

Propranolol may be given in conjunction with iodide and adrenal cortical steroids to prepare patients who are allergic to ATD for thyroidectomy (since most of these patients will be treated with ^{131}I, this is not a common indication).

Propranolol has greatly improved the treatment of thyroid storm. Most patients are better in less than 24 hours. The intravenous route of administration may be employed initially, with a switch to the oral route later.

Propranolol is most frequently used to relieve the tachycardia and tremor of patients with moderately severe hyperthyroidism. Depending upon the severity of the hyperthyroidism, I institute treatment with 20 to 40 mg of propranolol four times daily. The medication may be tapered to elimination over 4 to 6 weeks after high-dose ^{131}I therapy.

E. RADIOACTIVE IODINE THERAPY (^{131}I)

This is the treatment of choice for most patients with hyperthyroidism.

In terms of safety, simplicity, and economy the record of ^{131}I is clearly superior to that of alternative forms of treatment. Hence, the treatment of choice for most hyperthyroid patients is no longer the subject of serious dispute. Extensive

TABLE 2-16. INDICATIONS, ADVANTAGES, AND DISADVANTAGES OF RADIOACTIVE IODINE IN THE TREATMENT OF HYPERTHYROIDISM

INDICATIONS
1. Hyperthyroidism in most adults, whether TDG, TMNG, or toxic AFTA
2. Recurrent hyperthyroidism after thyroidectomy
3. Hyperthyroidism in children experiencing toxicity to ATD and for whom thyroidectomy is refused

ADVANTAGES
1. Safety—there should be no complications other than hypothyroidism
2. No hospitalization
3. Low cost
4. Rapid elimination of goiter and hyperthyroidism if high doses are given

DISADVANTAGES
1. Hypothyroidism occurs in 30 to 80 per cent, depending upon dosage and duration of followup
2. Prolonged illness and late relapse if low doses are given
3. Concern for possible but unrealized complications
4. Thyroid storm or exacerbation of hyperthyroidism in improperly prepared, severely toxic patients
5. Unwarranted lay and professional fear of radiation

experience reveals no increased incidence of thyroid cancer, leukemia, or genetic problems after ^{131}I therapy.

Hypothyroidism is the only complication inherently related to the treatment. It is to the reduction of this complication that principal attention has been paid in recent years. Suggestions to minimize hypothyroidism include external radiation, ^{125}I therapy, and smaller ^{131}I doses, followed by either ATD or stable iodide to maintain control of the hyperthyroidism in anticipation of a progressive decline in thyroid function that would permit ultimate withdrawal of the suppression drug. None of these methods has proved entirely satisfactory. Lower ^{131}I doses have been employed generally. After treating about 600 patients with small ^{131}I doses I reached the conclusion that this treatment results in a substantial increase in morbidity for many patients, often to the point of impracticality. Whether the ultimate incidence of hypothyroidism is thereby significantly reduced is unknown; but a substantial hypothyroid incidence is still seen in my patients. There is a growing feeling among thyroidologists (expressed freely orally, less often in print) that it might be better to treat routinely with high ^{131}I doses and warn the patients in advance that they will probably need replacement thyroid hormone for life. By this means one can virtually assure a prompt elimination of the hyperthyroidism with a single treatment, a minimal number of reevaluations, and minimum expense. These are persuasive arguments, and in practice I have found this approach acceptable and preferred by most patients.

Nevertheless, for patients who wish to take the risk of a prolonged illness with no guarantee of any real ultimate benefit in terms of reduced incidence of hypothyroidism, and for whom prolonged or recurrent hyperthyroidism constitutes no special risks (as would be the case with coexistent heart disease), then low-dose ^{131}I therapy might be employed. At this time it may be best to provide the patient with the facts and to permit him or her to participate in the final decision. The doctrine of informed consent would seem to oblige the physician to present a full discussion of alternative therapeutic methods employing ^{131}I in view of the possible differences in outcome.

TABLE 2-17. AGE AND SEX DISTRIBUTION OF 1092 PATIENTS WITH TDG

AGE (YEARS)	MALE	FEMALE	TOTAL
<20	29	70	99
20-29	32	205	237
30-39	46	213	259
40-49	41	211	252
50-59	35	116	151
60-69	15	62	77
70 +	3	14	17
Total	201	891	1092

Experience with TDG

Table 2-17 gives the age and sex distribution of 1092 patients with TDG seen between 1962 and 1973.

In 819 of these patients the initial treatment was ^{131}I. An additional 116 patients were given ^{131}I after unsatisfactory responses to treatment with ATD or Lugol's solution. Thus, 935 of 1092 patients with TDG (85 per cent) received therapeutic doses of ^{131}I. All 62 patients with TMNG, 21 of 25 patients with toxic AFTA, and 43 of 46 patients with TRG were treated with ^{131}I. (The remaining three TRG patients were not returned to Northland Thyroid Laboratory after the diagnosis was established.) Hence, a total of 1061 hyperthyroid patients received ^{131}I therapy.

By 1967 concern for the high incidence of hypothyroidism produced by conventional ^{131}I dosage was at its maximum. A number of authorities concluded that lower ^{131}I doses would reduce the incidence of this complication. Having by this time treated over 200 private patients (in addition to those I treated during my training and whose treatment I supervised during my tenure with the Thyroid Service at Wayne State University College of Medicine), I was hopeful that I might have had enough experience to be successful with small ^{131}I doses. Specifically, I had learned to be cautious with the following types of patients:

1. Patients with mild hyperthyroidism.
2. Patients with goiters of twice the normal size or smaller.
3. Patients with TRG.
4. Patients with RAI values of less than 50 per cent or over 70 per cent.

On the other hand, I found that patients with large TDG (e.g., three and a half times normal size or larger), those with TMNG, and those with toxic AFTA tolerated and required larger than usual ^{131}I doses.

Within these guidelines I employed reduced doses of ^{131}I for patients with TDG, barring those for whom prolonged hyperthyroidism might constitute a special hazard (e.g., thyrocardiacs, aged patients), for about 6 years, during which about 600 patients were treated. A detailed analysis of my methods and early results in comparison with those of others has been published previously.* The results of the most recently treated 197 patients are summarized in Table 2-18.

These patients were treated between 1972 and 1973 after several years experience with low ^{131}I doses; thus, the results should represent the best I can do.

From this experience the following conclusions were drawn:

---

*Hamburger JI: *Hyperthyroidism, Concept and Controversy.* Springfield, Illinois, Charles C Thomas, 1972, pp 92-137

TABLE 2–18. RESULTS OF LOW-DOSE ^{131}I THERAPY IN 197 PATIENTS

EUTHYROID AT 3 MONTHS			68 (34.5 per cent)
Still euthyroid		55	
Relapse—re-treated (at 6 and 10 months)		2	
Relapse—treated with Lugol's solution and again became euthyroid		5	
Relapse—still on Lugol's solution		2	
Relapse—mild, spontaneous recovery		1	
Possible relapse—under observation		1	
Euthyroid—treated with high serum TSH		2	
RE-TREATMENT			
(two doses—38; three doses—3; four doses—1)			42 (21.3 per cent)
Hypothyroid		20	
Recovered and became euthyroid	5		
Euthyroid after the second ^{131}I dose		16	
Still hyperthyroid more than 3 months later		3	
Incomplete followup		1	
Lost to followup after the second ^{131}I dose		2	
HYPOTHYROID AT 3 MONTHS			87 (44.2 per cent)
Recovered		35	
Again hypothyroid	2		
Nonsuppressible recovery with iatrogenic toxicosis	4		
Recovery followed by recurrent toxicosis, still on Lugol's solution	1		
Permanent hypothyroidism, not confirmed		17	
Permanent hypothyroidism, confirmed		35	
Partial nonsuppressible recovery with iatrogenic toxicosis	1		

1. Even with low ^{131}I doses a substantial incidence of hypothyroidism was produced, although the duration of followup was not more than 2 years.

2. About 20 per cent of patients failed to respond to the lower ^{131}I doses and received either repeated ^{131}I therapy or long-term treatment with Lugol's solution to control the hyperthyroidism.

3. The course of thyroid function after low-dose ^{131}I therapy is complex and unpredictable, and the therapeutic result achieved may be unstable.

4. The consequences of the unpredictable and unstable results of low-dose ^{131}I therapy include:

    a. Prolongation of the illness per se.

    b. Substantial increase in loss of time from work

        (1) Attributed to the debilitating effects of hyperthyroidism.

        (2) Because of extra visits to the physician.

    c. Increased cost to the patient

        (1) Loss of wages.

        (2) Charges for extra testing, drugs, and ^{131}I therapy.

Because of this experience I gradually became less satisfied with the low-dose regimen. The straw that broke the camel's back was a discussion with Dr. George Crile, Jr., early in 1973. He believed that using lower ^{131}I doses to try to avoid hypothyroidism was a foolish waste of effort and advised that I do what he had been doing for some time—i.e., attempt deliberate ablation of the thyroid gland followed by thyroid hormone. Of the first 100 patients I treated with large doses (8 to 30 mCi), elimination of hyperthyroidism was achieved with the initial ^{131}I dose within 3 months in 98 patients while the other 2 patients required only two doses. Within 3 months after the treatment, two thirds of the patients developed hypothyroidism, and one third were euthyroid. Some of the hypothyroid patients recovered later and had nonsuppressible function, making it necessary to discontinue replacement therapy. On the other hand, some who were euthyroid at 3 months became hypothyroid later. Therefore, my current routine treatment is as follows:

1. The dose of ^{131}I is empirical, ranging from 8 to 30 mCi depending primarily upon the size of the goiter and secondarily upon the RAI value, giving larger doses to patients with lower uptakes.

2. The initial followup visit is at 6 weeks. If there is evidence of hypothyroidism, either clinical or laboratory, at that time I will start treatment with LT$_4$, 0.1 to 0.15 mg daily.

3. The second followup visit is at 3 months.
   a. Those already on thyroid hormone, if still hypothyroid, will have the dose increased to full replacement levels (0.15 to 0.2 mg of LT$_4$ daily). If nonsuppressible thyroid function has recurred, as indicated by a normal RAI value in spite of the administration of LT$_4$, then thyroid hormone should be discontinued and the patient rechecked in 6 months.
   b. Those who did not require thyroid hormone at 6 weeks will start replacement therapy if needed (LT$_4$, 0.15 mg daily); or, if they are still euthyroid, they are advised to return for further followup in 3 months.
   c. The infrequent patient who is still hyperthyroid will be re-treated with ^{131}I.

4. The third followup visit is at either 6 months or 3 months.
   a. Six months for those on replacement therapy. The purpose is primarily to rule out recovery of nonsuppressible function.
   b. Three months for patients who were euthyroid at the 3 months check. The purpose is primarily to rule out declining function.

5. Once the situation is stable, annual examination is advised.
   a. For those on replacement thyroid hormone an FTI and TSH(RIA) are helpful to assure that the medication has been taken regularly and that the dose is neither too high nor too low. Recovery of nonsuppressible function may necessitate a reduction in the dose or even discontinuation of thyroid hormone. This would be suggested by either enlargement of the thyroid or tachycardia. An elevated FTI or a nonsuppressible RAI would confirm the diagnosis.
   b. If the patient had residual nonsuppressible but subnormal function for which a supplemental dose of thyroid hormone was given, the FTI and TSH(RIA) will be of value to assess the continued adequacy of the current dosage. If there is further deterioration in function it may be necessary to increase the dose of thyroid hormone. On the contrary, it is also possible for the residual function to increase, as noted above.
   c. For euthyroid patients the principal objective of the followup examination is to rule out late onset hypothyroidism. The FTI and TSH(RIA) are useful screening tests for this purpose.

Experience with TMNG

A number of years ago I wrote a paper entitled "Why Not Radioiodine Therapy For Toxic Nodular Goiter?" My point was that the arguments against this therapy were unsound. Results of ^{131}I therapy were not only good but better than those for TDG because there was much less hypothyroidism, even though high ^{131}I doses were employed. Many of these patients have coexistent heart disease and

TABLE 2-19. AGE AND SEX DISTRIBUTION OF PATIENTS WITH TMNG

AGE (YEARS)	MALE	FEMALE
30–39	0	1
40–49	1	5
50–59	1	13
60–69	2	18
70+	3	18
Total	7	55

should be prepared for ^{131}I therapy by 4 to 6 weeks of ATD pretreatment. In the absence of heart disease, one can treat with ^{131}I directly.

Since these are older patients, it may be advisable to administer propranolol prior to and for several weeks after the ^{131}I. A discharge of additional thyroid hormone could precipitate cardiac complications in marginally compensated patients. All of these patients were successfully treated with large doses of ^{131}I, e.g., 20 to 30 mCi or more. In 49 patients hyperthyroidism was eliminated with a single ^{131}I treatment, and 3 patients required two treatments. One patient had thyroidectomy subsequently for persistent obstruction.

Most of these patients do not require thyroid hormone after ^{131}I, although some pass through a temporary hypothyroid phase. Since late onset hypothyroidism is possible, annual followup is essential.

This experience supports my earlier suggestion that ^{131}I is an effective and safe method of treatment for patients with TMNG.

Reference

1. Hamburger JI: Why not radioiodine therapy for toxic nodular goiter? *Arch Intern Med* 119:75–79, 1967

Experience with Toxic AFTA

The toxic AFTA is an uncommon form of hyperthyroidism — the least common structural abnormality of the thyroid gland associated with hyperthyroidism in this country. It is a disease that is largely confined to the over 40 year old population, and more than half of our patients were over 60 years of age. For the older patient, ablation with ^{131}I is simple and successful. For patients under 40 years of age I prefer excision, unless there are contraindications. This recommendation is based upon a theoretical consideration for which there is only limited clinical support. The argument proceeds as follows:

1. Iodine-131 is concentrated almost exclusively by the AFTA, heavily irradiating this tissue and usually resulting in its functional ablation and death of most of the cells. The extranodular tissue is spared from the intense radiation since beta radiation, the principal emission of ^{131}I, travels only a few millimeters in tissue. However, ^{131}I also gives off some gamma radiation, which does irradiate the extranodular tissue, although much less intensely than the AFTA proper.

2. After ablation of the AFTA, the extranodular tissue, which previously was at rest by virtue of suppression of TSH by the autonomous secretion of the AFTA, becomes stimulated by TSH. It is now the thyroid tissue upon which the patient must depend for hormonal secretion.

TABLE 2-20. AGE AND SEX DISTRIBUTION FOR PATIENTS WITH TOXIC AFTA

AGE (YEARS)	MALE	FEMALE
30–39	0	3
40–49	0	4
50–59	0	3
60–69	3	5
70+	3	4
Total	6	19

3. The above conditions are almost precisely those created in the experimental animal if one wishes to induce thyroid cancer — i.e., low intensity radiation followed by TSH stimulation (in the animal the latter is induced by a low iodine diet or ATD).

4. One of my patients developed a multifocal cancer involving the extranodular tissue exclusively. A similar case has been published by an Italian worker.

5. These may have been coincidental phenomena, but the experimental and clinical circumstances seem too closely parallel to ignore.

Operation for a toxic AFTA is simpler than for TDG, since only nodulectomy rather than subtotal thyroidectomy is necessary. Hence, the risks of surgical complications are greatly reduced.

When ^{131}I is employed, a large enough dose should be given to deliver 15 to 20 mCi to the lesion. AFTA tend to be radioresistant, and failure to achieve ablation with the first dose may reduce ^{131}I uptake by the lesion, making it more difficult to deliver an adequate dose the second time. Furthermore, if AFTA function is totally eliminated, one can administer suppressive doses of thyroid hormone to prevent TSH stimulation of the less irradiated extranodular tissue.

The age distribution for toxic AFTA is similar to that for TMNG. Twenty-one patients were treated successfully with ^{131}I, while four had surgical treatment — three because they were less than 40 years old and the fourth because of obstruction.

References

1. Hamburger JI and Meier DA: Cancer following treatment of an autonomously functioning thyroid nodule with sodium iodide I[131]. *Arch Surg* 103:762–764, 1971
2. Scandelari C: [131]I treatment of toxic autonomous adenoma of the thyroid. In Fiorentino M, Vangelisto R and Grigolette E (eds): *Thyroid Tumors, Lymphomas, and Granulocytic Leukemia.* Piccin, Podova, 1972, p 89

SPECIAL PROBLEMS ASSOCIATED WITH HYPERTHYROIDISM

Hyperthyroidism Associated with Heart Disease

The term thyrocardiac has been coined to describe hyperthyroid patients with cardiac complications such as congestive heart failure and a cardiac arrhythmia other than sinus tachycardia (usually atrial fibrillation). Although hyperthyroidism may lead to cardiac decompensation at any age if the cardiac reserve is reduced by a primary disorder of the heart, for practical purposes this combination of problems is confined to the population over 40 years of age. The thyrocardiac is seriously ill and requires prompt and decisive treatment. With proper management rather remarkable clinical responses can be achieved, and rarely is it necessary even to hospitalize the patient.

Cardiac Measures. Rest, digitalis, and diuretics are important. It is correct that hyperthyroid patients are relatively resistant to digitalis, but it is incorrect that they do not respond. However, as thyroid function is progressively reduced to the euthyroid state the requirement for digitalis is likely to fall. Digitalis doses must then be reduced if toxicity is to be avoided.

The use of propranolol in patients with congestive heart failure is generally considered unwise. However, in hyperthyroidism, the cardiac failure may be aggravated or precipitated by the tachycardia per se, and the judicious use of propranolol may be acceptable and helpful. Having said this, I should add that propranolol should be used with caution under these circumstances and is seldom necessary; if the patient is sick enough to consider its use, then hospitalization is in order and so is consultation with a cardiologist.

Thyroid Management. The thyrocardiac should not be treated with ^{131}I until the hyperthyroidism has been controlled and the cardiac status stabilized. It is difficult to kill patients with ^{131}I, but this is the patient who may succumb if not properly prepared. The discharge of any stored hormone in response to the radiation injury of ^{131}I may be just enough to tip the balance of a marginally compensated patient. If in doubt, it is never wrong to prepare the patient.

One should not begin with less than 300 mg of PTU four times a day in such a patient. I do not use iodide in addition, for it is not necessary. Furthermore, these patients often have large multinodular goiters that conceivably could be induced to increase synthesis and secretion of thyroid hormone if iodides are given. Even the high PTU dose recommended may not completely block iodide uptake by the thyroid. I recall one patient with severe hyperthyroidism for whom I was concerned about impending storm. After 1 month of treatment with 1200 mg of PTU daily she was still quite hyperthyroid. The original RAI value was 72 per cent, and on PTU it was 38 per cent — far from a complete block.

The usual patient will be prepared in 1 month. PTU may be interrupted for 48 hours and ^{131}I given. I almost never give less than 30 mCi to patients who are this sick. I want to be as sure as possible that the hyperthyroidism will be definitively and permanently eliminated. Forty-eight hours after the administration of ^{131}I, I resume PTU, 150 mg four times a day for 3 weeks, then 100 mg four times a day for 3 weeks, after which it is usually possible to stop PTU. For the occasional resistant patient a second dose of ^{131}I may be needed, and full doses of PTU may have to be maintained until there is evidence of successful ablation.

Following ^{131}I therapy one should not assume that thyroid hormone will always be needed. Many of these patients have large TMNG and seldom develop permanent hypothyroidism. There may be a temporary period of hypothyroidism, but it usually lasts no more than a month or two, and the patient recovers. The recovered function is almost always nonsuppressible, so that inappropriate administration of thyroid hormone may precipitate an iatrogenic recurrence of hyperthyroidism. It is safer to observe the patient for a few months before deciding whether thyroid hormone is needed. When thyroid hormone is ordered, the dosage should be supplemental rather than total replacement. For example, if the patient seems to have significant, although subnormal, thyroid function, one might give LT_4, 0.1 mg daily, and check the TSH(RIA) in 1 month to see if suppression is achieved. If so, the dose should not be increased.

If the patient has a diffuse goiter no larger than three times normal size, it is almost certain that ablation of the hyperthyroidism will be achieved with 30 mCi of

TABLE 2-21. AGE AND SEX DISTRIBUTION OF 38 THYROCARDIAC PATIENTS

AGE (YEARS)	MALE	FEMALE
30–39	0	2
40–49	3	1
50–59	4	5
60–69	2	5
70–79	5	9
80+	0	2
Total	14	24

[131]I. Therefore, replacement therapy with thyroid hormone can be given as soon as there is beginning evidence of hypothyroidism. I start with LT_4, 0.15 mg daily, and check the patient in 4 to 6 months for recovery of nonsuppressible function. If this has not occurred, and the TSH(RIA) value is suppressed, then the patient is followed annually. Larger TDG may require more than one 30 mCi dose of [131]I.

The preponderance of elderly patients is, of course, expected. Twenty patients had TDG, 12 had TMNG, four had toxic AFTA, and two had TRG.

Nineteen patients had congestive heart failure, 15 had atrial fibrillation, and six had coronary artery disease (some had more than one of these problems—hence, the numerical discrepancy). Of those with atrial fibrillation, eight had recovery of normal sinus rhythm after correction of hyperthyroidism, four did not, and for three there was no opportunity to assess this point. Twenty-nine were treated as outpatients. Three were hospitalized only because the large dose of ^{131}I given necessitated hospitalization in keeping with Atomic Energy Commission regulations. Three were treated in the hospital because they had been hospitalized by their attending physicians before consultation was requested. Only two patients were hospitalized because of concern for the cardiac status per se.

These patients were prepared for ^{131}I with ATD in conjunction with routine care for the cardiac complications. Large ^{131}I doses were employed routinely, i.e, 30 mCi or more. No patient experienced a worsening of the heart disease as a result of the ^{131}I therapy, and improvement was the rule. One patient was not restored to the euthyroid state in spite of being given 75 mCi of [131]I. She refused further therapy and subsequently died.

On the basis of this experience it is concluded that ATD preparation followed by large-dose ^{131}I therapy is a safe and effective way to deal with hyperthyroid patients who have coexistent heart disease.

THE THYROCARDIAC—CASE REPORT

A 72 year old woman was hospitalized with atrial fibrillation, ventricular response 160, and congestive heart failure (Fig. 2–9). She had a history of goiter for many years. The RAI was 32 per cent.

Treatment was instituted with diuretics and Lanoxin, 0.25 mg twice a day. After 3 days there was improvement in the congestive heart failure, but the ventricular rate was still 140, and I was asked to see her in consultation. Lanoxin was increased to 0.25 mg four times a day. Reserpine (this patient was seen before propranolol was available), 0.25 mg four times a day, and PTU, 300 mg four times a day, were added to the regimen, with the plan that ^{131}I would be given when there was enough improvement to proceed safely.

Four weeks later the ventricular rate was 78, although the patient was still in atrial fibrillation (Fig. 2–9 D). The FTI value was 4.6. The RAI was 47 per cent

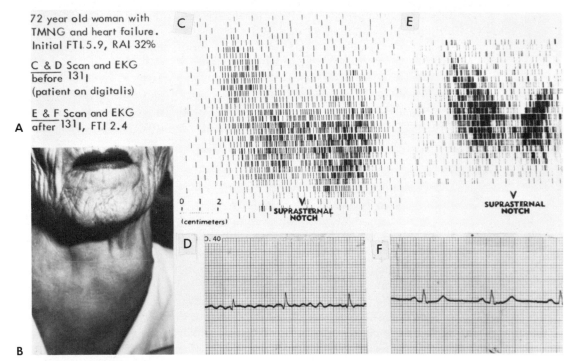

72 year old woman with TMNG and heart failure. Initial FTI 5.9, RAI 32%

C & D Scan and EKG before 131I (patient on digitalis)

E & F Scan and EKG after 131I, FTI 2.4

Figure 2–9. *The thyrocardiac. A,* The history. *B,* The patient. *C–F,* The scan and EKG before and after 131I therapy.

(PTU having been discontinued for 48 hours), and the scan confirmed the presence of a massive TMNG (Fig. 2–9 *C*). PTU preparation was continued for another 2 weeks and then stopped. Two days later, 100 mCi of 131I was given. PTU was resumed 2 days after the therapy. Reserpine and Lanoxin were, of course, continued. The 131I was tolerated without incident.

FTI values remained elevated for over 3 months after 131I, then gradually declined, permitting progressive reduction in PTU dosage. The PTU was discontinued 6 months after the therapy, when it was also possible to stop both reserpine and Lanoxin, since the patient was in normal sinus rhythm (Fig. 2–9 *F*).

Eight months after 131I therapy thyroid function tests were entirely normal. The scan (Fig. 2–9 *E*) showed that the goiter had been considerably reduced in size.

The patient did well until age 74 when she died of a stroke.

Jodbasedow's Disease

This is a very uncommon condition. Only four of more than 2000 hyperthyroid patients had jodbasedow's disease. The situation was the same for all: asthma plus multinodular goiter plus iodides resulted in hyperthyroidism. The cure consisted of discontinuing the iodides. If iodides are essential, 131I ablative therapy may render the thyroid incapable of producing toxicity. Of course, iodides would have to be discontinued for several weeks to permit 131I therapy.

Iatrogenic or Factitious Hyperthyroidism

The treatment is obvious — stop the thyroid hormone. Prevention is important. In my experience there are several distinct situations in which physicians tend to give excessive doses of thyroid hormone:

1. Failure to recognize that toxicity may result from the usual replacement doses if the patient has nonsuppressible function, e.g.:
   a. after ^{131}I or thyroidectomy for hyperthyroidism.
   b. if the patient has a multinodular goiter.
   c. if the patient has diffuse goiter, or euthyroid Graves' disease.
   d. if the patient has a solitary AFTA.
2. Treating fatigue without adequate evidence of thyroid disease.
3. Using desiccated thyroid preparations which may vary in potency from batch to batch. Unusually high doses may be well tolerated until a potent batch is given.
4. Failure to recognize that pure T_3-containing preparations will not restore a subnormal FTI to normal regardless of dosage.
5. Attempting to regulate the dosage by unreliable test methods. The most reliable test to confirm an impression of inadequate replacement is the TSH(RIA). If this value is not elevated, further increments in dosage are not going to help the patient.

Factitious hyperthyroidism — i.e., the covert self-administration of thyroid hormone — is uncommon. The only such patient I have seen was presented to me while I was a visiting professor in South Bend, Indiana. She was a nurse and had plagued her physicians for over 2 years with her hyperthyroidism and an unexplained suppression of the RAI. The diagnosis was really simple. Her FTI and T_3-(RIA) values were elevated, and her RAI was depressed but normally responsive to TSH. Of course, the same findings would be present with a toxic ovarian struma, so this point should be checked before making any accusations.

Of 52 patients with iatrogenic thyrotoxicosis seen at Northland Thyroid Laboratory, 46 were females and six were males. They ranged in age from 14 to 73, but most were between 16 and 20 years old.

Almost one third of the patients developed this problem when thyroid hormone was given for suspected hypothyroidism after treatment of hyperthyroidism. It is important to be alert to the possibility that any residual function after treatment of hyperthyroidism may be nonsuppressible, may remain nonsuppressible permanently, and may increase in hormonal secretory capacity.

Two patients were given thyroid hormone for small diffuse goiters. When features of hyperthyroidism ensued, it became clear that function was nonsuppressible. Without supplemental thyroid hormone the patients were euthyroid. It

TABLE 2-22. MECHANISMS UNDERLYING DEVELOPMENT OF IATROGENIC HYPERTHYROIDISM

	NO. PATIENTS
Recovery of nonsuppressible function after ^{131}I-induced hypothyroidism	13
Nonsuppressible function after operation for hyperthyroidism	4
Euthyroid Graves' disease	2
Excessive replacement of thyroid hormone after ^{131}I therapy	5
Excessive replacement of thyroid hormone after thyroidectomy	6
Excessive replacement of thyroid hormone for primary hypothyroidism	8
Excessive dosage for treatment of nontoxic goiter	1
Excessive dosage, no indication for treatment	4
Excessive dosage, indication for treatment unclear	9
Total	52

TABLE 2-23. DOSE RANGE AND TYPE OF THYROID HORMONE TAKEN BY PATIENTS WITH IATROGENIC HYPERTHYROIDISM

PATIENTS WITH NONSUPPRESSIBLE FUNCTION		19
LT_4, 0.1 to 0.3 mg	16	
Desiccated thyroid hormone, 120 to 180 mg	2	
Combination of desiccated thyroid hormone and synthetic T_3–T_4 mixture	1	
PATIENTS WITH SUPPRESSIBLE FUNCTION		34
LT_4, 0.3 to 0.75 mg	17	
T_3, 100 to 200 μg	3	
Desiccated thyroid hormone, 240 to 600 mg	10[a]	
Synthetic T_3–T_4 mixtures, 25 to 100 per cent excess	4[a]	
Total		53[a]

[a]One patient had two episodes of toxicity, once while taking 600 mg of desiccated thyroid hormone and once with a 100 per cent excess dose of synthetic T_3–T_4 mixture.

is a good practice to check an RAI on all goiter patients treated with thyroid hormone after they have taken the medication for 6 to 8 weeks. A value greater than 5 per cent is abnormal if the patient is on LT_4, 0.15 to 0.2 mg daily. If the RAI value is similar to that obtained prior to starting treatment, continued administration of thyroid hormone may lead to toxicity.

Twenty-nine patients were simply taking excessive doses of thyroid hormone. In some instances, the physician was not at fault, for the patient increased the dose without being advised to do so. However, four patients had been given toxic doses of thyroid hormone because of an erroneous diagnosis of hypothyroidism. Normal thyroid function tests were obtained after discontinuation of thyroid hormone.

For three patients the dose of thyroid hormone was increased to toxic levels in a vain effort to elevate the serum T_4 level by administering Cytomel. One patient was advanced to toxic levels of LT_4 on the basis of the ankle jerk test. It should be emphasized that the most reliable indicator of whether additional thyroid hormone is needed is the TSH(RIA) test. If the value for this test is not elevated, the patient neither requires nor will benefit from further increments in thyroid hormone dosage. I have observed one exception to this rule, and that is the patient who is developing hypothyroidism after ^{131}I therapy. Occasionally the rise in TSH(RIA) value may lag behind the fall in FTI and T_3(RIA) values by a week or so. (This discussion assumes that there is normal pituitary and hypothalamic function.)

Table 2–23 shows the types of thyroid hormone and the ranges of dosage which produced iatrogenic thyrotoxicosis in patients with either nonsuppressible or suppressible thyroid function.

T_3 Toxicosis

This entity has received considerable attention in the current medical literature. In T_3 toxicosis the thyroid gland secretes excessive quantities of T_3 without simultaneously producing enough T_4 to result in an elevated blood level.

The concept of T_3 toxicosis includes the implication that if one does not obtain the T_3(RIA) value the diagnosis may be missed. Frankly, I am not impressed. The few patients I have seen who might fulfill the criteria for this diagnosis were not difficult to recognize as having hyperthyroidism. If the diagnosis is doubtful in young patients, observation is safe and is usually conclusive. Nevertheless, a

TABLE 2-24. CLINICAL SETTINGS FOR T₃ TOXICOSIS

1. Toxic AFTA
2. Toxic multinodular goiter
3. Recurrent thyrotoxicosis after operation or ^{131}I therapy
4. Early in the development of toxic diffuse goiter

TABLE 2-25. CRITERIA FOR DIAGNOSIS OF T₃ TOXICOSIS

1. An elevated T_3(RIA) value
2. A normal FTI value
3. Clinical features of hyperthyroidism
4. A normal or elevated RAI value
5. A nonsuppressible RAI value
6. No abnormality of TBG concentration

striking elevation in T_3(RIA) value would be helpful and probably diagnostic. A lesser elevation would present problems, for one could not exclude a compensatory increase in T_3 output because of difficulties in synthesizing T_4.

The real problem exists with older patients with long-standing multinodular goiters in whom thyrotoxicosis may present primarily with cardiac symptoms. These same symptoms may be seen in patients with arteriosclerotic heart disease with coincidental multinodular goiter. An elevated T_3(RIA) value may represent only a compensatory process. Patients with TMNG usually do not have very high RAI values. Patients with heart disease are not good candidates for T_3 suppression testing, and a positive T_3 suppression test may be seen in patients with multinodular goiter whether toxicity is present or not. Hence, the diagnosis of hyperthyroidism may be difficult.

Nevertheless, the diagnosis is critical in terms of management. Even mild hyperthyroidism may be an important aggravating factor in the heart disease. Until the hyperthyroidism has been controlled, it may be difficult or even impossible to restore cardiac compensation. Over the years, I have seen half a dozen such patients and have been able to satisfy myself as to the presence of hyperthyroidism on the basis of the response to a month's treatment with PTU, 300 mg four times a day. If there is objective improvement (principally in the tachycardia), accompanied by a fall in the FTI and, more recently, in the T_3(RIA) also, I am then content to advise definitive therapy.

T₃ TOXICOSIS — CASE REPORT

A 57 year old woman with diabetes mellitus, hypertension, arteriosclerotic heart disease, chronic atrial fibrillation, and congestive heart failure was referred for evaluation and possible ^{131}I therapy. Thyroid function tests were normal, although the patient had had a large multinodular goiter for many years. Her attending physician had been treating her for 13 years and had noted weight loss of some 25 pounds over the previous 6 months. It was his opinion that she had hyperthyroidism even though testing did not show it. He had ordered digitalis and diuretics, which led to relief of congestive heart failure, but atrial fibrillation continued.

Physical examination revealed an elderly woman 67 inches in height and weighing 138 pounds. The blood pressure was 170/90, and the ventricular rate was irregular between 100 and 120. There was no evidence of congestive heart failure.

The RAI was 20 per cent, and the FTI was 3.0 (NR 1.1 to 3.4). The thyroid was multinodular and about six to eight times normal size. The T_3(RIA) was 230 ng per 100 ml (NR 50 to 150 ng per 100 ml). It was my opinion that the clinical findings in conjunction with the elevated T_3(RIA) value were consistent with a diagnosis of T_3 toxicosis. For further confirmation and to prepare the patient for ^{131}I therapy, she was given PTU, 300 mg four times a day for 4 weeks. At the end of this period the patient had gained 5 pounds and her ventricular rate had slowed to between 80 and 96. The T_3(RIA) had fallen to 139 ng per 100 ml. The patient was given ^{131}I, 30 mCi (PTU having been interrupted for 48 hours). Propranolol, 20 mg four times a day, was started 24 hours in advance of the ^{131}I and continued with graded reduction in dosage for 3 weeks. The patient improved progressively, and by 9 months after the ^{131}I therapy she was in normal sinus rhythm with a rate of 72. Her weight was 144 pounds, and she was feeling fine on no medication other than for diabetes.

References

1. Shafer RB and Nuttal FQ: Thyroid crisis induced by radioactive iodine. *J Nucl Med* 12:262–264, 1971
2. Parker JLW and Lawson DH: Death from thyrotoxicosis. *Lancet* 2:10–20, 1973
3. Rapoport B, Caplan R and DeGroot LJ: Low-dose sodium iodide I[131] therapy in Graves' disease. *JAMA* 224:1610–1613, 1973
4. Cevallos JL, Hagen GA, Maloof F and Chapman EM: Low-dosage ^{131}I therapy of thyrotoxicosis (diffuse goiters). *New Eng J Med* 290:141–143, 1974
5. Goolden AWG and Fraser TR: Treatment of thyrotoxicosis with low doses of radioactive iodine. *Brit Med J* 2:442–443, 1969
6. Sterling K, Refetoff S and Selenkow HA: T_3 thyrotoxicosis: Thyrotoxicosis due to elevated serum triiodothyronine levels. *JAMA* 213:571–576, 1970
7. Wahner HW and Gorman CA: Interpretation of serum triiodothyronine levels measured by the Sterling technic. *New Eng J Med* 284:225–230, 1971

Apathetic Hyperthyroidism (Masked Hyperthyroidism)

The apathetic form of hyperthyroidism is seen principally in elderly patients, who often have long-standing multinodular goiters which have become toxic after

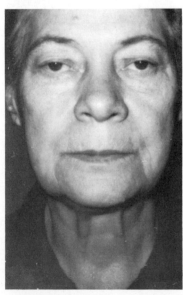

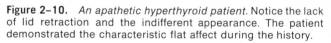

Figure 2-10. *An apathetic hyperthyroid patient.* Notice the lack of lid retraction and the indifferent appearance. The patient demonstrated the characteristic flat affect during the history.

years of quiescence. The principal clinical features often relate to the cardiovascular system — e.g., sudden onset of atrial fibrillation and congestive heart failure. Weight loss is also common and may be severe if anorexia is present, a common complaint in elderly thyrotoxic patients. The problem is overlooking the diagnosis. The solution is to consider hyperthyroidism under the circumstances just described. This is particularly important if there is an obvious goiter. One should not be distracted by the fact that the goiter has been present for many years. A case in point is an 86 year old woman who, when asked how long she had had her very large goiter, responded, "Sonny, I've had that goiter over 73 years, and it's never bothered me. Why is everyone making such a fuss over it now?"

Medical Treatment for Graves' Ophthalmopathy

Perhaps the most difficult problem with which the thyroidologist must deal is that of Graves' ophthalmopathy. These difficulties are not only therapeutic but also diagnostic.

Diagnostic Difficulties. Not every case of proptosis is part of the syndrome of Graves' disease. Most troublesome is the patient with unilateral or markedly asymmetrical proptosis. Most of these patients, barring those with obvious tumor as the cause, have Graves' ophthalmopathy. It is incorrect to think that patients with Graves' ophthalmopathy always have symmetrical proptosis. Symmetry is the exception, and prominent asymmetry is common. Unilateral proptosis may be followed months or years later with contralateral proptosis. However, when one encounters a patient with unilateral or markedly asymmetrical proptosis, the possibility of an orbital tumor requires careful consideration. A vascular lesion is also possible. In these patients auscultation of the eyeball may reveal a bruit. As formidable a problem as this may seem, it is only one of the diagnostic difficulties which the thyroidologist must face.

What should be said about the patient with bilateral proptosis of slight to moderate or even severe degree, who has no evidence of thyroid disease, present or past? Is this Graves' disease with the ophthalmopathy as an advance warning and the hyperthyroidism waiting in the wings? How can one tell? Of course, there is the T_3 suppression test. Most of these patients will have suppressible function, and those with nonsuppressible function do not usually progress rapidly to hyperthyroidism. In fact, this progression is the exception in my experience. It is my practice to advise serial measurements until it is clear whether the involvement is progressive. Thyroid function testing may be repeated if the clinical picture suggests the necessity. The usual sequence of events is a relatively rapid protrusion of the eyeball, followed by stability without subsequent development of hyperthyroidism.

Therapeutic Difficulties. Once having established the diagnosis of Graves' ophthalmopathy, one must face the fact that, in the absence of any fundamental understanding of the pathophysiology and with no specific remedy, all that can be offered are empirical and symptomatic measures. One hundred years from now physicians will laugh at our current therapy of Graves' ophthalmopathy, just as we laugh at our predecessors who used to paint the neck with iodine to treat goiter patients (perhaps that treatment is less laughable than ours).

With this brief introduction we can proceed to outline what is known about the management of Graves' ophthalmopathy.

Mechanical Methods. Periorbital edema and chemosis are usually worse in the morning after the patient has been in the horizontal position overnight. Elevation of the head of the bed, or at least sleeping on several pillows to elevate the head, will help to minimize the effects of gravity on fluid movement into the orbital area. It should be determined whether the patient's eyes close properly when asleep. A spouse, other relative, or friend may be asked to observe the patient for this purpose. If there is incomplete approximation of the lids a bland nocturnal ointment should be used in conjunction with eye patches of clear plastic wrap affixed with tape. Dark glasses are important when outside in sunlight. Also, it is useful to instruct the patient not to smoke and not to remain in closed areas with smokers.

Local Measures. If lacrimation and foreign body sensation are disturbing, local adrenal steroid preparations may be employed. These should be monitored by an ophthalmologist. Radiation therapy to the orbit using the linear accelerator is under investigation by Kriss. The preliminary results suggest that this treatment may have value, at least in improving the mobility of the globes.

Systemic Measures. Hyperthyroidism should be controlled and hypothyroidism strictly avoided. Both seem to be bad for the eyes. It makes no difference how the hyperthyroidism is treated. Restoration of the euthyroid state may improve the appearance, even though there is actually a measurable increase in proptosis. This is because upper lid retraction produces such a striking alteration of appearance (Fig. 2–11).

The use of adrenal steroids in large doses is an accepted form of treatment for severe progressive ophthalmopathy. The response to this treatment is unpredictable. At one time I thought that I might not be doing as well as others because I began treatment with 80 mg of prednisone daily rather than 100 or 150 mg. Use of the higher doses has not materially altered my success rate. Of course, the situation might have worsened without treatment. Actually, the disease is so unpredictable that one simply never knows.

I usually pursue treatment with graded reductions over a 3- to 6-month period, depending upon the response. I switch to an alternate day regimen after the first 2 weeks. Figure 2–12 shows the improvement in periorbital edema and ocular mobility achieved with steroid therapy.

If the involvement is not too severe, it may be best to take a watch and wait approach. The natural course of this disease is toward spontaneous improvement. On the other hand, occasionally there is an exceptional patient who develops

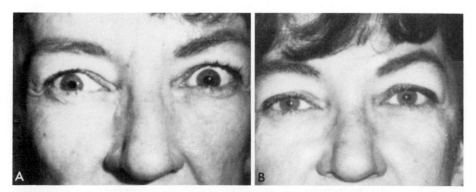

Figure 2–11. *The effect of a reduction in lid retraction on appearance. A,* Before treatment with ^{131}I, Hertel exophthalmometric measurements were 16 mm bilaterally. *B,* After ^{131}I therapy, the measurements increased to 19 mm bilaterally, but the appearance is greatly improved by the drop in the eyelids.

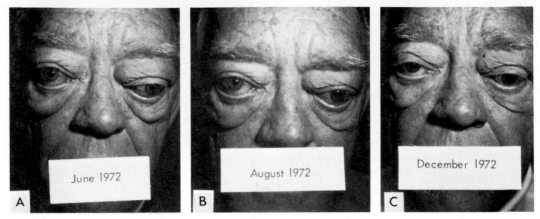

Figure 2-12. *Response of Graves' ophthalmopathy to prednisone. A,* Before treatment there is marked periorbital edema and deviation of the left eye laterally and inferiorly. *B,* Beginning improvement. *C,* After 6 months' treatment there is marked regression of edema, and the eyes are almost aligned.

worsening of the ophthalmopathy years after the hyperthyroidism has been eliminated (Fig. 2–13).

EXPERIENCE WITH MEDICAL MANAGEMENT OF GRAVES' OPHTHALMOPATHY

The initial ophthalmic findings in 204 consecutive patients with TDG (Graves' disease) are listed in Table 2–26.

For 118 patients exophthalmometric measurements were taken before and after correction of the hyperthyroidism. Table 2–27 summarizes the findings.

Regardless of the initial ocular measurements, most patients had no more than a 1 mm variation after treatment. The most common change was bilateral protrusion. The range of protrusion was 2 to 4 mm (average 2.5 mm) for those with unilateral protrusion, and 2 to 6 mm per eye (average 3.05 mm) for those with bilateral protrusion. In most patients the changes produced only a minimal effect on the appearance. In fact, the improvement in upper lid retraction easily masked a protrusion of 2 to 3 mm.

In the 7-year period between 1966 and 1973 I gave adrenal corticosteroids to 11 patients for severe ophthalmopathy. Table 2–28 summarizes this experience.

Only three patients experienced any improvement, and for one the improvement was minimal. Three patients had further proptosis in spite of treatment. Four patients had no change, and in one patient the steroids were discontinued because of peptic ulcer symptoms.

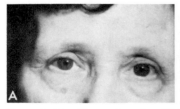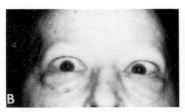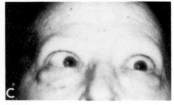

Figure 2-13. *Worsening of ophthalmopathy years after treatment of hyperthyroidism. A,* Immediately after restoration of euthyroidism. *B,* Three years later. Note upper lid retraction and periorbital edema. Upper lid retraction results from contracture of the inferior rectus muscles; as the patient attempts to look up, the lids also retract. Note that the left eye is deviated medially. *C,* The patient looking to the left. The left eye does not move laterally.

TABLE 2-26. INITIAL OPHTHALMIC FINDINGS IN TDG

No abnormality		95
Bilateral upper lid retraction only		42
Bilateral upper lid retraction, edema, chemosis		1
Unilateral upper lid retraction		9
with chemosis	1	
Chemosis only		1
Bilateral proptosis		37
with bilateral upper lid retraction	9	
with unilateral upper lid retraction	2	
with chemosis	1	
with muscular paresis	1	
with bilateral upper lid retraction, edema, and chemosis	8	
with bilateral upper lid retraction, chemosis, and paresis	2	
Unilateral proptosis		19
with bilateral upper lid retraction	6	
with bilateral upper lid retraction, edema, and chemosis	5	
Total		204

An additional patient not treated with adrenal steroids is of interest. In 1950 she had a thyroidectomy for toxic diffuse goiter. Eighteen years later she presented with bilateral proptosis (22 mm right, 20 mm left), severe periorbital edema, chemosis, paresis on convergence, and lateral gaze bilaterally. A 4-cm thyroid remnant which had nonsuppressible function was found on the right side of the neck. Although the patient was euthyroid, this remaining tissue was ablated with ^{131}I to permit full dosage replacement with LT_4 without concern for fluctuating nonsuppressible endogenous secretory activity. The LT_4, 0.2 mg daily, was begun 3 months after ^{131}I therapy and continued permanently thereafter. Over a 4-year followup period, the

TABLE 2-27. CHANGES IN EXOPHTHALMOMETRIC MEASUREMENTS IN GRAVES' DISEASE AFTER CORRECTION OF HYPERTHYROIDISM

INITIAL OCULAR MEASUREMENTS	NO. PATIENTS	CHANGES AFTER TREATMENT	NO. PATIENTS
Less than 18 mm bilaterally	78	No change[b]	55
		Bilateral protrusion	17
		Unilateral protrusion	5
		Unilateral regression	1
Unilateral proptosis[a]	11	No change[b]	7
		Bilateral protrusion	3
		Contralateral protrusion	1
Bilateral proptosis[a]	29	No change[b]	18
		Bilateral protrusion	4
		Unilateral protrusion	4
		Unilateral regression	2
		Bilateral regression	1
Total	118		118

[a]Measurements exceeding 18 mm were considered indicative of proptosis.
[b]No change includes those whose measurements varied by 1 mm or less.

TABLE 2–28. EXPERIENCE WITH ADRENAL CORTICOSTEROID THERAPY FOR GRAVES' OPHTHALMOPATHY

AGE SEX	INDICATION FOR TREATMENT	PRETREATMENT MEASUREMENT (mm)		INITIAL DOSE PRED- NISONE (mg)	DURA- TION TREAT- MENT (mo)	FINAL MEASUREMENT (mm)		COMMENT
		R	L			R	L	
21F	Sudden proptosis, episcleral hemorrhage	22	20	80	6	16	13	Prompt regression in proptosis
21M	Increase in proptosis 5 mm bilaterally	24	25	80	30	28	27	Progression of proptosis
26F	Increase in proptosis 4 mm bilaterally	20	19	75	3.5	23	23	Progression of proptosis
42F	Immobile globes	18	18	100	2.5	20	20	No improvement in mobility
44F	Increase in proptosis 7 & 3 mm, paresis	22	18	80	10	25	22	Progression of proptosis
44M	Severe unilateral proptosis, paresis	31	20	60	1	no change		Treatment DC, peptic ulcer
47M	Severe proptosis, chemosis, & paresis	30	30	100	6	31	29	No improvement
58M	Increase in proptosis unilateral 4 mm, chemosis	22	24	80	20	24	25	Less chemosis
59F	Proptosis, chemosis, periorbital edema	25	24	80	6	25	25	No improvement
63M	Severe proptosis, periorbital edema and paresis	32	31	100	10	30	29	Decreased edema, improved movement
69M	Severe chemosis	17	20	80	6	20	21	Surgery for control of herniation of conjunctiva

proptosis regressed 8 mm bilaterally, the periorbital edema cleared, and ocular movement became normal (Fig. 2–14).

Boris Catz might claim that the ^{131}I ablative therapy was the key to success in this patient. It is more likely, in my opinion, that the improvement was simply the result of the natural tendency of some patients to improve spontaneously. Others, of course, do not.

SURGICAL MEASURES FOR GRAVES' OPHTHALMOPATHY

For Lid Retraction. Persistent retraction of the upper eyelid can be corrected by freeing the levator palpebrae from the tarsal plate. Tarsorrhaphy, although often employed, is usually ineffective for this purpose. Tarsorrhaphy will reduce a widened lateral palpebral fissure and elevate the lower lid, but it will not bring down a retracted upper lid.

For Muscular Imbalance. The usual muscular involvement is characterized by swelling and contracture which limit the movement of the globe in response to the

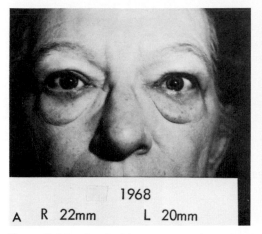 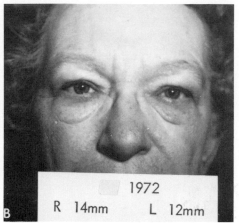

Figure 2-14. *Gradual improvement in periorbital edema and proptosis over a 4 year period. A,* After treatment with ^{131}I and establishment of the euthyroid state with thyroid hormone. *B,* Four years later.

opposing muscle. Recession of the tendon may be effective but should not be undertaken until the condition has been stable for 1 to 2 years. Lesser degrees of muscular imbalance producing diplopia may be improved with prisms.

For Severe Proptosis. Proptosis that fails to respond to adrenal steroids may be corrected by orbital decompression, preferably antral. The principal indication is visual deterioration. The procedure also may be considered for cosmetic reasons.

References

1. Donaldson SS, Bagshaw MA and Kriss JP: Supervoltage orbital radiotherapy for Graves' ophthalmopathy. *J Clin Endocrinol* 37:276–285, 1973
2. Brown J, Coburn JW, Wigod RA, Hiss JH, Jr and Dowling JT: Adrenal steroid therapy of severe infiltrative ophthalmopathy of Graves' disease. *Am J Med* 34:786–795, 1963
3. Catz B and Perzik SL: Subtotal versus total ablation of thyroid: Malignant exophthalmos and its relation to remnant thyroid. *In* Cassano C and Andreoli M (eds): *Current Topics in Thyroid Research.* New York, Academic Press, 1965, p 1183
4. Pequenat EP, Mayberry WE, McConahey WM and Wyse EP: Large doses of radioiodine in Graves' disease: Effect on ophthalmopathy and long-acting thyroid stimulator. *Mayo Clin Proc* 42:802–811, 1967
5. Werner SC, Feind CR and Aida M: Graves' disease and total thyroidectomy. *New Eng J Med* 276:132–137, 1967

PART V. SELF-ASSESSMENT

CASE 2-1. EUTHYROID GRAVES' DISEASE

February, 1967. A 34 year old woman was referred for possible hyperthyroidism. She had been taking thyroid hormone for 1 year in increasing doses; her current dose of levothyroxine was 0.4 mg daily. Her complaints included palpitation, staring gaze, nervousness, and a 4-pound weight loss.

Examination revealed a heart rate of 100, hyperactive reflexes, a mild hand tremor, bilateral lid lag, and a minimally enlarged firm goiter. The RAI on levothyroxine, 0.4 mg daily, was 26 per cent. The scan revealed diffuse symmetrical function. Thyroid hormone was discontinued.

June, 1967. The patient was clinically euthyroid. The serum T_4 by column chromatography was 3.6 μg per 100 ml (normal), and the RAI was 29 per cent. The diagnosis was euthyroid Graves' disease.

With which of the following statements do you agree?

a. The patient will become hyperthyroid soon.
b. Do not be surprised if she becomes hypothyroid.
c. Do not be surprised if her function becomes suppressible in time.
d. She should be treated with ^{131}I prophylactically.
e. Give Lugol's solution.
f. Antithyroid drugs should be given.

Case 2–1 — Followup

May, 1970. The patient returned for reevaluation. She was taking 3 grains of desiccated thyroid hormone daily. The thyroid gland was small. The patient was clinically euthyroid. The FTI was 1.6 and the RAI was 2 per cent.

It was recommended that she continue to take thyroid hormone but preferably levothyroxine, 0.15 mg daily. She has remained euthyroid on this medication, and the RAI has remained suppressed through 1976.

Euthyroid Graves' disease — i.e., diffuse nonsuppressible thyroid function without hyperthyroidism — is seen in our practice about ten times each year. Almost never do these patients progress to frank hyperthyroidism. I am sorry that I have not had antibody studies done on these patients, for it seems possible that this type of information would be of value in understanding why these patients do not develop hyperthyroidism.

In any event, the lesson is clear. No treatment is needed. Observe and anticipate no problems.

Selected Current References for Case 2–1

1. Wyse EP, McConahey WM, Woolner LB, et al: Ophthalmopathy without hyperthyroidism in patients with histologic Hashimoto's thyroiditis. *J Clin Endocrinol* 28:1623–1629, 1968

    Ten patients with ophthalmic findings typical of Graves' disease are reported, none of whom had hyperthyroidism at any time. Some had nonsuppressible RAI values, others did not. All had histologic evidence of Hashimoto's disease, and three ultimately became hypothyroid.

2. Gharib H and Mayberry WE: Diagnosis of Graves' ophthalmopathy without hyperthyroidism: Long-acting thyroid stimulator (LATS) determination as laboratory adjunct. *Mayo Clin Proc* 45:444–449, 1970

    This article describes 34 patients with euthyroid Graves' disease. T_3 suppression tests revealed nonsuppressible function in two thirds. The article contains a good discussion and extensive bibliography of earlier literature.

CASE 2–2. EUTHYROID GRAVES' DISEASE

June, 1970. A 50 year old woman noted retraction of the left upper eyelid. There were no clinical features of hyperthyroidism. Examination of the thyroid revealed no abnormalities.

Exophthalmometry measurements were 13.5 mm right and 15 mm left. Most normal patients have measurements of 18 mm or less. Measurements of between

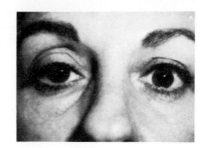

Figure 2-15. Left upper lid retraction.

18 and 20 mm are equivocal evidence for proptosis, whereas measurements greater than 20 mm are abnormal.

The FTI was 2.3, and the RAI was 18 per cent. A repeat RAI after 1 week of treatment with T_3, 50 μg twice a day, was 11 per cent. Observation without treatment was advised.

June, 1971. There was no change in the ocular status. The patient remained euthyroid, and there were no palpable abnormalities. A repeat T_3 suppression test revealed an initial RAI of 17 per cent and a value of 3 per cent at the end of 1 week of T_3 administration. Observation without treatment was advised once again.

June, 1972. The ocular findings were unchanged. However, the patient reported a 4-pound weight loss in spite of increased appetite over the previous 2 months. She also noted palpitation, mild hand tremor, and minimal heat intolerance. The thyroid gland was now one and a half times normal size. The FTI was 4.3, the T_3(RIA) 190 ng per 100 ml, and the RAI 49 per cent. After T_3 administration there was no suppression of the RAI.

How would you treat this patient?

a. [131]I.
b. ATD.
c. Thyroidectomy.
d. Lugol's solution.

Case 2-2—Followup

This patient was treated with Lugol's solution, three drops daily for 9 months. She remained euthyroid, and the eyelid returned to the normal position. Lugol's solution was discontinued, and the patient has remained euthyroid for 2 years with no further treatment. The eyes have been normal.

This patient had only mild hyperthyroidism and minimal enlargement of the thyroid. Most physicians would treat such a patient with ^{131}I, while some would try ATD. Instead, I

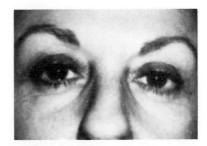

Figure 2-16. Note that lid positions are normal.

elected to try an old-fashioned treatment, one that is scorned by most thyroid experts and all but forgotten by many physicians—i.e., stable iodine in the form of Lugol's solution.

Modern textbooks suggest that stable iodine will only suppress hyperthyroidism for a period of a few weeks, following which there will be escape from its suppressant effects and a recrudescence of hyperthyroidism. In many instances this is correct. However, some patients with very mild hyperthyroidism and minimal thyroid enlargement may be successfully treated with this method until the condition goes into remission.

This approach has decided advantages when used appropriately. These include simplicity, economy, and safety. Three drops of Lugol's solution daily in a single dose is all that is needed. This small amount of iodine is exceedingly unlikely to give rise to any adverse reactions.

In the event of an escape ^{131}I may be given. The frequently expressed opinion that the iodine will lead to a prolonged suppression of ^{131}I uptake by the thyroid is incorrect. An uptake adequate for ^{131}I treatment will regularly be obtained in 1 to 2 weeks. During this time the patient may be maintained in reasonable comfort on propranolol.

This patient exemplifies an uncommon but not rare initiation of Graves' disease with ophthalmic abnormalities—in this instance, unilateral upper lid retraction. In other patients proptosis, unilateral or bilateral, may be the presenting feature.

A diagnosis of euthyroid Graves' disease is usually made after the discovery of either ophthalmic abnormalities or goiter in a patient without other clinical findings suggestive of hyperthyroidism. One may back into the diagnosis as in Case 2–1, in which administration of thyroid hormone produced hyperthyroidism and then nonsuppressible function was recognized. However, for euthyroid patients with ophthalmic findings suggestive of Graves' disease, the T_3 suppression test will be helpful in confirming the diagnosis if there is no fall in the baseline RAI value. Unfortunately, as often as not, there is good suppression. Occasionally, one may observe a lesser degree of suppression than that usually seen in normal patients but more than that seen with active Graves' disease, when no significant fall in the RAI would be expected. A blunted response to TRH has similar significance to a nonsuppressible RAI.

Demonstration of nonsuppressible function is diagnostic of Graves' disease, but suppression does not exclude this diagnosis as the explanation for either the ophthalmic findings or the goiter. This patient shows that an initially suppressible RAI may become nonsuppressible as the disease advances. Prolonged observation is essential.

The magnitude of the nonsuppressible RAI provides a general indication of the probability of the development of hyperthyroidism only when it is high. For example, a value greater than 30 per cent may indicate that the full hyperthyroid syndrome is likely to ensue within a matter of months. By contrast, when the baseline RAI value is less than 25 per cent, whether or not it is suppressible is of little prognostic value with respect to the immediacy of the onset of hyperthyroidism. Most of these patients do not become hyperthyroid. The ophthalmopathy usually remains stable, but we have observed the spontaneous regression of unilateral lid retraction.

One might ask why these patients develop lid retraction prior to hyperthyroidism, particularly unilaterally. I have no answer.

Selected Current References for Case 2–2

1. Chopra IJ and Solomon DH: Graves' disease with delayed hyperthyroidism: Onset after several years of euthyroid ophthalmopathy, dermopathy and high serum LATS. *Ann Intern Med* 73:985–990, 1970

   Our patient did not have dermopathy, nor did we have the LATS assay; otherwise, the cases are strikingly similar.

2. Michaelson ED and Young RL: Hypothyroidism with Graves' disease. *JAMA* 211:1351–1354, 1970

   In this case Hashimoto's disease had advanced to the point where hypothyroidism developed. The patient had not only Graves' ophthalmopathy but also pretibial myxedema.

3. Friend DG: Iodide therapy and the importance of quantitating the dose. *New Eng J Med* 263:1358–1360, 1960

   This is a classic article, brief but loaded with pearls about the therapeutic uses for iodide. For example, one drop of SSKI contains as much iodide as the entire body (50 mg) and eight times as much iodide as one drop of Lugol's solution. One drop of either SSKI or Lugol's solution daily is enough to suppress the hyperfunctioning thyroid gland (of Graves' disease). More than this does not enhance the therapeutic effect. I usually give two or three drops just to be sure. Doses of 30 or 40 drops daily only increase the chances for toxic reactions.

CASE 2–3. A CHILD WITH A MASSIVE TDG UNCOOPERATIVE IN TAKING ATD IN PREPARATION FOR THYROIDECTOMY

July, 1974. A 12 year old girl was referred for treatment of TDG. For 9 months she had been taking methimazole, 10 mg three times a day, and desiccated thyroid hormone, 2 grains daily. In spite of this treatment the goiter had progressively enlarged, and the parents requested consultation.

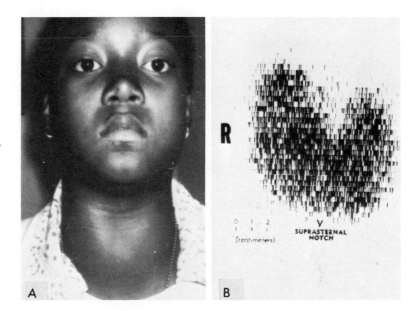

Figure 2-17 *A massive TDG. A, The patient. B, The scan.*

The patient weighed 165 pounds and was 62 inches tall. The heart rate was 104. There was a mild hand tremor. The thyroid gland was massively enlarged.

The FTI was 3.9. In view of the size of the goiter and the age of the patient, it was advised that after a further period of ATD treatment, thyroidectomy should be performed. Methimazole, 10 mg three times a day, was continued, and the supplemental thyroid hormone was stopped.

October, 1974. The FTI was 10.3 and the T_3(RIA) 245 ng per 100 ml. Careful questioning made it clear that the patient was taking her medication only sporadically. Her parents both worked and could not closely supervise her.

With which of the following statements do you agree?

a. Hospitalize the patient for as long as necessary to control the hyperthyroidism and then perform thyroidectomy.

b. Prepare her with stable iodine and operate. The goiter is too large for radioiodine.

c. Prepare her with stable iodine, propranolol, and adrenal steroids and operate. The goiter is too large for radioiodine.

d. Give radioiodine therapy.

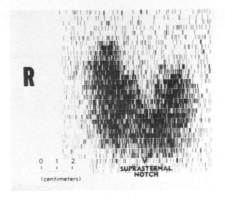

Figure 2-18. The scan 3 months after the initial dose of 30 mCi of [131]I.

Case 2-3—Followup

The parents were reluctant to permit surgical treatment with the increased risk that less than optimal preparation might entail and agreed to a trial of [131]I.

October, 1974. 30 mCi of ^{131}I was given.

January, 1975. The patient had improved in that the goiter was less than half its original size. However, the patient was still clinically hyperthyroid. The FTI was 7.6, and the RAI was 48 per cent.

A second dose of 30 mCi of ^{131}I was given.

April, 1975. The patient was now clinically euthyroid, and the thyroid gland was normal in size. Rechecks at 6-month intervals revealed persistent euthyroidism.

COMMENT: There is increasing interest in the use of ^{131}I as the primary treatment for hyperthyroidism in children. We have not accepted this position because there is not yet enough experience to be sure that the radiation exposure to growing children will not prove carcinogenic. The data are adequate to permit the conclusion that the risk, if any, must be small; however, when alternative treatments are suitable we prefer to employ them. We advise long-term ATD when the goiter is not so large that it is disfiguring. Otherwise, we prefer thyroidectomy after adequate preparation. Often unexpected developments or special situations dictate deviations from this general program. These include:

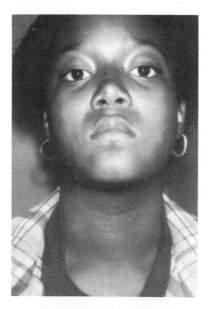

Figure 2-19. The patient after successful ^{131}I therapy.

1. Poor cooperation is a common problem with children and is understandable when one realizes that the medication must be taken for years, often several times daily. Although a remission may be achieved within 1 to 2 years in some patients, hyperthyroidism persists for at least 50 per cent of patients. ATD failure may be expected for almost all who have large goiters — i.e., three and a half times normal size or larger. For these patients we advise continued ATD therapy until they are fully grown, and then ¹³¹I administration.

2. Toxic reactions have occurred in 14 per cent of our juvenile hyperthyroid patients, necessitating a change in treatment.

3. Occasionally the patient or the parents will become disgruntled with repeated rechecks (even as infrequently as every 3 months) and demand some alternative form of management.

4. In some cases dissatisfaction relates to enlargement of the goiter and teasing by other children. This may indicate overtreatment with ATD. A rising serum TSH concentration will expose this problem. This patient's enlarging goiter reflected an increasing severity of the hyperthyroidism itself.

5. For some patients long-term ATD therapy may be unsuitable because of associated illnesses. We have seen six patients who were both mentally retarded and hyperthyroid. Radioiodine was considered a simpler and more appropriate form of treatment for these patients. Children with diabetes (often brittle), heart disease, or liver disease also are not ideal candidates for ATD therapy. Because of less than perfect cooperation, hyperthyroid children treated with ATD will have periods during which thyroid function may be somewhat high or a bit too low. This is not a problem if the patient is otherwise well. If the patient has other illnesses that may be aggravated by thyroid dysfunction, long-term ATD treatment would be a poor choice.

The principal alternatives are ¹³¹I and thyroidectomy. Neither treatment is ideal. Although it has been well established that ¹³¹I does not promote the development of thyroid cancer in adults, the situation may be different in children. This risk can be virtually eliminated by using ablative doses of ¹³¹I. However, thyroid function ablation produces the necessity for lifelong replacement therapy with thyroid hormone. It is of interest that two large doses failed to eliminate the function of this child's thyroid gland. She will be followed at 6-month intervals for both observation of thyroid function and examination for the development of thyroid nodules.

The question of genetic risk from incidental radiation to the gonads has been raised. To this author it seems to have received unjustified emphasis. The risk, by all calculations, is exceedingly small and is one that does not significantly exceed that which has been accepted for many years without question for diagnostic radiographic studies. Furthermore, any potential genetic risk is much less than the minimum mortality that must be anticipated from thyroidectomy. At this point, it should be recalled that complications of thyroidectomy in children are more frequent than in adults. Therefore, ¹³¹I is our usual choice of treatment for children for whom ATD are unsuitable.

We advise operation if the goiter is particularly large. This is not because we cannot eliminate it with ¹³¹I (as was clearly accomplished in this case) but because the dose of ¹³¹I which would be required may prove to be quite large. Nevertheless, we do not believe the facts dictate that either thyroidectomy or ¹³¹I is mandatory under these circumstances. We advocate a full discussion of the advantages and risks — real and potential — of both forms of treatment with the parents and the patient (if old enough), so that they may participate in the selection of treatment if they wish.

Selected Current References for Case 2–3

1. Vaidya VA, Bongiovanni AM, Parks JS, et al: Twenty-two years' experience in the medical management of juvenile thyrotoxicosis. *Pediatrics* 54:565–570, 1974

   The authors treated 95 hyperthyroid children with ATD, and considered the results "eminently satisfactory." However, of 73 who were adequately followed, 32 ultimately underwent thyroidectomy, 18 were still on ATD, and only 23 were in remission after an average of 3.2 years of treatment. The duration of the remissions ranged from 4 to 151 months (average 50 months); hence, it can be anticipated that some of the patients will experience relapses. The major problem they encountered was – right you are – patient noncompliance. Children often have difficulty accepting the idea that they are sick and thus different from other children. Their failure to take medication is actually a denial of the illness. I have observed that children from lower socioeconomic strata generally have the most trouble (hardly an original observation). Unfortunately, there is no easy solution to the problem. Alternative treatments also require patient cooperation – i.e., preparation for thyroidectomy and treatment of hypothyroidism and occasionally hypoparathyroidism afterwards, or treatment of hypothyroidism after [131]I. I have several children whom I see every few months in a continuing battle to convince them of the necessity for taking thyroid hormone. They may cooperate for a while, but require regular reinforcement.

2. Sheline GE, Lindsay S and Bell HG: Occurrence of thyroid nodules in children following therapy with radioiodine for hyperthyroidism. *J Clin Endocrinol Metab* 19:127–137, 1959

   This is the report which is frequently cited as evidence that hyperthyroid children treated with ^{131}I have an increased risk of developing neoplastic nodules. This happened to three of 18 patients treated before the age of 20 years. The authors suggest that if children are treated with ^{131}I they should be given doses large enough to produce hypothyroidism, and this should preclude the development of nodules later. We shall see that this thesis has gained support from other workers (including me).

3. Starr P, Jaffe HL and Oettinger L: Later results of ^{131}I treatment of hyperthyroidism in 73 children and adolescents: 1967 followup. *J Nucl Med* 10:586–590, 1969
4. Hayek A, Chapman EM and Crawford JD: Long-term results of treatment of thyrotoxicosis in children and adolescents with radioactive iodine. *New Eng J Med* 283:949–953, 1970
5. Safa AM, Schumacher OP and Rodriguez-Antunez A: Long-term followup results in children and adolescents treated with radioactive iodine (^{131}I) for hyperthyroidism. *New Eng J Med* 292:167–170, 1975

   These three reports deal with the elective use of ^{131}I therapy for hyperthyroidism in children. In all, 190 patients were treated. All of the authors agree that the treatment has important advantages of simplicity and effectiveness. Starr was particularly disturbed to learn that two of his patients whose hyperthyroidism failed to respond to an initial dose of ^{131}I were then operated upon and failed to survive the thyroidectomy.

   Followup studies revealed that these children in turn had 193 pregnancies of which 16 miscarried and one was a molar pregnancy. Of the 176 live births, 171 were normal. The five abnormalities included one with club foot, one with patent ductus arteriosus, one with pancreatic cystic fibrosis, one with hydrocephalus, and one born prematurely who developed retrolental fibroplasia. This incidence of abnormalities is no greater than that anticipated in a similar number of random births.

CASE 2–4. A "HOT" NODULE

May, 1973. A 15 year old girl was found to have a 3- × 2-cm nodule in the right lobe of the thyroid on a routine checkup. She was clinically euthyroid. The FTI was 2.1, and the RAI was 23 per cent. The scan showed a "hot" nodule. After TSH stimulation there was activation of the suppressed contralateral lobe and portions of the ipsilateral lobe also, confirming the diagnosis of an autonomously functioning thyroid adenoma (AFTA).

With which of the following statements do you agree?

a. Any thyroid nodule in a 15 year old should be removed because of an unacceptable risk of cancer.

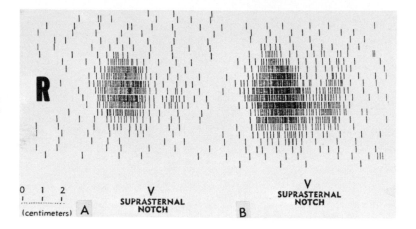

Figure 2–20. *An AFTA A,* The preliminary scan. *B,* The scan after TSH administration.

b. This lesion is almost certainly benign.

c. Although this lesion is benign, the potential for future hyperthyroidism is so great that surgery is mandatory.

d. It may be satisfactory to observe this nodule, deferring judgment as to therapy pending future developments.

e. Spontaneous degeneration commonly occurs in these nodules, reducing the capacity for future toxicity.

f. A normal FTI does not exclude T_3 toxicosis, a common problem with these lesions.

g. Although the AFTA is undoubtedly benign, carcinoma of the thyroid may occur elsewhere in the thyroid more often than might be expected on the basis of chance alone. Therefore, routine thyroidectomy should be considered for patients less than 50 years old who have AFTA.

h. If ^{131}I therapy is needed in the near future, a small dose (usually less than 10 mCi) will be satisfactory for a nodule which so avidly concentrates ^{131}I.

i. If thyroidectomy is the treatment chosen, not only should the nodule be removed but also a generous subtotal thyroidectomy should be performed. There are often other microscopic areas of autonomous function that will rapidly grow to maturity after the initial nodule is removed.

Case 2–4—Followup

Observation was advised.

May, 1974. The nodule had grown slightly, but the patient was still euthyroid.

April, 1975. The nodule had more than doubled in size, and the patient was now hyperthyroid. The heart rate was 110, and a mild tremor, fine warm skin, and hyperactive reflexes were present. The FTI was 4.6, the T_3(RIA) 240 ng per 100 ml, and the RAI 41 per cent. The nodule was removed surgically after 3 weeks preparation with PTU, 200 mg four times a day. The nodule was benign, and there was no evidence of cancer elsewhere in the thyroid.

COMMENT: The autonomously functioning thyroid adenoma is an uncommon thyroid lesion. My series includes only about 250 patients from more than 20,000 thyroid patients seen in my laboratory. Of these patients, this one is exceptional in several respects. She is younger than usual — the average age is 42 years. Also, most nontoxic AFTA remain nontoxic for many years. This is the

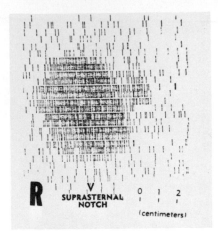

Figure 2-21. Enlargement of the AFTA confirmed by scanning.

only patient I have observed who progressed from euthyroid to hyperthyroid, and she did it in only 2 years. Finally, this is by far the youngest patient I have seen with a toxic AFTA. Prior to this case all toxic patients seen in my laboratory were over 30 years of age, and most were older than 50 years. My recommendation for observation was based upon my prior favorable experience with nontoxic AFTA, and I was surprised by the subsequent course.

The AFTA is generally believed to have too low a potential for malignancy to justify the risks of thyroidectomy on that account. However, reports of associated thyroid cancer occurring elsewhere in the gland and even buried within the otherwise benign AFTA are common enough to suggest that the association may be more than a chance phenomenon. This matter has been reviewed in some detail recently (Reference 1, p 103). Nevertheless, the risk of associated cancer would not seem great enough to justify more than observation.

It is true that most thyroid nodules in teenagers are best removed, but not all. Some are hyperplastic nodules in a thyroid gland that has impaired function. Others may represent ectopic thyroid that has failed to descend to the proper location and will render the patient athyreotic if removed. These nodules respond to thyroid hormone. Finally, there are the uncommon but occasional nontoxic AFTA. These lesions may not require removal if they remain stable or if they undergo spontaneous degeneration, a very common occurrence. Occasionally their size produces cosmetic problems that require treatment.

These lesions may produce T_3 toxicosis, but this is the exception. One need not be overly concerned about T_3 toxicosis in a patient without clinical evidence of hyperthyroidism.

I do not advise ^{131}I therapy for toxic AFTA in patients less than 40 years old. They tend to be relatively resistant to treatment. To be reasonably certain of successful ablation, one must deliver 15 to 20 mCi of ^{131}I to the nodule. Since the RAI value is often no greater than 25 to 50 per cent, a sizeable ^{131}I dose may be needed (e.g., to deliver 20 mCi to a nodule with a 33 per cent RAI value would require a 60 mCi dose). I prefer not to give such large doses of ^{131}I to younger patients for benign disease. Hence, surgical treatment is usually advised.

It is true that a high incidence of microscopic foci of autonomous function has been associated with macroscopic AFTA. However, removal of just the nodule is all that is necessary. The microscopic lesions generally tend not to progress rapidly, although there has recently been a report of a recurrent AFTA in the same lobe as that from which an earlier AFTA had been excised (Reference 4, p 103).

Selected Current References for Case 2–4

1. Hamburger JI: Solitary autonomously functioning thyroid lesions: Diagnosis, clinical features and pathogenetic considerations. *Am J Med* 58:740–748, 1975

   This paper summarizes my experience with 164 patients with AFTA, emphasizing the relative stability of untreated nontoxic lesions followed up to 12 years.

2. Burman KD, Earll JM, Johnson MC, et al: Clinical observations on the solitary autonomous thyroid nodule. *Arch Intern Med* 134:915–919, 1974

   These workers had similar experiences with a series of 54 patients. They confirmed my observations (and those of many others) that spontaneous degeneration occurs frequently and may preclude the development of toxicity.

3. Blum M, Shenkman L and Hollander CS: The autonomous nodule of the thyroid: Correlation of patient age, nodule size and functional status. *Am J Med Sci* 269:43–50, 1975

   Their experience was slightly different. They observed progression from euthyroidism to hyperthyroidism in four of 17 patients. They also observed a correlation between advancing age, increasing nodule size, and toxicity.

4. Weiner JD: A systematic approach to the diagnosis of Plummer's disease (autonomous goiter), with a review of 224 cases. *Neth J Med* 18:218–233, 1975

   This European study includes 224 patients. His data are consistent with those of other Europeans but at variance with American reports in that one third of his hyperthyroid patients had toxic autonomous nodules. These lesions account for less than 5 per cent of our hyperthyroid patients. Of particular interest is one patient who progressed from the nontoxic state to fatal thyroid crisis in only 3 months. Another unique experience was that with a patient who developed a recurrent toxic AFTA in the same lobe from which another toxic AFTA had been removed surgically less than 2 years earlier.

5. Sterling K, Refetoff S and Selenkow HA: T_3 thyrotoxicosis: Thyrotoxicosis due to elevated serum triiodothyronine levels. *JAMA* 213:571–576, 1970

   This early report on T_3 toxicosis reveals a disproportionate number of patients with toxic AFTA. One should not conclude from this data that most or even many AFTA tend to secrete T_3 preferentially over T_4. My paper contains data to the contrary. However, I tested consecutive patients with AFTA, whereas Sterling dealt with patients who demonstrated preferential T_3 hypersecretion. Therefore, of those patients who have T_3 toxicosis (a rare occurrence in our experience), a disproportionate percentage may have toxic AFTA, but most patients with AFTA do not have preferential hypersecretion of T_3.

6. Evered DC, Clark F and Petersen VB: Thyroid function in euthyroid subjects with autonomous thyroid nodules. *Clin Endocrinol* (Oxford) 3:149–154, 1974

   Six patients with nontoxic AFTA had high serum T_3 concentrations, contrary to our experience. Nevertheless, perhaps the European AFTA is different than the American variety. Blum's patients also seemed to develop hypersecretion of T_3 initially. As frank hyperthyroidism developed, both T_3 and T_4 were secreted in excess. So far, we have seen this only once. However, New York is closer to Europe than Detroit.

7. Marsden P, Facer P, Acosta M, et al: Serum triiodothyronine in solitary autonomous nodules of the thyroid. *Clin Endocrinol* (Oxford) 4:327–330, 1975

   These British workers again suggest that T_3 toxicosis is the common form of hyperthyroidism in these patients. We just do not find that to be the case here.

CASE 2–5. A 15 YEAR OLD GIRL WITH A LARGE TDG

July, 1968. A 15 year old girl was referred for treatment of hyperthyroidism. The clinical features were classic and had been increasingly evident over the previous 3 months. The thyroid gland was visibly enlarged, about four times normal size.

The FTI was 9.4, and the RAI was 87 per cent. The patient was 64 inches tall and fully developed. Menarche had taken place at age 11 years.

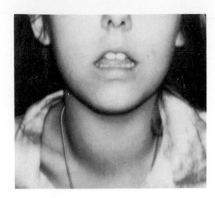

Figure 2-22. The patient.

What would you advise?

a. She is old enough for [131]I.

b. Why not try ATD for up to 2 years, and then if there is no remission ^{131}I can be given?

c. Preparation with ATD followed by thyroidectomy will control hyperthyroidism and eliminate the goiter most efficiently.

Case 2-5—Further Data

After a discussion of the alternatives it was decided that a trial of ATD would be undertaken even though the chances for obtaining a remission in the hyperthyroidism seemed small because of the size of the goiter. After 6 months' treatment, during which the hyperthyroidism had been controlled, the patient and her mother objected to a continuation of ATD because the patient's schoolmates had been teasing her about the goiter. After a discussion of the advantages and disadvantages of ^{131}I and thyroidectomy, the patient requested the latter because a friend had done well with surgical treatment.

With which of the following statements do you agree?

a. Do not permit the patient to make this decision, since she is not qualified to do so.

b. Iodine-131 therapy carries too great a potential risk to this patient's future progeny and should not be used electively in so young a patient.

c. The risks of thyroidectomy are greater in children than in adults.

d. Recurrent hyperthyroidism is very uncommon after a successful thyroidectomy.

e. If the patient remains euthyroid for 5 years after the thyroidectomy, one need no longer be concerned about recurrent hyperthyroidism.

f. If the patient remains euthyroid for 5 years after the thyroidectomy, one need not be concerned about late onset hypothyroidism.

g. After thyroidectomy an annual serum calcium determination is mandatory indefinitely, even if there is no evidence of hypoparathyroidism in the first 2 years of followup.

h. If the patient is hypothyroid after thyroidectomy the dose of thyroid hormone required for proper replacement may require adjustment in the years to come.

Case 2–5—Followup

January, 1971. Thyroidectomy was uneventful.

April, 1971. The patient returned with recurrent hyperthyroidism. The goiter was twice the normal size, the FTI was 5.2, and the RAI was 42 per cent. An ablative dose of ^{131}I was given, and the patient has remained euthyroid on levothyroxine, 0.2 mg daily.

COMMENT: There is no reason not to allow the patient to participate in the selection of the form of treatment. In fact, the physician has the legal obligation to inform the patient or parent (in the case of a minor) of the advantages and disadvantages of the possible methods of management, and having done so, the final decision should be theirs. To be sure, the physician may and should express his preference, but the patient has the final say, subject only to the physician's right to refuse to care for her if he believes strongly that her choice is inappropriate.

A case in point is a 35 year old hyperthyroid school teacher who came to me from Chicago for treatment. She wanted to be treated with ATD and could not find a physician there who would do it. They all advised ^{131}I. I told her that I, too, would advise ^{131}I, because her chances for success with ATD were probably no greater than 20 per cent. I suggested that it would be more prudent and more efficient for her to return to Chicago and take the ^{131}I. However, she was adamant and was willing to come to see me as often as necessary if I would treat her with ATD. On this basis I agreed. Needless to say, after 18 months' treatment she went into a remission which has been maintained for 6 years.

My point is that the best treatment for hyperthyroidism in many situations is arguable. Therefore, physicians should be flexible enough (and indeed secure enough) to accept a patient's selection of a method that might not be the physician's first choice.

Much has been written about the potential for genetic damage from ^{131}I if given to patients who may bear children. These fears are based upon calculations derived from animal experimentation. The data indicate that the risk is exceedingly small. From the practical standpoint these discussions have little bearing upon the management of patients. No treatment for hyperthyroidism or any other disease is without risks. When more than one therapeutic option is available, obviously one should select the safest. From the standpoint of human as well as genetic considerations it seems absurd to me to prefer the known mortality of thyroidectomy (probably no less than 0.1 per cent at the very best) to a potential ^{131}I-induced genetic problem with a far lower statistical possibility.

Complications of thyroidectomy are more common in children than in adults. The structures in the neck are smaller and more subject to injury. The trachea is smaller and more likely to collapse, leading to respiratory obstruction.

Recurrent hyperthyroidism after thyroidectomy is more common than one might conclude from the surgical literature. I have seen recurrences as long as 50 years after the initial operation, and more than half the patients in my series of recurrent hyperthyroidism developed recurrences 10 or more years after the thyroidectomies. Similarly, hypothyroidism and hypoparathyroidism may both occur many years after thyroidectomy. They are both more common when a bilateral operation is performed, as is generally the case for hyperthyroid patients.

Any functioning thyroid tissue that remains after thyroidectomy for hyperthyroidism may have or may develop nonsuppressible function, or it may undergo gradual functional deterioration. Hence, the replacement dose of thyroid hormone may require periodic adjustment unless a total thyroidectomy is performed.

Selected Current References for Case 2–5

1. Evered D, Young ET, Tunbridge WG, et al: Thyroid function after subtotal thyroidectomy for hyperthyroidism. *Brit Med J* 1:25–27, 1975

   This series of hyperthyroid British patients treated surgically experienced only a 4 per cent recurrence in up to 7 years of followup. However, 15 per cent were hypothyroid, and an additional 50 per cent, although euthyroid clinically, had subnormal serum T_4 concentrations and elevated serum TSH concentrations. Serum T_3 concentrations were normal, and in the authors' opinion these were adequate to maintain the euthyroid state. Most American thyroidologists would conclude that these patients should be treated with thyroid hormone.

2. Hamburger JI: Recurrent hyperthyroidism after thyroidectomy. *Arch Surg* 111:91–92, 1976

   This study showed that recurrent hyperthyroidism occurred on the average 12.4 years after the original operation, and 19 per cent of recurrences were from 20 to 50 years later. Hence, the low recurrence rate in Evered's series (followed only up to 7 years) is probably an underestimate.

3. Hedley, AJ, Flemming CJ, Chesters MI, et al: Surgical treatment of thyrotoxicosis. *Brit Med J* 1:519–523, 1970

   This is a British report of a retrospective analysis of the results of thyroidectomy for hyperthyroidism after an average of 9.3 years (up to 21 years). Hyperthyroidism recurred in 6.2 per cent of these patients. Almost half developed recurrences between 10 and 20 years after the operation. Thirty-six per cent of their patients were hypothyroid. They found 14 patients with untreated hypothyroidism and six with untreated hyperthyroidism. This study supports our recommendation for life-long followup of all patients after treatment of hyperthyroidism.

CASE 2–6. A 16 YEAR OLD GIRL WITH HYPERTHYROIDISM AND A HISTORY OF RADIATION THERAPY TO THE THYMUS AT BIRTH

November, 1975. A 16 year old girl was referred for treatment of hyperthyroidism of moderate severity. The clinical picture had progressively evolved over the previous 4 months. She had received x-ray therapy at birth to shrink an enlarged thymus gland.

She was 63 inches tall, weighed 110 pounds, had a heart rate of 108, and was fully developed, having experienced menarche at age 12 years. The thyroid gland was twice the normal size, there were no palpable nodules, and a high resolution ^{99m}Tc gamma camera image revealed no filling defects that might have suggested nodules.

The FTI was 4.6, the T_3(RIA) 280 ng per 100 ml, and the RAI 46 per cent.

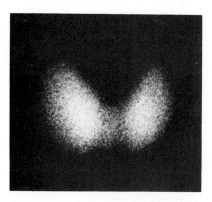

Figure 2–23. A gamma camera image reveals a diffuse goiter with no filling defects.

With which of the following statements do you agree?

    a. Thyroidectomy will eliminate the hyperthyroidism and also concern for occult thyroid cancer as a result of the thymic radiation.

    b. Advise ATD. She is too young for ^{131}I, and thyroidectomy has greater risks in children.

    c. An ablative dose of ^{131}I will eliminate the hyperthyroidism and also may reduce any cancer potential.

    d. ATD therapy may increase the potential for cancer development.

    e. The thymic radiation is too remote to be of concern as a cause of thyroid cancer.

Case 2–6 — Followup

Usually we advise ATD for someone this young with a relatively small goiter and only moderately severe hyperthyroidism. These patients have the best chance of achieving a remission following ATD suppression. However, the history of thymic radiation presents a problem. This treatment does increase the risk of thyroid cancer development, although the incidence of cancer in the first 1000 irradiated patients I checked was only 2 per cent. Most thyroid cancers caused by such treatment to the head, neck, and upper chest have been detected between 20 and 30 years after the radiation therapy.

In the experimental induction of thyroid cancer in the rat, one irradiates the thyroid and then provokes increased endogenous TSH stimulation of the irradiated thyroid tissue by giving ATD. If we were to treat this patient with ATD might we not be reproducing the very conditions shown to favor cancer production in the rat? This would seem at best an imprudent choice.

One might argue that this risk could be obviated by the administration of fully blocking doses of ATD, with full replacement doses of supplemental thyroid hormone to assure suppression of TSH. We do not advocate this method of treatment, for the supplemental thyroid hormone obscures the best indication of improvement — i.e., the progressive reduction of the ATD dose without a recurrence of hyperthyroidism. Also, the use of supplemental thyroid hormone makes it necessary to give a larger ATD dose, thus reducing the chances for administering the drug in a single daily dose. Finally, combined thyroid ATD treatment is more complex, making it more difficult to obtain sustained patient cooperation.

The choice between thyroidectomy and an ablative dose of ^{131}I cannot be made on the basis of a scientific mandate. However, if one wishes to ablate the thyroid totally it is probable that ^{131}I will do the job more certainly and with less likelihood of any complications. In this instance, ^{131}I was the selection. A dose of 20 mCi produced complete ablation of the thyroid. This treatment should eliminate any potential for future development of thyroid cancer; after all, if the cells are destroyed, they should not become malignant.

This patient has remained euthyroid on levothyroxine, 0.2 mg daily.

Selected Current References for Case 2–6

1. Arnold JE and Pinsky S: Comparison of ^{99m}Tc and ^{123}I for thyroid imaging. *J Nucl Med* 17:261–267, 1976
2. Favus MJ, Schneider AB, Stachura ME, et al: Thyroid cancer occurring as a late consequence of head-and-neck irradiation. *New Eng J Med* 294:1019–1025, 1976

   These two papers are the latest in a series of reports on the Michael Reese callback of irradiated patients to search for thyroid cancer. Among 1056 patients the authors found 60 cancers, a somewhat higher yield than our 16 cancers in 844 patients. However, they dealt primarily with patients who had had tonsillar radiation, which delivers a higher dose to the thyroid than thymic radiation. This may account for the difference.

3. The National Cancer Institute: Information for physicians on irradiation-related thyroid cancer. *Ca* 26:150–159, 1976

   This is a report of the proceedings of a workshop on this subject attended by a number of leading thyroidologists, oncologists, and representative specialists from associated fields. The paper is a clear example of the fact that committees do not practice medicine very well. Nevertheless, this article contains a great deal of useful information. Just beware of the conclusions.

4. Hamburger JI and Stoffer SS: Late thyroid sequelae of radiation therapy to the upper body. In *Radiation-Associated Thyroid Carcinoma.* DeGroot LJ, ed. New York, Grune and Stratton, 1977, pp 17–31.

This article summarizes our experience with 814 irradiated patients. Two per cent had cancer.

CASE 2–7. A 17 YEAR OLD GIRL WHO EXPERIENCED A REMISSION IN HYPERTHYROIDISM AFTER 2½ YEARS' TREATMENT WITH PTU, ONLY TO RELAPSE 6 MONTHS LATER

August, 1970. A 17 year old girl was referred for treatment of hyperthyroidism. The diagnosis had been made 1 year earlier, and ATD had been advised. However, the medication was used irregularly, and none had been taken in the past 3 months. The clinical features of hyperthyroidism were obvious and included a diffuse goiter three times normal size. The laboratory data confirmed the diagnosis, and treatment was reinstituted with PTU, 100 mg four times a day.

March, 1973. In the intervening 2½ years the dose of PTU was gradually reduced, and the medication was finally discontinued in February, 1973. The thyroid gland was still about twice normal size.

September, 1973. The patient returned with a relapse of the hyperthyroidism. She was now 20 years old and 63 inches tall. The thyroid gland was twice normal size, the FTI was 4.8 and the RAI 74 per cent. However, the heart rate was only 92, and the patient weighed 126 pounds, having lost only 2 pounds in the preceding 6 months. The patient is single and has no plans for marriage in the immediate future.

With which of the following statements do you agree?

    a.   The patient should be given ^{131}I therapy.

    b.   Resume ATD therapy. The hyperthyroidism is very mild and a second course of ATD may be followed by a lasting remission.

    c.   Advise thyroidectomy. This thyroid will be resistant to any medical management.

    d.   The previous ATD therapy will increase resistance to [131]I.

    e.   If she were planning to have children in the next few years this would be a point against ATD treatment.

Case 2–7—Followup

One might choose ^{131}I as a more decisive treatment. It is true that ATD therapy increases the resistance of the thyroid to ^{131}I but not greatly. Our current method of ^{131}I therapy utilizes large ^{131}I doses to assure prompt and certain elimination of the hyperthyroidism, so this ATD effect is of no consequence. If the patient had plans for marriage and childbearing in the near future, we would certainly advise ^{131}I therapy rather than ATD. In our series of 32 pregnant hyperthyroid patients, the diagnosis of hyperthyroidism in 20 had been made months to years before the patient became pregnant. Had definitive therapy (^{131}I or thyroidectomy) been employed initially, this complicated condition could have been avoided.

Since hyperthyroidism reduces fertility, ATD may actually promote the probability of pregnancy complicating the hyperthyroidism. Many of our pregnant hyperthyroid patients had been infertile prior to control of the hyperthyroidism.

In this instance we were impressed by the mildness of the hyperthyroidism and offered the patient the option of another trial of PTU. After 1 additional year of treatment, another remission was obtained, and this has persisted for 2 years. The patient has been advised to return annually indefinitely. Should there be another episode of hyperthyroidism we would surely recommend [131]I.

CASE 2–8. ATD TREATMENT OF HYPERTHYROIDISM

July, 1972. A 19 year old girl reported recent onset of tremor, heat intolerance, nervousness, and an 8-pound weight loss. The heart rate was 100, the reflexes were hyperactive, and the thyroid gland was diffusely enlarged to twice normal size. There were no eye signs of hyperthyroidism.

The FTI was 7.0, and the RAI was 48 per cent. Treatment was begun with PTU, 150 mg four times a day.

August, 1972. The patient was much better. The heart rate was now 84, and other features of hyperthyroidism had subsided. The thyroid gland was two and a half times normal size. The FTI was 1.5.

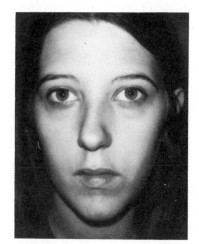

Figure 2–24. The patient.

With which of the following statements do you agree?

a. The patient has experienced a dramatic remission. Stop PTU.

b. The enlarging thyroid gland is an ominous sign suggesting that PTU will fail.

c. Add levothyroxine to the program and maintain the present dose of PTU.

d. Add Lugol's solution. This will reduce the size of the goiter.

e. Discontinue PTU and treat with [131]I.

f. Reduce the dose of PTU to 100 mg three times daily and recheck the patient in 3 months.

g. There is a 50 per cent chance that this patient will obtain a remission if PTU is continued for 12 to 18 months.

h. If a remission is obtained and the patient remains euthyroid for 6 months, a relapse is unlikely.

i. The best indication of satisfactory progress is the ability to reduce the dose of PTU gradually and progressively without a recurrence of hyperthyroidism.

j. The PTU can be given as a single daily dose of 300 mg. This will reduce the potential for omission of medication.

k. The initial total dose of 600 mg daily was probably unnecessarily high.

l. Thyroid hormone should have been given from the beginning. This would have prevented the goiter from enlarging.

Case 2–8—Followup

The rapid clinical improvement accompanied by an unusually marked drop in the FTI and a modest increment in goiter size suggests the following:

1. The initial dose of PTU was probably higher than necessary. I generally start with no less than 100 mg three times a day for patients with mild hyperthyroidism, and use increasing initial doses up to 300 mg four times a day for more severe involvement. In this instance the patient's clinical features were relatively mild, but I was impressed by the rather high FTI of 7.0. Therefore, I began with a larger PTU dose than I might have ordered otherwise. The initial PTU dose is really a test dose of the patient's sensitivity. A recheck in 4 weeks permits the assessment of the initial response and the determination of whether an adjustment in the dose is needed.

2. The enlargement of the thyroid gland also probably means that the PTU dose is too high and can be substantially reduced. An enlarging thyroid gland in spite of a reduced PTU dose and a rise in the FTI to the mid or upper normal level would be an unfavorable prognostic sign.

3. The patient will probably do well on PTU. The chances for a remission should be as high as 50 per cent.

4. A substantial reduction in the PTU dose should be well tolerated.

With respect to the other suggestions, I would offer the following comments. I do not agree with those who use combined ATD–thyroid hormone therapy for these patients. I object for the following reasons:

1. The best indicator of successful ATD management is a progressive reduction in the ATD dose without a relapse in the hyperthyroidism. In this regard, the FTI is one of the best objective indicators of favorable progress. Supplemental thyroid hormone obscures the usefulness of this test.

2. If supplemental thyroid hormone is given, the patient must take two drugs instead of one. This is a needless complication of the treatment.

3. When supplemental thyroid hormone is used a higher ATD dose is necessary. If a full replacement dose of thyroid hormone is given (as usually advised by those who advocate this approach), then one must give enough ATD to fully block the thyroid secretory activity. Otherwise, the additive effects of any endogenous secretion plus the supplemental thyroid hormone would restore the hyperthyroidism. The higher dose of ATD that is required has the added drawback of reducing the chances that a single daily dose of ATD will be practical.

To give thyroid hormone along with PTU when treatment is initiated is absurd. The patient already has too much thyroid hormone, and giving more will only make matters worse. (Nevertheless, I have seen patients for whom this was done.)

I usually split the total daily quantity of PTU into two to four doses until I can control the patient's condition with 150 mg per day or less. Then I employ a single daily dose. This seems to be satisfactory for most patients. Of course, the higher the dose required, the more severe the hyperthyroidism, and it stands to reason that more severe hyperthyroidism will be more easily controlled with a multiple dose regimen.

Lugol's solution sometimes will reduce the size of the goiter in Graves' disease. However, in this patient the enlargement was probably related to an overdosage of PTU. Although there may be a good chance for a remission, there is no guarantee that a remission once achieved will be sustained. Most relapses seem to occur within the first 2 years of followup. Nevertheless, these patients should be followed indefinitely. Our routine is to see the patient 1 month after discontinuation of ATD, then at 6 months, and then annually.

For this patient the PTU dose was decreased to 100 mg three times a day. The subsequent course can be followed in Table 2–29.

TABLE 2-29. FOLLOWUP DATA ON CASE 2-8

DATE	FTI	GOITER SIZE	PTU DOSE
Jul, 1972	7.0	$2 \times N$	150 mg q.i.d.
Aug, 1972	1.5	$2\frac{1}{2} \times N$	100 mg t.i.d.
Nov, 1972	2.3	$2\frac{1}{2} \times N$	100 mg b.i.d.
Feb, 1973	3.2	$2 \times N$	100 mg b.i.d.
May, 1973	2.4	$2 \times N$	150 mg daily
Aug, 1973	2.8	$1\frac{1}{2} \times N$	100 mg daily
Nov, 1973	2.9	$1\frac{1}{2} \times N$	50 mg daily
Jan, 1974	2.2	$1\frac{1}{2} \times N$	Stop PTU
Feb, 1974	2.6	$1\frac{1}{2} \times N$	—
Jul, 1974	1.9	Normal	—
Jul, 1975	2.1	Normal	—

Selected Current References for Case 2–8

1. Wartofsky L: Low remission after therapy for Graves' disease. *JAMA* 226:1083–1088, 1973

   A disappointing 13.7 per cent remission rate after ATD treatment of hyperthyroidism is the point of this article. We share the author's conclusion that long-term ATD administration is likely to be employed much less often in the future.

2. Wiberg JJ and Nuttall FQ: Methimazole toxicity from high doses. *Ann Intern Med* 77:414–416, 1972

   Nine of 25 patients treated with high doses of methimazole developed toxic reactions: cutaneous for seven but agranulocytotic for two. The authors advise that high doses of ATD should be employed only when prompt control of hyperthyroidism is essential. Some thyroidologists have had the impression that methimazole may be more toxic than PTU. Unfortunately, I cannot prove it (although for this reason I use PTU principally).

3. Geffner DL, Azukizawa M and Hershman JM: Propylthiouracil blocks extrathyroidal conversion of thyroxine to triiodothyronine and augments thyrotropin secretion in man. *J Clin Invest* 55:224–229, 1975

   This study shows that PTU has a peripheral effect that interferes with the conversion of T_4 to T_3, thus decreasing the metabolic effectiveness of T_4 in animals. This action is probably of no clinical importance in humans.

4. Marsden P, Howorth PJN and Chalkley S: Hormonal pattern of relapse in hyperthyroidism. *Lancet* 1:944–947, 1975

   Elevated serum T_3 levels may precede elevated serum T_4 levels in relapses of hyperthyroidism after initially successful ATD therapy.

5. Wise PH, Marion M and Pain RW: Single-dose, "block-replace" drug therapy in hyperthyroidism. *Brit Med J* 4:143–145, 1973

   They claim that since methimazole has a longer duration of action than PTU, the use of methimazole may more often permit control with a single daily dose. However, in my experience with PTU, most patients who are maintained on less than 200 mg per day can be treated with a single daily dose. Hence the proposed advantage of methimazole may be largely theoretical.

6. Lowry RC, Lowe D, Hadden DR, et al: Thyroid suppressibility: Followup for two years after antithyroid treatment. *Brit Med J* 2:19–22, 1971

   British workers from Glasgow have championed the idea that a T_3 suppression test will help determine whether ATD-treated patients will remain in remission after withdrawal of the drug. These Irish physicians disagree. They found too many exceptions both ways (suppressible patients who relapsed and nonsuppressible patients who remained in remission) for the test to be useful. I agree. The best guideline to success is gradual withdrawal of the ATD without a relapse of hyperthyroidism. The best index of a permanent remission is continued euthyroidism on followup.

CASE 2–9. HIGH DOSE ^{131}I THERAPY FOR TDG

June, 1975. A 20 year old man had hyperthyroidism for about 3 months, during which he noted a progressive swelling in the neck. His clinical picture was classic. The thyroid gland was estimated to be eight times normal size, i.e., 150 to 200 grams.

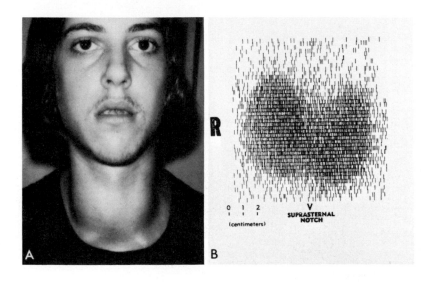

Figure 2–25. *A,* The patient. *B,* His thyroid scan.

The FTI was 10.6, the T$_3$(RIA) 400 ng per 100 ml, and the RAI 73 per cent. He was treated with 30 mCi of ^{131}I.

September, 1975. He was hypothyroid. The FTI was 0.2, the TSH(RIA) 28 μU/ml, and the T$_3$(RIA) 13 ng per 100 ml. However, the RAI was 17 per cent, and the thyroid gland was still enlarged, about three and a half times normal size.

He was treated with levothyroxine, 0.1 mg daily, and asked to return in 3 months.

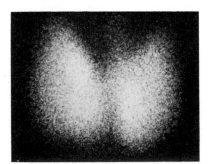

Figure 2–26. The thyroid image 3 months after treatment with 30 mCi of ^{131}I.

December, 1975. The patient was feeling fine. The heart rate was 76, and the weight was stable at 175 pounds (having increased from 146 to 175 pounds between June and September of 1975). The thyroid gland was now only twice normal size. Nevertheless, the FTI was 4.2, and the T$_3$(RIA) was 230 ng per 100 m.. Thyroid hormone was discontinued.

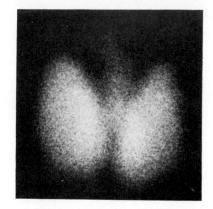

Figure 2-27. The thyroid image 6 months after treatment with 30 mCi of ^{131}I.

March, 1976. The patient was still feeling fine. The heart rate was 92, the weight stable, and the thyroid gland was only one and a half times normal size. The FTI was 5.2, the T_3(RIA) 390 ng per 100 ml, and the RAI 28 per cent. Although the laboratory data were worse, the patient seemed to be doing well.

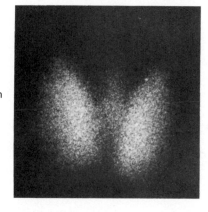

Figure 2-28. The thyroid image 9 months after treatment with 30 mCi of ^{131}I.

With which of the following statements do you agree?

a. The goiter was too large for treatment with ^{131}I. Thyroidectomy would have been simpler and quicker.

b. He needs more ^{131}I now.

c. Don't treat the laboratory. Observe this patient for a few more months. He is getting better.

d. Add Lugol's solution to the program.

e. His early hypothyroidism signifies that he will ultimately be hypothyroid.

Case 2-9—Followup

June, 1976. The patient was given no treatment and continued to improve. At this point he was euthyroid. The thyroid gland was normal in size. The FTI was 3.2, and the T_3-(RIA) was 180 ng per 100 ml.

I do not think that his initial hypothyroidism means very much. Transient hypothyroidism is seen rather commonly after high-dose ^{131}I therapy for patients with large toxic diffuse goiters, a point I made a number of years ago. Most of them recover and remain euthyroid. Naturally, this young man has many years to go, and there is no alternative to continued annual followup.

True enough, this patient required a few extra visits, but I do not see that surgical treatment would have been simpler. It would have taken a long time to prepare him for thyroidectomy, and a goiter this size may prove a bit challenging to the surgeon. The patient remained on the job throughout his treatment and at no time was willing to consider a thyroidectomy as long as it was possible to avoid it.

Using our current higher dose ^{131}I therapy (10 to 30 mCi as the initial dose), we are successful in eliminating hyperthyroidism with a single ^{131}I treatment in 96 per cent of patients. Most of the time when more than a single treatment is required an initial 30 mCi dose was given, rather than a smaller dose. This simply indicates that larger goiters that are given larger ^{131}I doses may be more resistant to [131]I. However, we have not had to give more than two treatments even to these patients. If one reads the older literature dealing with ^{131}I therapy, he will find occasional patients who remained hyperthyroid for 2 years or more and received six to eight treatments before success was achieved. For some, ^{131}I was abandoned for thyroidectomy because of poor results.

It is important to recognize those patients for whom relative resistance to ^{131}I may be anticipated. The most important criterion is goiter size. Any thyroid that is more than three times normal size will probably require a large ^{131}I dose. I would not use less than 20 mCi (20 mCi might be adequate if the thyroid is three and a half to four times normal size *and* the RAI is more than 70 per cent). Most of the time I give 30 mCi as the initial dose. A second criterion that calls for a larger initial ^{131}I dose is multinodularity.

Selected Current References for Case 2–9

1. Hamburger JI and Paul S: When and how to use higher ^{131}I doses for hyperthyroidism. *New Eng J Med* 279:1361–1365, 1968

   In 1964, 1967, and earlier in 1968 we proposed essentially the same message. Larger ^{131}I doses were more decisive for selected hyperthyroid patients (especially the elderly and those with heart disease). Small doses, far from being conservative, could lead to disastrous cardiovascular consequences from prolonged hyperthyroidism.

2. Mills DH: Whither informed consent? *JAMA* 229:305–310, 1974

   Mills repeatedly refers to the treatment of hyperthyroidism to exemplify the necessity for surgeons to inform their patients not only of the risks of thyroidectomy but also of the availability of nonsurgical alternatives. I recently saw a patient who sought another opinion, hoping that his hyperthyroidism could be treated without an operation. When he asked his surgeon about ^{131}I, the surgeon allegedly professed ignorance about that treatment. Other patients have told me that physicians had warned them that ^{131}I could make them sterile or might cause cancer or leukemia. On the other hand, I have seen patients who were unreasonably fearful of thyroidectomy for equally absurd reasons.

   Biased and inaccurate statements are obviously a disservice both to the public and to the medical profession. Less obvious is the frequency with which they ultimately reflect badly upon their source. The public is becoming more and more sophisticated and aggressive about obtaining more than one opinion before choosing an elective ablative treatment (whether surgery or ^{131}I).

   Sometimes the truth comes out after the fact. In this case, the physician who failed to obtain informed consent by misleading the patient about the risks of alternatives or not even discussing them, may find himself the subject of litigation even if a satisfactory therapeutic result was obtained; and if a complication occurs, look out!

3. McDougall IR: Thyroid cancer after iodine-131 therapy (editorial). *JAMA* 227:438, 1974

   This short letter to the editor is important reading for all who treat hyperthyroid patients. A table summarizes data from 15 reports of patients in whom thyroid cancer was discovered after ^{131}I therapy for hyperthyroidism. This is the world-wide published experience and is a small yield considering the hundreds of thousands of patients so treated — even if all of these cancers could be directly attributed to the treatment. In fact, in view of autopsy studies indicating a 2 per cent incidence of thyroid cancer in all thyroid glands and the U.S. Public Health Service data revealing a prevalence of 25 thyroid cancer cases per million population per year, the small number of reported cancers after ^{131}I therapy seems almost to suggest that the treatment may reduce the potential for future thyroid cancer.

McDougall observed that six of the patients had received small ^{131}I doses (less than 6 mCi), probably to try to avoid hypothyroidism. I agree with McDougall that this is futile. I also agree with his suggestion that ablative ^{131}I doses not only have the advantage of producing a rapid one-dose cure but also may prevent the subsequent development of thyroid cancer by "sterilization of follicular cells." I heard George Crile, Jr, say essentially the same thing in Pontiac, Michigan, in 1973.

4. Saenger EL, Thoma GE and Tompkins EA: Incidence of leukemia following treatment of hyperthyroidism. *JAMA* 205:147–154, 1968
5. Dobyns BM, Sheline GE, Workman JB, et al: Malignant and benign neoplasms of the thyroid in patients treated for hyperthyroidism: A report of the cooperative thyrotoxicosis followup study. *J Clin Endocrinol* 38:976–998, 1974

These two reports have served to dispel concern for either cancer or leukemia as complications of ^{131}I therapy for hyperthyroidism.

CASE 2–10. LOW-DOSE ^{131}I THERAPY FOR TDG

October, 1972. A 30 year old woman with hyperthyroidism was referred for ^{131}I therapy. She had been sick for about 4 months with classic features of the disease, including a goiter about two and a half times normal size. The FTI was 6.5, and the RAI 70 per cent. A 3 mCi dose of ^{131}I was given, a low dose in the hope that hypothyroidism would be avoided.

January, 1973. By 3 months the patient was experiencing symptoms of hypothyroidism, including muscle cramps, paresthesias, and lack of pep. The thyroid was one and a half times normal size. The FTI was 0.1, the RAI 12 per cent. Because of the RAI value, I suspected that the hypothyroidism might only be temporary. Therefore, levothyroxine, 0.1 mg daily, was ordered, and the patient was asked to return in 3 months.

April, 1973. The patient appeared to be euthyroid, although the heart rate was 98 at rest. The FTI was 4.4, and the RAI (while the patient was taking 0.1 mg of levothyroxine daily) was 42 per cent. I congratulated myself on my foresight in anticipating recovery, discontinued thyroid hormone, and asked the patient to return in 3 months.

July, 1973. She was feeling quite well and had gained 2 pounds in the 3 months. Her heart rate was 96/minute. The thyroid was slightly enlarged. The FTI was 4.2, and the RAI 43 per cent. Observation with reevaluation in 6 months was advised.

September, 1973. The patient returned prematurely, complaining of intense nervousness. She had gained another 2 pounds, and her heart rate was 80/minute. The FTI was 4.0, and the RAI 31 per cent. Some action seemed desirable, and I was reluctant to give more ^{131}I to a patient with minimal clinical evidence of hyperthyroidism. Hence, she was asked to take Lugol's solution, 2 drops daily.

January, 1974. The patient seemed somewhat worse. The heart rate was 108, the skin was moist and warm. She had gained 1 additional pound. She had not been taking Lugol's solution regularly. The FTI was 4.2. I asked her to be more responsible about taking her Lugol's solution and to return in 3 months.

April, 1974. She was feeling well, had gained another 1½ pounds, and the heart rate had slowed to 80. The thyroid was normal in size. The FTI was 2.5, normal at last. A recheck in 6 months was requested.

January, 1975. The patient was euthyroid clinically and biochemically. By dieting she had lost 4 pounds (which she did not really need). Her current weight was 142 pounds, which for her height of 67 inches was acceptable. Lugol's solution was discontinued.

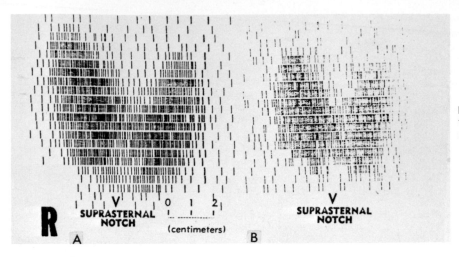

Figure 2-29. *A,* The original thyroid scan, October, 1972. *B,* The scan of March, 1975.

March, 1975. She had lost 5 pounds (still dieting) and the heart rate was 98. The FTI was 4.9. Additional ^{131}I was considered. However, the RAI was only 28 per cent, and the scan looked normal. Once again, observation was advised with a recheck planned for 6 months.

August, 1975. The patient was clinically hyperthyroid. The heart rate was 120, and moderate hand tremor and hyperactive reflexes were present. The FTI was 4.6, and the RAI was 45 per cent. Seven millicuries of ^{131}I was given.

November, 1975. The patient was hypothyroid, and replacement with levothyroxine, 0.15 mg daily, was instituted.

With which of the following statements do you agree?

a. Admittedly, this patient had quite a prolonged illness, but other patients treated as she was do well and remain euthyroid indefinitely.

b. Higher doses of ^{131}I do not guarantee prompt and decisive elimination of hyperthyroidism. After all, when most therapists were using initial doses of 7 to 12 mCi for patients like this, they obtained remissions in the hyperthyroidism with one dose of ^{131}I in only 60 to 70 per cent of patients.

c. Thyroidectomy would have been so much simpler and quicker and also much cheaper, considering the cost of all that testing and all those examinations.

Comment — Case 2-10

All of the statements are correct but irrelevant in my opinion. This patient is a perfect example of the average, run-of-the-mill hyperthyroid patient in terms of age, sex, goiter size, and severity of hyperthyroidism. She had the usual thyroid function test values. There was no discernible difference between her and many others I treated who responded quite differently to similar doses of ^{131}I. Some remained euthyroid for a number of years. About 25 per cent became hypothyroid within the first 2 years of followup. Another 25 per cent had persistent hyperthyroidism requiring one to three additional doses of ^{131}I. Many of the initially euthyroid patients ultimately became hypothyroid after a variable number of years, whereas others developed recurrent hyperthyroidism. In the long run the proportion of patients successfully treated and remaining euthyroid was small.

It is true that higher doses of ^{131}I as employed in the past provided no guarantee of success in terms of the elimination of hyperthyroidism. A careful review of the literature affirms this fact. In most reports only 50 to 70 per cent of patients were free of hyper-thyroidism after a single treatment. The only explanation for this poor showing that I can discern is failure to appreciate which patients will be particularly resistant to ^{131}I therapy—e.g., those with goiters more than three times normal size, especially if multinodular.

At any rate, I am doing better with my second thousand patients than I did with the first. Since I gave up small doses and began employing 8 to 30 mCi of ^{131}I as the initial treatment, I have been successful in eliminating hyperthyroidism in 96 per cent of patients with one dose. Most of the failures were patients who took more than one 30 mCi dose because the goiter was extremely large. No patient has required more than two doses.

For this patient, thyroidectomy would certainly have been quicker, simpler, and pos-sibly even cheaper, although hospital bills today are out of sight, and one must also in-clude the costs of preparation for thyroidectomy. Nevertheless, this patient is presented because she represents about the poorest result obtainable from ^{131}I therapy. This case is not unique. I have had other patients with similarly prolonged hyperthyroidism. Even if they represent a minority of the total treated, it makes the prospects for ^{131}I therapy less appealing than if higher doses are given. To be sure, after the higher doses most patients require thyroid hormone (about 80 per cent); but that is a small price for the benefits ob-tained. At least that is the opinion of the patients, for I give them the option of a low or high dose of ^{131}I when this treatment is indicated.

Selected Current References for Case 2–10

1. Cevallos JL, Hagen GA, Maloof F, et al: Low-dosage ^{131}I therapy of thyrotoxicosis (diffuse goiters). *New Eng J Med* 290:141–143, 1974

   This is a further report from the Massachusetts General Hospital on experience with low ^{131}I doses in an attempt to avoid hypothyroidism. The authors state that "the yearly increment of hypothyroidism appears greater with lower than with higher doses, which is at variance with a plateau described by others." A comparison of the tone of this article with that inferred from a reading of their 1967 report (Hagen GA, Ouellette RP, and Chapman EM: Comparison of high and low dosage levels of ^{131}I in the treatment of thyrotoxicosis. New Eng J Med 277:559–562, 1967) suggests declining enthusiasm for low ^{131}I doses, and almost (but not quite) an admission that the end result will be only an insubstantial reduction in the incidence of hypothyroidism. The price for this reduction is a substantial increase in the morbidity of the hyperthyroidism.

2. Rapoport B, Caplan R and DeGroot LJ: Low-dose sodium iodide I[131] therapy in Graves' disease. *JAMA* 224:1610–1613, 1973

   These authors have progressed a bit further along the road to advocacy of high routine ^{131}I doses. They found that low doses were unsatisfactory for many patients. Some were under treatment for 2 years or longer and ultimately required two or three treatments. The authors still look forward to solving the problem with greater precision in dosage. Apparently they do not agree with Cevallos et al that there are inherent limitations in our ability to predict individual biologic variations in responsiveness of thyroid tissue to radiation.

3. Safa AM and Skillern PG: Treatment of hyperthyroidism with a large initial dose of sodium iodide I[131]. *Arch Intern Med* 135:673–675, 1975

   Penn Skillern (whose clinical acumen I have always admired) has been employing large ^{131}I doses routinely since 1966 (7 years before I woke up, although I had used them for high risk cases since 1961). Ninety per cent of his patients were successfully treated with one dose. I do better at 96 per cent, but his early large doses were not really so large — as low as 6 mCi. More recently, he has been giving no less than 10 mCi, and his one dose cure rate will probably rise.

   It is remarkable that only 1 per cent of his patients stopped taking replacement thyroid hormone. My patients are not that dependable.

   Even more remarkable is the fact that he has not observed hyperthyroidism resulting from the combined effect of replacement thyroxine and recovery of nonsuppressible endogenous secretory activity. I respectfully suggest that he has not checked carefully enough. If one relies on the clinical findings alone, some of these patients may be missed. Even on clinical grounds the diagnosis is obvious for several of my patients every year.

   The statement that ATD "as a definitive treatment for hyperthyroidism is no longer indicated" seems too strong to me. However, just as I trailed behind him in appreciating that low-dose ^{131}I therapy was a bad way to treat hyperthyroid patients, perhaps I will some day be willing to abandon ATD for all the young adults and children I am now treating.

CASE 2–11. PREGNANCY DIAGNOSED 3 WEEKS AFTER ^{131}I THERAPY FOR HYPERTHYROIDISM

November, 1974. A 26 year old woman with hyperthyroidism was referred for treatment. The menstrual history was normal, and a pregnancy test was negative. She was given 8 mCi of [131]I. Three weeks later her family physician called to tell us she was pregnant.

With which of the following statements do you agree?

  a. Advise immediate abortion.

  b. Permit the patient to carry to term, checking her monthly to assure that thyroid function is normal and adding supplemental thyroid hormone if necessary.

  c. Forget it, the family physician is wrong. After all, the pregnancy test was negative.

  d. Iodine-131 does not cross the placenta.

  e. Supplemental thyroid hormone will protect the fetus.

  f. Although ^{131}I crosses the placenta, the fetal thyroid does not concentrate iodine until the third trimester; thus, it is no problem.

  g. The fetal thyroid begins to concentrate iodine at between 10 and 12 weeks of intrauterine life.

  h. The urine pregnancy test does not become positive until the second trimester.

  i. The urine pregnancy test becomes positive by the sixth week of intrauterine life.

Case 2–11 — Followup

About three times yearly we receive phone calls from worried physicians who face this problem. The problem is no problem if the physician had taken the simple precaution of performing a routine pregnancy test prior to administering the therapeutic dose of [131]I. Although this does not exclude very early stages of pregnancy, the fetal thyroid is not mature enough to take up ^{131}I until the end of the first trimester. Therefore, a negative pregnancy test provides reassurance that one has not delivered ^{131}I to the fetal thyroid even if the patient happens to have been a few weeks pregnant on the day the therapy was given. When a pregnancy test has not been done, it is impossible to be sure how far along the mother was, and therapeutic abortion may be considered justifiable.

A normal menstrual history or a history of use of birth control measures will not substitute for a pregnancy test. We have had positive pregnancy tests in women who were menstruating or had been "taking" birth control pills. After a positive pregnancy test the latter patient admitted having missed some of her pills in the previous few months. In this instance we permitted the patient to carry to term. The baby was normal.

Until 1975 our response to this type of question was based upon our own limited experience and our knowledge of fetal physiology. In 1975 we undertook a survey of 963 physicians who were actively engaged in the treatment of thyroid patients to determine what recommendations they make when inadvertent ^{131}I therapy is given within the first trimester of pregnancy and what problems they had with any infants that were carried to term.

Of 517 physicians who responded, 116 had seen 237 such patients. Twenty-two physicians advised therapeutic abortion for 55 patients. From the remaining 182 pregnancies, there were six fetal abnormalities other than hypothyroidism—a frequency not greater than that expected in a similar number of random pregnancies. In addition, six hypothyroid infants were reported. However, it was clear that three of the mothers had received ^{131}I in the second trimester. None of the mothers had been given pregnancy tests prior to ^{131}I therapy. One infant had only temporary hypothyroidism, possibly the result of trans-placental passage of ATD given to the mother when the ^{131}I failed to eliminate the hyper-thyroidism.

Since pregnancy tests become positive before the fetal thyroid will accumulate ^{131}I, a negative pregnancy test virtually eliminates concern for harmful effects of ^{131}I on the fetal thyroid. If one cannot be certain of the timing of the ^{131}I therapy with respect to the age of a pregnancy discovered after the treatment (because of failure to do a routine pretherapy pregnancy test), therapeutic abortion may have to be considered.

Selected Current Reference for Case 2–11

1. Stoffer SS and Hamburger JI: Inadvertent ^{131}I therapy for hyperthyroidism in the first trimester of pregnancy. *J Nucl Med* 17:146–149, 1976

    This article should be required reading for every physician who administers ^{131}I therapy. All right, if you are too busy to read it I will give you the punch line. You had better routinely perform a pregnancy test before administering ^{131}I therapy to a woman who could conceivably be pregnant (i.e., any woman between puberty and menopause who has not had a hysterectomy). If the pregnancy test is negative and the menstrual history normal, you need not be concerned if pregnancy is diagnosed several weeks later. The data provide no evidence of any special risk to the fetus from ^{131}I therapy. I realize that this summary may raise questions. They are answered in the article.

CASE 2–12. MANAGEMENT OF THE PREGNANT HYPERTHYROID PATIENT

September, 1970. A 31 year old hyperthyroid woman 3 months pregnant, was referred for treatment. She had been hyperthyroid for about 2 years, the hyper-thyroidism having been controlled by PTU, 100 mg three times daily, for the previous 9 months. An urticarial eruption had developed 1 week earlier, and PTU was discontinued, with prompt subsidence of the skin lesions. The patient was 63 inches tall and weighed 118 pounds. The heart rate was 110, there was a moderate hand tremor, and the thyroid gland was three times normal size. The FTI was 5.2, the CBC was normal. The patient was placed on methimazole, 10 mg four times a day, and asked to return in 1 month.

October, 1970. The patient was clinically euthyroid, her weight was 124 pounds, and the heart rate was 88. The thyroid gland was unchanged in size. The FTI was 2.8.

With which of the following statements do you agree?

a. Add Lugol's solution, 5 drops three times a day for 10 days, and operate. Another drug reaction is likely, and then you will not be able to prepare the patient adequately for operation.

b. Continue methimazole, adjusting the dose downward as the course permits. If there is another reaction, the patient may still be prepared for surgical treatment, and thyroidectomy is best avoided early in pregnancy.

c. Continue the same dose of methimazole but add levothyroxine, 0.2 mg daily, to the regimen to prevent maternal hypothyroidism and protect the fetus from the goitrogenic effects of the transplacental passage of methimazole.

d. Same as c, but use T_3, 75 μg daily, instead of levothyroxine (T_4) because T_4 does not cross the placenta as readily as T_3.

Case 2–12—Followup

There is no need to panic over a drug reaction in a pregnant patient, particularly if the reaction is simply of the cutaneous type, with no hematologic abnormalities. Most of the time the other ATD will be suitable for the balance of the pregnancy. If another reaction occurs, it is still possible to prepare the patient for operation using iodides, propranolol, and adrenal steroids. Therefore, we elected to continue methimazole without supplemental thyroid hormone.

The administration of the smallest possible dose of ATD is essential for the successful management of the pregnant hyperthyroid patient (i.e., both mother and fetus are euthyroid and there is no fetal goiter). Since hyperthyroidism tends to improve as pregnancy advances, it is possible to reduce progressively the ATD dose for most patients, and for some even to discontinue ATD by the third trimester.

The patient should be seen and examined every 4 weeks, and blood taken for an FTI and TSH(RIA). Dosage reductions should be made in anticipatory fashion, assuming that the functional indices will drop from visit to visit.

If (as some authorities recommend) one gives supplemental thyroid hormone, the usefulness of the FTI as an index of progress will be negated. The value will not fall even if the patient is improving because the supplemental thyroid hormone will prevent this. Any ATD dosage reduction will have to be made without laboratory guidance. Since supplemental thyroid hormone is no more effective than endogenous thyroid hormone in preventing maternal hypothyroidism, it is unnecessary as long as care is taken to maintain the FTI at the upper level of normal.

Furthermore, a normal level of thyroid hormone in the mother does not necessarily prevent fetal goiter and hypothyroidism. ATD cross the placenta readily, whereas thyroxine does so only with difficulty.

The suggested use of T_3 instead of T_4 presents a new problem rather than providing a solution. T_3 also does not cross the placenta as freely as ATD. Furthermore, if full doses of T_3 are given to a mother whose thyroid function is blocked by ATD, T_3 will replace T_4 as the principal circulating thyroid hormone in the blood. Since T_3 is less well bound to carrier protein than T_4, maternal thyroid-binding proteins will become relatively desaturated. This will create conditions favoring transfer of thyroid hormone from the fetus to the mother rather than vice versa. Adherence to the principles of using the smallest ATD dose possible, making anticipatory reductions in ATD dose, and avoiding supplemental thyroid hormone will greatly simplify the management of pregnant hyperthyroid patients. However, careful followup and a reliable laboratory are essential. Here is the subsequent course of this patient:

DATE	FTI[a]	TSH(RIA) μU/ml	METHIMAZOLE DOSE
Oct, 1970	2.8	2.5	10 mg q.i.d.
Nov, 1970	2.6	3.0	10 mg b.i.d.
Dec, 1970	3.2	2.0	10 mg b.i.d.
Jan, 1971	2.4	2.0	5 mg b.i.d.
Feb, 1971	1.8	2.5	Discontinued
Mar, 1971	2.0	2.5	None
Apr, 1971	Normal nongoitrous infant delivered		

[a]NR: 1.1 to 3.4.

July 1971. The patient returned with a relapse of the hyperthyroidism. The thyroid gland was two and a half times normal size. The FTI was 5.2 and the RAI 61 per cent.

Now what do you do?

a. Resume methimazole.

b. Give ^{131}I.

c. Advise thyroidectomy.

I believe that no patient should be required to endure more than one episode of hyperthyroidism during pregnancy. Resuming treatment with ATD is an invitation to a recurrence of this dual disease. In fact, the first episode could probably have been prevented if the patient had been treated either with ^{131}I or thyroidectomy rather than with ATD. In my opinion the use of long-term ATD administration for hyperthyroidism in women planning to have children is a prime example of poor medical judgment. For reasons already discussed, and in accordance with the preponderance of informed opinion on the subject, I treat these patients with ^{131}I. I have no strong objection to thyroidectomy providing that the patient understands and prefers the surgical risks (including the small but definite risk of mortality) to the questionable risks of ^{131}I.

Selected Current References for Case 2–12

Few problems with which thyroidologists must deal generate as much controversy as treatment of hyperthyroidism in the pregnant patient. Frankly, our experience is not great and would be even less if we had had the opportunity of determining the treatment for the patients we did see at the onset of the disease. I believe that our policy of advising definitive therapy (^{131}I or thyroidectomy, as the patient prefers) for all young women who contemplate child bearing within 3 years has materially reduced the number of women who have had to deal with hyperthyroidism complicating pregnancy in the Detroit area. Since I saw to it that any woman who I treated for this problem was subsequently treated definitively after delivery if still hyperthyroid, contrary to the experiences reported in most of the papers cited, I have yet to deal with this problem more than once in any patient.

A careful review of the literature on this subject reveals that there is an increased risk to the fetus of the pregnant hyperthyroid patient, even in the hands of experts. Therefore, thoughtful physicians should take steps to prevent the problem. A large proportion of patients face this difficult situation only because they received what I consider bad advice from their physicians when the diagnosis of hyperthyroidism was made — i.e., long-term ATD therapy. That treatment increases fertility while at the same time perpetuating the disease, thereby requiring continued ATD administration.

1. Bullock JL, Harris RE and Young R: Treatment of thyrotoxicosis during pregnancy with propranolol. *Am J Obstet Gynecol* 121:242–245, 1975
2. Langer A, Hung CT, McA'Nulty JA, et al: Adrenergic blockade: A new approach to hyperthyroidism during pregnancy. *Obstet Gynecol* 44:181–186, 1974

These two reports deal with the use of propranolol as the sole treatment of hyperthyroidism during pregnancy. This might be worth considering as an alternative to thyroidectomy for a patient with mild hyperthyroidism who has developed toxic reactions to both antithyroid drugs. ATD remains the preferred initial treatment for the rather obvious reason that it not only relieves symptoms (as does propranolol) but also restores the euthyroid state.

3. Hayek A and Brooks M: Neonatal hyperthyroidism following intrauterine hypothyroidism. *Pediatrics* 87:446–448, 1975

A nice demonstration of how poor treatment of the mother led to fetal hypothyroidism. PTU dosage was not reduced progressively in anticipation of the improvement in the maternal status which so often occurs in the last half of the pregnancy. As a result, from the twenty-eighth week on, the PTU dose was higher than necessary, as shown by a progressive decline in the serum T_4 value from 17.8 µg per 100 ml (a level only slightly higher than optimal during pregnancy) to 9.6 µg per 100 ml, a level clearly indicative of ATD overdosage. In pregnancy one should follow the patient with the FTI. If the T_4 value alone is employed, one should aim for a level about 25 per cent higher than the upper level of normal for the nonpregnant individual.

Incidentally, the administration of propranolol throughout the pregnancy was not only unnecessary but also undoubtedly made the clinical followup more difficult, since the significance of the heart rate was thereby eliminated.

4. Worley RJ and Crosby WM: Hyperthyroidism during pregnancy. *Am J Obstet Gynecol* 119:150–155, 1974

A small series suggesting that medical management (without supplemental thyroid hormone) is preferable to thyroidectomy.

5. Talbert LH, Thomas CG, Jr, Holt WA, et al: Hyperthyroidism during pregnancy. *Obstet Gynecol* 36:779–785, 1970

A larger series suggesting that thyroidectomy is preferable to medical management (they also emphasize that supplemental thyroid hormone is inappropriate).

It is amusing to read the literature on this subject because you can find support for any position you wish. (Of course, there is the paper I co-authored which tells it like it is.)

6. Goluboff LG, Sisson JC and Hamburger JI: Hyperthyroidism associated with pregnancy. *Obstet Gynecol* 44:107–116, 1974

The lessons are clear. Use ATD in the lowest possible doses (this is possible when supplemental thyroid hormone is avoided). Follow patients closely from the clinical standpoint and by obtaining FTI and TSH(RIA) values. Anticipate improvement by advance reductions in ATD dosage, preferring mild hyperthyroidism to any degree of hypothyroidism. Expect to be able to discontinue ATD in about 25 per cent of patients in the last trimester because they will be in remission — usually temporary but occasionally sustained.

7. Mujtaba Q and Burrow GN: Treatment of hyperthyroidism in pregnancy with propylthiouracil and methimazole. *Obstet Gynecol* 46:282–286, 1975

These physicians really had trouble. However, they violated most of the rules stated above. They saw their patients irregularly and too infrequently, did not obtain FTI or TSH(RIA) values, and generally flew by makeshift means.

In my opinion their carelessness is epitomized by the fact that their patients were allowed to remain on ATD through two and even three pregnancies, a sin shared by the authors of the next paper, which is cited only because they had the good sense to appreciate that supplemental thyroid hormone makes bad sense.

8. Ayromlooi J, Zervoudakis IA and Sadaghat A: Thyrotoxicosis in pregnancy. *Am J Obstet Gynecol* 117:818–823, 1973
9. Mestman JH, Manning PR and Hodgman J: Hyperthyroidism and pregnancy. *Arch Intern Med* 134:434–439, 1974

These authors compared the results of treatment with ATD alone and with supplemental thyroid hormone. Control was possible with lower doses of ATD when supplemental thyroid hormone was not given. Logical, isn't it? At least, that is what I said in 1972.

10. Hamburger JI: Management of the pregnant hyperthyroid. *Obstet Gynecol* 40:114–117, 1972

In an afterword to this article, Engbring accused me of trying to refute the data (of Selenkow) with logic that he did not consider logical. Engbring, where are you now? The troops are deserting you and your mentor, as even a casual perusal of the literature will confirm.

11. Horger EO, III, Kenimer JG, Azukizawa M, et al: Failure of triiodothyronine to prevent propylthiouracil-induced hypothyroidism and goiter in fetal sheep. *Obstet Gynecol* 47:46–49, 1976

This recent article provides more evidence against the concept that supplemental thyroid hormone will protect the fetus from undesirable effects of antithyroid drugs.

12. VanHerle AJ, Young RT, Fisher DA, et al: Intrauterine treatment of a hypothyroid fetus. *J Clin Endocrinol* 40:474–477, 1975

This patient had been given a therapeutic dose of ^{131}I in the twenty-fourth week of pregnancy (see reference for Case 2–11). There is no excuse for such an error. Nevertheless, the fetus was successfully treated by transuterine injections of LT_4 into the fetal buttock, believe it or not. This is one way to cover an infant exposed to ATD. A simpler and better way is to give the smallest dose of ATD possible.

CASE 2–13. A PREGNANT HYPERTHYROID PATIENT WHO DEVELOPS TOXIC REACTIONS TO BOTH PTU AND METHIMAZOLE

May, 1972. A 24 year old woman was diagnosed as having hyperthyroidism in November of 1971 when she was about 6 weeks pregnant. PTU, 50 mg twice daily, was given, and 3 months later she developed a cutaneous reaction that cleared promptly when PTU was stopped. No treatment was given subsequently, and she was clearly hyperthyroid when first seen by us. Laboratory studies were all positive. Methimazole, 5 mg four times a day, was prescribed. In 2 weeks a recurrence of the cutaneous reaction took place.

With which of the following statements do you agree?

a. Prepare her for thyroidectomy with propranolol, 20 mg four times a day, Lugol's solution, 5 drops three times a day, and an adrenal steroid preparation.

b. Treat with propranolol for the balance of the pregnancy.

c. Treat with Lugol's solution throughout the balance of the pregnancy.

d. She is in her sixth month, and the hyperthyroidism will go into a remission, so no treatment is necessary other than mild tranquilizers — e.g., phenobarbital.

e. Propranolol is contraindicated in pregnancy.

f. There is a higher risk to the fetus when thyroidectomy is performed in later stages of pregnancy.

g. Thyroidectomy without ATD preparation will probably be followed by thyroid storm.

h. This is one time when ^{131}I should be given during pregnancy. Of course, the mother will require supplemental thyroid hormone, and thyroid hormone should also be given to the infant by injection into the amniotic fluid.

Case 2–13—Followup

The patient was prepared for thyroidectomy with propranolol and Lugol's solution for 1 week. Cortisone acetate was given intramuscularly in doses of 100 mg the night before and the morning and afternoon of the operation, and half that amount was given the evening of the operation and the next morning.

The thyroidectomy was uneventful, as was the balance of the pregnancy. Supplemental thyroid hormone was instituted beginning 3 weeks after the operation and has been maintained ever since.

Surprisingly, thyroid storm is uncommon even when unprepared hyperthyroid patients have major surgical procedures. Nevertheless, there is no need to take chances with less than optimal preparation ordinarily. Although ATD could not be utilized for this patient, considerable alleviation of the hyperthyroidism was obtained with Lugol's solution and propranolol. The cortisone offered further protection against thyroid storm. Certainly the operative risks were not great enough to justify ^{131}I therapy.

Long-term Lugol's solution is a poor choice for pregnant patients, since iodine crosses the placenta and rarely may cause goitrous fetal hypothyroidism and, if the goiter is large enough, asphyxiation.

The operative risks to the fetus are least late in the second trimester.

Propranolol may be given for the few days necessary in such a case.

Selected Current Reference for Case 2–13

1. Michie W, Hamer-Hodges DW, Pegg CAS, et al: Beta-blockade and partial thyroidectomy for thyrotoxicosis. *Lancet* 1:1009–1011, 1974

This article shows that propranolol alone (for 37 patients, mean age 34 years) can be used to prepare hyperthyroid patients for thyroidectomy. This is the type of study which deserves to be condemned.

They didn't do it because they had to. (The circumstances under which one would have to are hard to imagine. Have they not heard of ^{131}I?) They did it to see if they could get away with it. After all, only the lives of their patients were at risk.

In addition to questioning the judgment of these physicians, their ethics also might be subjected to review. Can one really get informed consent for this type of experimentation? I would not give my consent, and I cannot imagine anyone who was informed of a possible increased risk of mortality giving his consent.

Having done their human experimentation, they felt obliged to indicate to the reader when such treatment might be appropriate. They note that preparation for thyroidectomy can be accomplished in 5 to 6 days rather than the 2 to 3 months required with ATD (longer than I usually require). To the natural question as to what is the hurry, they reply that this method is cheaper and more convenient for patients coming long distances. To this one may respond that ^{131}I is quicker, cheaper, and undoubtedly safer. If thyroidectomy is the patient's choice, to me it makes no sense to operate on a poorly prepared patient. I have heard some anecdotal reports of very stormy events when this method was employed.

CASE 2–14. TOXIC RECURRENT GOITER

1967. A 20 year old hyperthyroid woman was treated surgically. Three months after the operation she was euthyroid.

1969. After 2 years of good health she experienced a recurrence of tachycardia, heat intolerance, and a weight loss of 5 pounds in the previous 3 months. The patient was 65 inches tall and weighed 135 pounds. There was a mild hand tremor, a heart rate of 110 per minute, and the right lobe of the thyroid was enlarged to about twice normal size. The FTI was 4 (NR: 1.4 to 3.8), the RAI was 43 per cent, and there was no suppression in response to T_3 administration, 50 μg twice a day for 1 week. A scan showed essentially all of the activity to be in the enlarged right lobe.

With which of the following statements do you agree?

a. If the patient was initially treated with a unilateral lobectomy this may be an important factor in the recurrence of her hyperthyroidism.

b. This asymmetrical enlargement would best be treated surgically.

c. Iodine-131 therapy would be the safest and most definitive method of treatment.

d. ATD therapy would be suitable because the patient has only mild hyperthyroidism.

e. Why not try long-term Lugol's solution?

Case 2–14—Followup

Unilateral lobectomy for hyperthyroidism is a procedure that has fallen into disuse because of a high incidence of recurrence. A repeat operation is more likely to result in damage to adjacent structures, especially the parathyroids and recurrent nerves.

The usual treatment for recurrent hyperthyroidism after unsuccessful thyroidectomy is ^{131}I. However, this patient had mild hyperthyroidism and was so young that there was time for a trial of suppression with Lugol's solution in the hope that after a period of control a remission might occur. ATD could have been tried, but the simplicity and safety of Lugol's solution are advantages that deserve attention.

After 2 years' treatment with 2 drops of Lugol's solution daily, during which she remained euthyroid, withdrawal of the medication was possible, and she has been well since then. In November of 1975 the FTI value was 1.8.

Selected Current Reference for Case 2–14

1. Hamburger JI: Recurrent hyperthyroidism after thyroidectomy. *Arch Surg* 111:91–92, 1976

    Again note that recurrent hyperthyroidism after thyroidectomy may occur many years later.

CASE 2–15. "HYPERTHYROIDISM" TREATED WITH METHIMAZOLE

March, 1973. A 37 year old woman had been treated for hyperthyroidism with methimazole for 2 years. The diagnosis had been suspected on clinical grounds and confirmed by an elevated RAI only. She was then referred for reevaluation and recommendations for further treatment.

Her weight had fluctuated between 98 and 120 pounds during the 2 years of treatment, and now is 105 pounds. In the 6 weeks prior to examination she had gained 4 pounds, after having lost 15 pounds in the previous 3 months. Additional complaints were intermittent palpitation, tremor, loose bowels, and excessive hair loss. She was 64 inches tall, the heart rate was 72, the skin was cool and dry, the reflexes were normal, and there was no tremor. The thyroid gland was diffusely enlarged to twice the normal size. There were no ophthalmic abnormalities. Her medications included methimazole, 5 mg three times a day, and conjugated estrogen. The FTI was 0.8, the T_3(RIA) 100 ng per 100 ml, and the TSH(RIA) 128 $\mu U/ml$.

The problem is to determine whether this patient still has hyperthyroidism (if she ever did, for the original diagnosis may be open to serious doubt).

With which of the following statements do you agree?

   a. Stop methimazole for 6 weeks and recheck the FTI and T_3(RIA).

   b. The T_3(RIA) of 100, in the face of an FTI which is subnormal, suggests that stopping methimazole will lead to T_3 toxicosis.

   c. Stop methimazole and give T_3, 50 μg twice daily, for 5 days, and on the fourth and fifth days perform an RAI. A value of greater than 45 per cent would suggest that the patient will have a recurrence of hyperthyroidism if no further action is taken; whereas a value of less than 10 per cent would indicate that she is in remission. Intermediate values would be less specific.

   d. Frankly hypothyroid values for the FTI and TSH(RIA) on such a small dose of methimazole mean that the patient will not experience a recurrence of hyperthyroidism in the near future if methimazole is discontinued.

Case 2–15—Further Diagnostic Data

The T_3 suppression test is helpful in such a patient. If methimazole is just discontinued, it cannot be predicted how rapidly hyperthyroidism might recur. Furthermore, there is no need to allow this to happen. In most cases a high RAI value while on T_3 will alert the physician that a recurrence of hyperthyroidism is probable. If no T_3 is given, a high RAI value after withdrawal of methimazole would be expected as a rebound effect. This may persist for more than a month. The administration of T_3, by suppressing the pituitary TSH release, prevents a high RAI whenever the patient no longer has active Graves' disease. The T_3-(RIA) level has no prognostic significance. A T_3(RIA) level relatively higher than the FTI level simply reflects an attempt by the thyroid to compensate for suppressed T_4 output by a relative increase in T_3 secretion. Furthermore, the value is artificially elevated by the high TBG concentration produced by the estrogens the patient is taking.

In this instance the RAI at the end of 5 days of T_3 administration (50 μg twice daily) was 38 per cent. The patient experienced no adverse symptoms and actually felt better in terms of pep and energy.

With which of the following statements do you agree?

a. Resume methimazole for another 2 years but give a smaller dose.

b. Observe the patient with no treatment, rechecking in 1 month initially; if she is euthyroid, recheck at 6 months and then annually as long as the euthyroid state persists.

c. Give T_3 for 10 days and see whether there is a further fall in RAI (suggesting a remission) or no further fall in RAI (suggesting active Graves' disease requiring ^{131}I or thyroidectomy).

d. Give ^{131}I therapy. The probability of a recurrence of hyperthyroidism is great.

e. The 38 per cent RAI value is abnormally high but does not necessarily mean that hyperthyroidism is imminent.

f. Without a baseline RAI, the 38 per cent value has no meaning.

Case 2–15—Followup

The 38 per cent RAI value on T_3 was high enough to suggest that hyperthyroidism would soon return if no action were taken. Since the patient was young, there was no urgency to begin definitive treatment; hence, I decided to observe and wait. At this age, ^{131}I would have been my choice initially, and the failure of a 2-year trial of methimazole only confirmed this preference. A longer period of T_3 suppression would add nothing and might be poorly tolerated. We already knew that the RAI was less than normally suppressible, and a nonsuppressible RAI does not prove that hyperthyroidism will recur—it just increases the probability. Of course, the higher the RAI value (on T_3) the more nearly certain is a relapse of hyperthyroidism.

April, 1972. One month after stopping methimazole the patient was euthyroid, clinically and by testing. She was asked to return in 6 months, unless she thought that hyperthyroidism was recurring sooner.

June, 1972. She had lost 6 pounds and noted palpitation and increasing nervousness. The heart rate was 110. The FTI was 4.1, the T_3(RIA) 200 ng per 100 ml, and the RAI 52 per cent. Iodine-131 therapy was given.

Having earlier discounted the value of the T_3 suppression test to determine whether a remission had been obtained after ATD treatment, it may seem contradictory to suggest its use in this patient for what might appear to be the same purpose. However, there is a difference. In the first instance, I am referring to a patient for whom I had confirmed the diagnosis and instituted ATD therapy. For such a patient, I would progressively reduce the ATD dose, condition permitting, until it is discontinued. It is axiomatic that the patient should remain euthyroid, clinically and by testing, throughout the treatment period. A T_3 suppression test at the endpoint, whether positive or negative, would not influence choice of further treatment. By contrast, this patient had already taken ATD for 2 years. The original diagnosis was suspect. Had I seen her initially and made a diagnosis of hyperthyroidism, I would have treated her with ^{131}I, not ATD (for reasons amply discussed already). In her case, a T_3 suppression test may provide confirmation of the present level of disease activity (e.g., the higher the RAI on T_3, the more certain it is that hyperthyroidism will follow ATD discontinuation), and may (if the RAI is well suppressed) suggest prompt discontinuation of ATD. If the RAI on T_3 were high it would indicate a switch from ATD to ^{131}I therapy.

CASE 2–16. HYPERTHYROIDISM TREATED WITH A LOW DOSE OF ^{131}I

July, 1971. A 32 year old hyperthyroid woman was referred for treatment. The clinical features were typical and included a goiter of twice the normal size. The FTI was 4.4, and the RAI was 55 per cent. The patient was given 4 mCi of ^{131}I, a dose calculated to deliver 50 μCi per gram of thyroid tissue in the hope that hyperthyroidism could be eliminated without the subsequent development of hypothyroidism.

October, 1971. The patient appeared clinically euthyroid. The FTI was 1.0, the TSH(RIA) 32 μU/ml, and the RAI 3 per cent. The patient was given levothyroxine, 0.1 mg daily, and asked to return in 3 months to exclude either recovery of nonsuppressible function, which would necessitate a reduction in the levothyroxine dose (if not its discontinuation), or a further drop in endogenous thyroid function, which would necessitate an increase in the dose of levothyroxine.

January, 1972. The patient appeared euthyroid. The FTI was 1.2, the TSH(RIA) 19 μU/ml, and the RAI 5 per cent. The levothyroxine dose was increased to 0.15 mg daily. The patient was asked to return in 1 year.

January, 1973. The patient returned complaining of palpitation, tremor, heat intolerance, and a weight loss of 5 pounds in the previous 3 months. The heart rate was 104, the reflexes were hyperactive, and there was a mild hand tremor. The thyroid gland was normal in size by palpation. The FTI was 5.2, and the RAI was 22 per cent. Thyroid hormone was discontinued, and the patient was asked to return in 6 weeks to be sure that supplemental thyroid was no longer needed. At that time she was again hypothyroid, complaining of cold intolerance, muscle cramps, and paresthesias. The FTI was 0.8 and the TSH(RIA) 50 μU/ml. Levothyroxine, 0.1 mg daily, was reinstituted. The patient was rechecked in 6 weeks and was euthyroid clinically and by testing.

With which of the following statements do you agree?

a. Hyperthyroidism may yet recur, as she has a relatively resistant gland.

b. After this length of time no further changes are very likely.

c. It is unsafe to predict the future. Regular reevaluation and testing will be needed for life.

d. Thyroid function can be expected to decline progressively until the patient requires a larger dose of thyroid hormone.

e. A large initial ^{131}I dose given with the aim of ablating the function of the thyroid gland would have greatly simplified the management of this patient, while also reducing the cost of her treatment by eliminating the necessity for much of the repeated testing.

f. Although this patient had problems, the avoidance of post-^{131}I hypothyroidism is important enough to justify the inconvenience and added expense.

g. Lower dosage ^{131}I therapy for hyperthyroidism has clearly reduced the long-term incidence of hypothyroidism and is gaining in popularity.

Case 2–16—Followup

This patient did experience a gradual further deterioration in thyroid function, requiring a return to the previously untolerated dose of 0.15 mg levothyroxine daily. However, the course of thyroid function in these patients is unpredictable. We have seen recurrent hyperthyroidism several years after the initial treatment, even though the patient had been temporarily hypothyroid in the interim. Other patients remain euthyroid for several years and then gradually drift into hypothyroidism.

The important thing to remember is that any functioning remnant of the thyroid gland after ^{131}I therapy for hyperthyroidism is abnormal and unpredictable in terms of its future behavior. For this reason we believe it is preferable to advise deliberately ablative doses of ^{131}I as the most efficient and effective method of dealing with this disease. This avoids much repeated testing and many office visits. It also virtually eliminates the necessity for more than a single ^{131}I dose. The price is a requirement for life-long replacement therapy with thyroid hormone. Most patients readily accept this as the lesser evil when the alternatives are explained. Other authorities here and abroad are also coming to this conclusion.

Long-term followup studies suggest that lower ^{131}I doses may only delay the onset of hypothyroidism, not prevent its development. Any minor reduction in the incidence of hypothyroidism is more than counterbalanced by the disadvantages of prolongation of hyperthyroidism for many patients and the instability of the thyroid functional status after treatment for others, as this case so well demonstrates.

CASE 2–17. RECURRENT GOITER, POSSIBLE IATROGENIC THYROTOXICOSIS

August, 1972. A 55 year old woman had undergone thyroidectomy for an obstructing goiter in Germany in 1956. She now has a recurrent goiter and characteristic clinical features of hyperthyroidism. Two weeks earlier she had been hospitalized for an acute episode of atrial fibrillation without congestive heart failure, but she converted to normal sinus rhythm in response to the usual dose of Lanoxin. Lanoxin was continued in a dose of 0.25 mg daily. She has been taking levothyroxine, 0.3 mg daily, for 2 to 3 years.

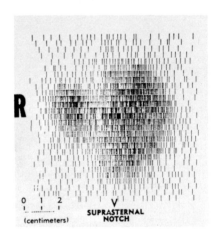

Figure 2–30. The scan reveals most of the tracer in an enlarged left thyroid lobe.

She was 61 inches tall and weighed 188 pounds. There had been no weight loss. The heart rate was 92 and regular. The left lobe of the thyroid was enlarged and nodular and measured about 3 by 6 cm.

The FTI was 7.1 (NR: 1.1 to 3.4), the T_3 (RIA) 195 ng per 100 ml, and the RAI 20 per cent, with most of the tracer taken up by the nodular left lobe.

With which of the following statements do you agree?

a. She has thyrotoxicosis; give [131]I.

b. This toxic nodule will be resistant to [131]I. Thyroidectomy will be quicker and more certain.

c. Since the RAI is only 20 per cent, perhaps she is only hyperthyroid because of the combined effect of the nonsuppressed endogenous secretion and the supplemental levothyroxine.

d. This is iatrogenic thyrotoxicosis. If thyroid hormone is discontinued, all will be well.

e. A dose of 0.3 mg of levothyroxine daily is usually excessive.

f. If her atrial fibrillation was due to hyperthyroidism she would not have responded to the "usual dose" of Lanoxin.

Case 2-17—Further Data

Levothyroxine was discontinued and the patient rechecked in 1 month.

September, 1972. She had gained 3 pounds; however, her palpitations had increased. Atrial fibrillation had recurred.

The FTI was 3.9, the T_3(RIA) 205 ng per 100 ml, and the RAI 40 per cent. A short course of PTU was given to prepare her for ^{131}I therapy. After 4 weeks she was euthyroid and considered ready for [131]I.

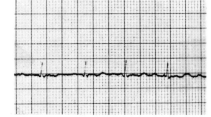

Figure 2-31. The EKG shows atrial fibrillation.

How much ^{131}I should be given?

a. A small dose (3.5 mCi). Patients with recurrent hyperthyroidism after surgery are usually overly sensitive to [131]I.

b. An intermediate dose (10 mCi). The thyroid is nodular, and a small dose will be inadequate. However, the patient has an unstable cardiac status, and a large ^{131}I dose may not be safe.

c. A large dose (30 mCi). Not only is this a nodular goiter, but the cardiac complication makes it essential to eliminate the hyperthyroidism as quickly as possible. The PTU preparation will protect her from any important discharge of preformed thyroid hormone. Supplemental propranolol may be given if needed in the first few weeks after ^{131}I therapy.

Case 2-17—Followup

It is correct that recurrent hyperthyroidism after thyroidectomy is often sensitive to ^{131}I, and even small doses may produce hypothyroidism promptly. However, this is the case when only a rather small amount of functioning thyroid tissue remains. Large nodular recurrences are often resistant and should be treated generously. The faint of heart are likely to find that a smaller ^{131}I dose not only will fail to eliminate the hyperthyroidism but will produce a lower uptake of ^{131}I, so that further treatment may be more difficult. Your first shot is the best you will have. With preparation, these patients tolerate large ^{131}I doses, and also usually do not become hypothyroid. In this instance, a 30 mCi dose of ^{131}I restored the patient to the euthyroid state in 6 weeks. Sinus rhythm returned. She subsequently remained euthyroid.

There is confusion on the matter of the response of atrial fibrillation to digitalis when the patient is hyperthyroid. It is correct that some hyperthyroid patients are relatively resistant to the effects of digitalis. It is incorrect to conclude that hyperthyroid patients with atrial fibrillation do not respond to the drug, or that they never respond to the usual doses.

CASE 2–18. IATROGENIC (IN PART) THYROTOXICOSIS

December, 1968. A 58 year old man was treated with ^{131}I 9 years previously for hyperthyroidism. Seven years later a diagnosis of hypothyroidism was made, and he was given a thyroid hormone product containing both T_4 and T_3. In the 3 months prior to examination he noted increasing nervousness, palpitation, and heat intolerance. The heart rate was 110. The thyroid gland was normal in size. There was mild hand tremor and brisk reflexes.

You would expect the following laboratory values:

a. Elevated FTI and T_3(RIA) values, and an RAI of less than 5 per cent. The patient is taking an overdose of thyroid hormone.

b. Elevated FTI and T_3(RIA) values with an elevated RAI also. The patient has a recurrence of hyperthyroidism resulting primarily from a resumption of excessive endogenous secretory activity.

c. The FTI and T_3(RIA) are elevated, but the RAI is normal. The patient is taking the usual replacement dose of thyroid hormone but has developed recovery of endogenous nonsuppressible function. Hyperthyroidism results from the combined effects of endogenous and exogenous hormone.

Case 2–18 — Further Data

The FTI was 6.2, the T_3(RIA) 200 ng per 100 ml, and the RAI 12 per cent.

Now what do you do?

a. Discontinue thyroid hormone and recheck in 6 weeks. The patient may be euthyroid or hypothyroid then.

b. Give a large ^{131}I dose (the RAI is only 12 per cent) to ablate the residual tissue; then thyroid hormone can be given without difficulty.

c. If the patient had been treated surgically in the first place this would not have happened.

Case 2–18—Followup

Thyroid hormone was discontinued.

January, 1969. Six weeks later the FTI was 1.1, and the TSH(RIA) was 42 μU/ml. Thus, although the remaining thyroid tissue was not suppressible, the secretory capacity was inadequate to maintain the euthyroid state. The patient was given levothyroxine, 0.1 mg daily, and has remained euthyroid since then.

The problem of subnormal but nonsuppressible thyroid function after treatment of hyperthyroidism, whether with ^{131}I or by thyroidectomy, has received inadequate attention in the literature. Any remaining thyroid function after treatment of hyperthyroidism may be, or in the future may become, nonsuppressible. Recommendations for routine administration of full doses of thyroid hormone to all treated hyperthyroid patients are based upon inadequate experience. Life is not so simple. For this patient a supplemental dose was proper. Furthermore, periodic reevaluation is necessary, for the residual nonsuppressible endogenous function may increase or decrease as the years go by.

Selected Current Reference for Case 2–18

1. Meier DA and Hamburger JI: Problems resulting from suppressible and nonsuppressible thyroid function. *Mich Med* 69:29–32, 1970

This is one of the earlier of my frequent warnings about unexpected nonsuppressible function. Selected cases are briefly presented to exemplify the clinical settings in which one must be on the alert.

CASE 2–19. TOXIC NODULAR GOITER

October, 1973.   A 44 year old man had been treated for hyperthyroidism with ATD for 12 years, during which there was progressive enlargement of the right lobe of the thyroid gland. There was persistent palpitation and heat intolerance in spite of treatment. The heart rate was 120, and there was a 4 × 8 cm mass on the right side of the neck. No thyroid tissue was palpable on the left side.

The FTI was 4.5, and the RAI (48 hours after discontinuation of ATD) was 36 per cent. The scan is shown in Figure 2–32. The patient was given propranolol, 20 mg four times a day, to control his tachycardia.

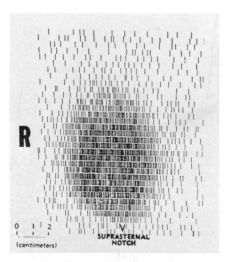

Figure 2-32. The initial scan.

A 30 mCi dose of ^{131}I was given.

January, 1974.   The thyroid mass was only slightly smaller. The patient was still toxic. The FTI was 4.8, and the T_3(RIA) 205 ng per 100 ml. However, the RAI was now only 15 per cent.

With which of the following statements do you agree?

a.   Administer ATD for 1 month, and then give another 30 mCi dose of [131]I.

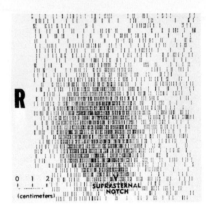

Figure 2–33. The scan 3 months after ^{131}I therapy.

    b.   Advise operation. The RAI is too low for effective ^{131}I therapy.

    c.   Since the RAI is so low, give 100 mCi of ^{131}I.

    d.   Wait a few months. He may yet improve without further treatment.

    e.   Administer ATD in the hope that in 1 or 2 years the long-term effects of the initial ^{131}I treatment will produce a satisfactory result.

    f.   Give stable iodine (Lugol's solution) as a temporary measure while waiting for the full effects of the first ^{131}I dose.

    g.   These toxic AFTA do poorly with ^{131}I therapy.

Case 2–19—Followup

With this much goiter remaining the likelihood of further significant benefit from the initial ^{131}I dose is too small for serious consideration. Therefore, observation, with or without ATD, would not be my choice. Stable iodide may add fuel to the fire, enhancing the output of thyroid hormone in this nodular goiter.

The patient did not wish an operation, and operations are seldom (if ever) needed, even for large toxic nodular goiters of this type. The 100 mCi dose of ^{131}I would probably have done the job, but such a large dose would have necessitated hospitalization, and this was a busy executive who had no time for such nonsense. Furthermore, 100 mCi is a substantial dose of radiation and should not be given for benign thyroid disease unless there is no alternative.

In this case there was an alternative. A month's treatment with PTU, 300 mg four times daily, produced a state of relative thyroidal iodide depletion, so that upon withdrawal of the PTU the RAI value rebounded to 39 per cent. A second 30 mCi dose of ^{131}I was given and successfully restored the patient to the euthyroid state.

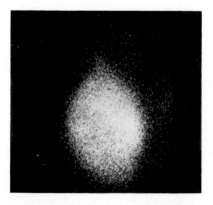

Figure 2–34. The gamma camera image after two treatments with ^{131}I.

May 1974. The mass was much smaller than it had been originally, and the patient has remained euthyroid for 2 years.

These large, toxic nodular goiters often take more than a single dose of [131]I. This should be anticipated and the patient so advised if disappointment is to be avoided. In almost every instance, persistence will be rewarded.

Initially I was not sure whether this was a large toxic autonomous adenoma or a toxic hemithyroid. Failure of any recovery of function on the left side suggested that the latter diagnosis was correct. In this instance, it made no difference in terms of treatment, for a large toxic thyroid mass requires a large ^{131}I dose.

Selected Current References for Case 2–19

1. Burman KD, Adler RA and Wartofsky L: Hemiagenesis of the thyroid gland. *Am J Med* 58:143–146, 1975

   These authors tell of three patients with this uncommon but not rare anomaly. One of their patients had hyperthyroidism. They review the literature on the subject and note that 17 of 21 patients had absent left lobes.

2. Harada T, Nishikawa Y and Ito K: Aplasia of one thyroid lobe. *Am J Surg* 124:617, 1972

   Five of seven patients had hyperthyroidism.

3. Hamburger JI and Hamburger SW: Thyroidal hemiagenesis. *Arch Surg* 100:319–320, 1970

   This is the first modern report on the subject in English. Our case had cancer, and we thought that it might not have been coincidental.

CASE 2–20. THE THYROCARDIAC

July, 1974. A 48 year old male businessman was referred for treatment of hyperthyroidism. He had noted increasing nervousness, palpitation, heat intolerance, and a 30-pound weight loss over the previous 6 months. He was 70 inches tall and weighed 129 pounds. The BP was 130/60, and the temperature was 99° F. He was in atrial fibrillation with a ventricular response of 140 per minute. There was striking muscular atrophy readily visible in the pectoral and scapular areas. The thyroid gland was five times normal size and multinodular. There was no evidence of congestive heart failure. The FTI was 14, the T_3(RIA) 400 ng per 100 ml, and the RAI 72 per cent.

With which of the following statements do you agree?

a   Hospitalize him as an emergency.

b.   Administer adrenal steroids to prevent thyroid crisis.

c.   Give Lugol's solution orally to block release of any further thyroid hormone.

d.   Give propranolol to help control the peripheral response to the excess thyroid hormone.

e.   Give him digitalis.

f.   Administer ^{131}I immediately.

g.   Order PTU, 100 mg four times a day.

h.   Order PTU, 300 mg four times a day.

i.   Alert house staff to avoid use of propranolol — it might precipitate heart failure.

j.   Give sodium iodide, 1 gram intravenously stat.

k.   After 10 days' preparation with PTU, Lugol's solution, and propran-

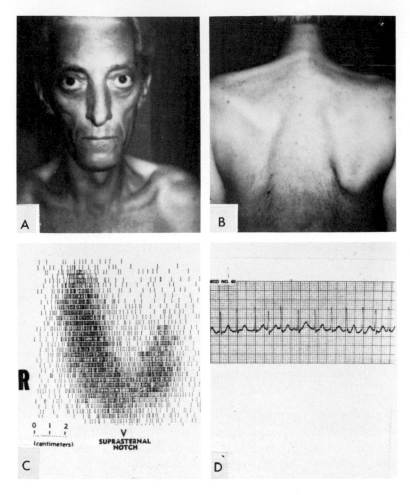

Figure 2–35. *A* and *B*, The patient. Note the evidence of weight loss and the atrophy of shoulder muscles. *C*, The scan. *D*, The EKG.

olol he should be in shape for thyroidectomy, and this is the most decisive way to correct this life-threatening condition.

l. Order a high caloric diet with vitamin supplements.

m. After a suitable period of preparation ^{131}I will be given.

n. Preparation for ^{131}I therapy will probably take no more than 2 weeks.

o. Preparation for ^{131}I therapy may require 4 to 6 weeks.

Case 2–20—Followup

This is a very sick man. The duration of his untreated illness (6 months) is longer than the average we see these days. Most hyperthyroid patients are treated within 2 to 3 months from the onset (at least by history) of the disease. Furthermore, the severity of the hyperthyroidism is greater than average.

The size of the goiter roughly correlates with the secretory activity in younger patients because most of the thyroid tissue is functional, and the more functioning tissue there is, the more hormone can be produced. In older patients hyperthyroidism may become engrafted upon a largely degenerated goiter, and size is therefore of less significance.

The degree of weight loss, the striking muscular atrophy, and the atrial fibrillation with a very rapid ventricular response all indicated severe and long-standing disease. The fact that the patient had not gone into heart failure was a tribute to his capacity to tolerate this severe illness.

In view of these findings prompt and vigorous action was indicated.

The first decision that must be made is whether or not to hospitalize. Hospitalization is not mandatory if one can be certain that the patient is able and willing to cooperate with a rather complex regimen and is also willing to return rather frequently for rechecks in the first 2 weeks. This businessman was capable and pleased to try outpatient management because this permitted him to continue to manage his affairs on a part-time basis. He was advised that if his condition failed to improve rather promptly, hospitalization might still be necessary. A patient with less intellectual capacity might better be hospitalized. However, it should be borne in mind that hospitalization may result in delay in obtaining medication, given the sluggish responses of the hospital nursing—pharmacy—nursing chain of command that must be activated before medication reaches the patient. For the outpatient medication is much more readily available from the local pharmacy.

The critical organ requiring urgent support in this patient was the heart. Control of the ventricular response and, if possible, restoration of sinus rhythm were essential to prevent heart failure. Measures to reduce thyroid hormonal secretion take days or even weeks to achieve their goal. The combination of beta blockade and digitalis has a favorable effect in a matter of hours. In the absence of heart failure there is no reason to withhold propranolol. In some instances this drug may produce a beneficial response even in the presence of congestive heart failure if the failure is largely attributable to the tachycardia of hyperthyroidism. (Obviously such a patient would only be treated in the hospital under close and continual supervision.) In this patient we began with propranolol, 40 mg stat and four times a day. Lanoxin, 0.5 mg, was given every 6 hours for four doses, and then 0.25 mg daily.

The next portion of the initial regimen was directed at curtailing thyroid hormonal synthesis and secretion. PTU, 300 mg four times a day, was ordered. A lesser dose would only delay response. Iodides, orally or intravenously, should not be given to patients with toxic multinodular goiters. Multinodular goiters may be induced to become toxic by the administration of iodide (jodbasedow's phenomenon), and they seem to be less sensitive to the suppressant effects of iodide than the smaller diffuse goiters of Graves' disease.

Iodine-131 should not be given until the hyperthyroidism is under reasonable control. There may be a discharge of preformed hormone in response to the radiation, and this could tip the balance into thyroid crisis or precipitate congestive heart failure. Our plan was to give ^{131}I after the patient had been restored to the euthyroid state. For a patient this ill it will take 4 to 6 weeks for optimal preparation.

The patient was advised to increase his caloric intake and to take supplemental vitamins, for adequate nutrition is important if he is to rebuild the body tissues that have been lost. This patient (as is often the case in severe thyrotoxicosis) had a poor appetite. He was thus encouraged to eat small amounts at frequent intervals rather than large amounts at any one time.

Adrenal steroids are not necessary at this point. They are used only in thyroid crisis and then only for the first few days.

In summary, the initial regimen included: (1) digitalis, (2) propranolol, 40 mg four times a day, (3) PTU, 300 mg four times a day, and (4) augmented nutrition.

In 24 hours his ventricular response had slowed to 100, and he was much more comfortable. In 2 weeks he spontaneously converted to normal sinus rhythm. Table 2–30 summarizes the further course of the patient and the adjustments in medication.

May, 1975. He was euthyroid on levothyroxine, 0.1 mg daily. His EKG was normal. His muscular atrophy was repaired. He was asked to return for annual reevaluation.

The question of whether to prepare patients for ^{131}I therapy or to treat them without preparation is raised rather frequently. Some physicians prepare all patients with ATD before giving ^{131}I. This needlessly prolongs the illness and increases costs for the vast majority. We prepare less than 10 per cent of the hyperthyroid patients we see. Criteria indicating the desirability of preparation include the following:

1. Severe long-standing hyperthyroidism with extreme weight loss and obvious muscular atrophy.

2. Atrial fibrillation with or without congestive heart failure.

3. Congestive heart failure alone.

4. Elderly patients with more than moderately severe hyperthyroidism.

It is clear that these criteria are in part subjective. However, there is one overriding rule: If in doubt, it is never wrong to prepare.

TABLE 2-30. TREATMENT OF THE THYROCARDIAC

TIME	WEIGHT (lb)	HEART RATE	CARDIAC RHYTHM	FTI	T$_3$(RIA) (ng per 100 ml)	TSH(RIA) (μU/ml)	PTU (DOSE mg)	PRO-PRANOLOL (DOSE mg)	LANOXIN (DOSE mg)	COMMENT
Initial visit	129	140	A.F.[a]	14	400		300 q.i.d.	40 q.i.d.	0.5 q.i.d., then 0.25 daily	Treatment initiated
24 hours later		100	A.F.				Same	Same	Same	
4 weeks later		98	Sinus	4.6	200		Same	Same	Same	PTU stopped for 48 hours and 30 mCi ^{131}I given; PTU resumed 48 hours later
10 days after ^{131}I therapy	135	80	Sinus	5.8	285		Same	Same	Same	Mild exacerbation of hyperthyroidism following ^{131}I therapy was well tolerated
6 weeks after ^{131}I therapy	140	120[b]	Sinus	3.4	150		150 q.i.d.	20 q.i.d.	Same Same	
9 weeks after ^{131}I therapy	147	98	Sinus	1.1	50	2.5	Stop	Stop	Same	
12 weeks after ^{131}I therapy	149	78	Sinus	0.4	35	28	—	—	Stop	Add levothyroxine, 0.1 mg daily

[a]A.F. = atrial fibrillation.
[b]Patient was not taking propranolol.

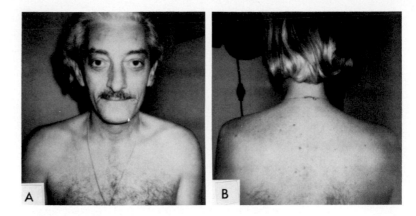

Figure 2-36. The patient after treatment. Note restoration of shoulder musculature.

Selected Current References for Case 2-20

1. Hamburger JI and Paul S: When and how to use higher ^{131}I doses for hyperthyroidism. *New Eng J Med* 279:1361–1365, 1968

   This article provides details on preparation of patients for ^{131}I therapy with ATD.

2. Shafer RB and Nuttall FQ: Thyroid crisis induced by radioactive iodine. *J Nucl Med* 12:262–264, 1971

   This is a report of a patient with severe long-standing hyperthyroidism and a large goiter who was given a large dose of [131]I. The authors emphasize treatment of thyroid crisis in their discussion. They should have mentioned its prevention by adequate preparation with large doses of ATD.

COMMENT: I have just seen a very unusual patient from whom I have learned something that you may want to know some day. She was breast feeding an infant and taking 2.3 mg of levothyroxine daily (about 15 times the usual daily replacement dose of 0.15 mg). I wondered how much thyroid hormone might get into the breast milk. The breast milk T_4(RIA) value was 0.4 μg per 100 ml, but the T_3-(RIA) concentration was 525 ng per 100 ml, essentially the same as the patient's serum concentration. Assuming that an infant might take 1500 ml of breast milk per day, he would receive 7875 ng, or about 8 μg of T_3 daily, not very much actually.

CASE 2-21. RECURRENT HYPERTHYROIDISM AND COLON CANCER

A 63 year old woman had undergone thyroidectomy for hyperthyroidism 42 years earlier. She had been well up to 6 months prior to her referral for evaluation of possible recurrent hyperthyroidism. During that 6-month period she developed rather typical features of hyperthyroidism, including a 10-pound weight loss. Physical examination revealed fine textured warm skin, moderate hand tremor, hyperactive reflexes, and a heart rate of 100. The thyroid gland was diffusely enlarged to about twice normal size. The FTI was 4.2, the T_3(RIA) 210 ng per 100 ml, and the RAI 43 per cent. A diagnosis of toxic recurrent goiter was established. However, she also had cancer of the colon for which surgical intervention was considered urgent.

With which of the following statements do you agree?

a. The hyperthyroidism is mild. Proceed with the abdominal operation immediately.

b. Why not do the thyroid and bowel operations at the same time?

c. A large dose of ^{131}I followed 48 hours later by Lugol's solution, 5 drops twice daily, will restore this patient to the euthyroid state within 3 weeks. The bowel operation can then be performed without additional risk.

d. ATD in large doses will prepare this patient for the bowel operation in a few weeks.

e. Propranolol will be adequate preparation for the immediate bowel operation. The thyroid can be taken care of later.

Case 2–21 — Followup

The patient's hyperthyroidism was not very severe. Therefore, I chose to prepare her for the bowel operation while simultaneously eliminating the recurrent hyperthyroidism by giving a large ^{131}I dose (20 mCi), followed 48 hours later by Lugol's solution, 5 drops twice daily. Two weeks later the heart rate was 80, and the patient was clinically euthyroid. The FTI was 3.4 and the T_3(RIA) 140 μg per 100 ml. The bowel operation was successful and uneventful 1 week later.

There is no need to take the risks of operation in an unprepared hyperthyroid patient for the sake of a few weeks. One could probably get away with propranolol preparation, and unquestionably the patient could have been prepared with ATD. Both of these choices have less appeal to me. One cannot be sure how sick this patient will be after the operation, and this may make the necessity for medication for the thyroid aspect of her problem inconvenient. Remember, there is no intravenous preparation of either PTU or methimazole. However, the tablets may be crushed, placed in capsules, and given rectally. By giving a large dose of ^{131}I followed by Lugol's solution, the problem was simplified. Incidentally, thyroid hormone also can be given rectally.

Does option b really require comment?

We should not pass over the fact that this patient developed recurrent hyperthyroidism 42 years after thyroidectomy. Surgeons tell us that we need not worry if the patient remains euthyroid for 5 years after thyroidectomy. However, our patients with recurrent hyperthyroidism relapsed on the average more than 10 years after thyroidectomy. Hence, lifelong followup is necessary.

CASE 2–22. CONSEQUENCES OF LOW-DOSE ^{131}I THERAPY FOR HYPERTHYROIDISM IN THE ELDERLY

November, 1974. A 70 year old woman developed hyperthyroidism in December of 1973. There was intermittent rapid atrial fibrillation alternating with sinus tachycardia but no evidence of congestive heart failure. She was treated initially with propranolol and PTU, 100 mg three times daily, for a period of 5 months and then given 5 mCi of ^{131}I in May of 1974. A second dose of ^{131}I (10 mCi) was given in September of 1974 for persistent hyperthyroidism. In spite of these two treatments she remained hyperthyroid, and consultation was requested.

The patient noted the recent onset of exertional dyspnea and peripheral edema, in addition to the usual features of hyperthyroidism.

Examination revealed atrial fibrillation with a ventricular response of 110 per minute. The blood pressure was 200/80. The thyroid gland was twice normal size. Her weight was 105 pounds, and her height 61 inches. There were bilateral basilar rales in the chest and pitting edema to the knees bilaterally.

The FTI was 8.4, the T_3(RIA) 225 ng per 100 ml.

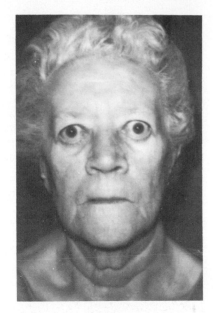

Figure 2-37. An elderly hyperthyroid woman.

With which of the following statements do you agree?

a. The patient should be given an additional dose of 5 mCi of ^{131}I.

b. The patient should be given 30 mCi of ^{131}I.

c. The patient requires PTU at this point, along with digitalis and diuretics.

d. This is an excellent example of how not to treat an elderly thyrotoxic patient who has evidence of cardiac instability.

Case 2-22—Followup

The patient had been treated with a total lack of appreciation of the significance of her initial intermittent atrial fibrillation. Preparing her for ^{131}I therapy with PTU was fine, but a dose of 100 mg three times a day was woefully inadequate. How well she was prepared after 5 months' treatment could not be determined, since the data available were incomplete.

The problem was further compounded by giving an inadequate dose of 5 mCi of ^{131}I. A 5-month course of treatment with PTU will probably produce some degree of resistance to the effects of ^{131}I, so this alone should have suggested a larger dose. Furthermore, the last thing that this patient needed (from the cardiac standpoint) was prolonged hyperthyroidism. She had demonstrated previously a propensity to respond to hyperthyroidism with atrial fibrillation. Was it really necessary to stress this marginal system with prolonged hyperthyroidism until frank congestive failure intervened? The second dose of 10 mCi of ^{131}I was another example of too little, too late.

Our first priority was to control her hyperthyroidism and improve her heart failure. This was accomplished by a combination of PTU, 300 mg four times a day, digitalis, and diuretics. In 6 weeks she was ready for ^{131}I. Her heart failure had cleared, she was in sinus rhythm and euthyroid. PTU was interrupted for 48 hours. Thirty mCi of ^{131}I was given and the PTU resumed 48 hours later. Between 4 and 8 weeks after the ^{131}I therapy, PTU was gradually phased out of the program. Thyroid hormone was begun on the tenth week after ^{131}I therapy. She has done very well subsequently.

Elderly people do not tolerate prolonged hyperthyroidism with impunity. They should be treated decisively and without unnecessary delay.

CASE 2–23. AN ELDERLY PATIENT WITH A LARGE MULTINODULAR GOITER, HYPERTHYROIDISM, AND A RELATIVELY LOW RAI VALUE

April, 1974. A 73 year old woman presented with a 6-month history of increasing nervousness, palpitation, tremor, heat intolerance, and a loss in weight from 120 to 108 pounds. The heart rate was 118 and regular, the reflexes were hyperactive, the skin warm and moist, and there was a moderate hand tremor. The thyroid gland was multinodular and about six times normal size. There was no clinical evidence of cardiac decompensation.

The FTI was 6.1, the T_3(RIA) 210 ng per 100 ml, and the RAI 22 per cent.

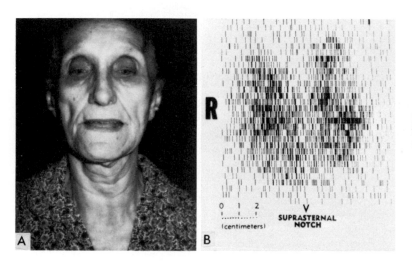

Figure 2–38. *A*, An elderly patient with toxic multinodular goiter. *B*, The scan.

With which of the following statements do you agree?

a. The RAI of only 22 per cent suggests that this patient has subacute thyroiditis rather than hyperthyroidism.

b. The RAI of only 22 per cent suggests that this patient received iodides in some unrecognized form.

c. This is the usual presentation of the toxic multinodular goiter.

Case 2–23—Further Data

The RAI is characteristically lower in TMNG than in TDG, but in general levels are higher than 22 per cent. Nevertheless, about one fourth of the patients I see with TMNG have values of this general magnitude, and this may be a limiting factor in their response to treatment. In the hyperthyroid phase of subacute thyroiditis the RAI is always less than 5 per cent, and is usually essentially zero. There are two reasons for this. First, the inflammatory reaction impairs the thyroid's ability to concentrate [131]I. If the discharge of thyroid hormone is enough to produce hyperthyroidism, then pituitary TSH release will be suppressed, even when the involvement is patchy. Hence, the function of the uninvolved (lesser involved may be more nearly correct) portions of the thyroid gland will also be suppressed. Therefore, the patient has TMNG. The problem is how to treat her.

With which of the following statements do you agree?

a. Give her 30 mCi of ^{131}I immediately. Propranolol, 20 mg four times a day, should be added to protect her heart from any strain resulting from the release of stored thyroid hormone because of the radiation effect on the goiter.

b. The RAI is too low for optimal ^{131}I therapy. The maximum permissible outpatient dose of 30 mCi will deliver only 6.6 mCi to the goiter (22 per cent uptake), and this is too small a dose to be effective.

c. Because the RAI is so low, thyroidectomy should be considered in spite of her age (of course, after suitable preparation).

d. Although the RAI is low, ^{131}I (30 mCi) followed by Lugol's solution will do the job for her.

e. This elderly patient should be treated cautiously with small doses of ^{131}I (5 mCi) at monthly intervals until she becomes euthyroid. Since she has no evidence of cardiac decompensation, there is no rush. The safest approach is a cautious one.

f. She should be treated with PTU, 300 mg four times a day, for 1 month. This will reduce the severity of her hyperthyroidism and prepare her for ^{131}I. When PTU is withdrawn the rebound RAI may well be more than double the present 22 per cent, thus improving chances for a single dose cure with ^{131}I.

g. Give 30 mCi of ^{131}I now, but 48 hours later start treatment with PTU, 300 mg four times a day for 1 month, and then progressively lower the PTU dose as the clinical condition permits. If the initial ^{131}I treatment is effective, the supplemental PTU will hasten the return to the euthyroid state. If the initial dose of ^{131}I is not effective, the supplemental PTU will prepare the patient for a second ^{131}I treatment by virtue of the higher RAI value that is probable when PTU is discontinued. The patient may be given propranolol as needed for the first few weeks to control her tachycardia.

h. Hospitalize the patient and give her 100 mCi of ^{131}I. With a 22 per cent RAI this will deliver 22 mCi to the thyroid and should do the job nicely. Supplemental propranolol should be given for a few weeks as necessary to control the heart rate.

Case 2-23—Followup

One could find proponents for almost every one of the therapeutic options suggested (even thyroidectomy). I do not like the idea of giving Lugol's solution to a patient with TMNG because this may aggravate the hyperthyroidism by supplying fuel for the fire (jod-basedow's phenomenon). The low RAI value does reduce the probability of a one-dose cure with ^{131}I; however, this would not suggest thyroidectomy to me. Nor would I ever consider using repeated small doses of ^{131}I. Repeated small doses of ^{131}I would simply permit the hyperthyroidism to persist long enough to increase the probability of serious complications, especially cardiac complications. Hyperthyroidism in the elderly should be treated with the respect due a potentially life-threatening illness. Prompt control and decisive elimination of the disease will produce the best results. I would favor PTU preparation followed by ^{131}I (30 mCi).

Initial treatment with ^{131}I followed by PTU (with or without propranolol) might work out all right too. If the ^{131}I proves effective the problem is over. If not, the PTU has prepared the patient for a second ^{131}I dose that should have a better chance for success, since the RAI should be higher. Occasionally the initial ^{131}I dose may lead to a lower RAI value that may persist for some time. Hence, this is probably a less desirable method.

Hospitalization with a high ^{131}I dose (100 mCi) would probably be satisfactory except for the disadvantage of hospitalization of an elderly patient. I have done this on occasion with patients in the late 70's and early 80's and have had problems with unacceptable behavior by a disoriented patient. When very large ^{131}I doses are given, the patients must be able to cooperate with an isolation regimen for about 48 hours. In my experience, elderly patients do best at home.

This patient was actually given 30 mCi of ^{131}I without preparation and without any supplemental treatment. Her hyperthyroidism was not materially improved over the next 3 months. She lost another 9 pounds, and both the patient and her family were concerned about her course. The heart rate was 110, but there was still no evidence of cardiac decompensation.

The FTI was 13, the T$_3$(RIA) 360 ng per 100 ml, and the RAI 55 per cent. The scan showed a much more uniform distribution of the tracer, suggesting that a second dose of ^{131}I might have a better chance for success.

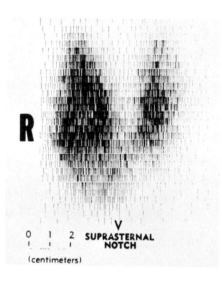

Figure 2-39. The thyroid scan after the first 30 mCi dose of ^{131}I therapy.

R

0 1 2 **SUPRASTERNAL NOTCH**

(centimeters)

A second 30 mCi dose of ^{131}I was given, followed in 48 hours by PTU, 300 mg four times a day. The PTU was gradually withdrawn over 8 weeks. Three months after the second ^{131}I therapy dose the patient was euthyroid. The FTI was 1.5, the T$_3$(RIA) 53 ng per 100 ml, and the TSH(RIA) 2.5 μU/ml. The patient has remained euthyroid for 2 years.

In retrospect I am not overly impressed with my treatment of this patient. I should have known enough to prepare her with ATD in the first place. I was lucky that the RAI increased to 55 per cent after the initial treatment; it could have decreased. Had this happened, I would have had to prepare her with PTU for 1 to 2 months and then given ^{131}I, further prolonging the course of her illness. My only defense (and it is not very good) is that my previous experience with TMNG patients indicated that most of them did respond to a 30 mCi dose, even when the RAI was relatively low. Direct ^{131}I treatment is simpler and, when it works, shortens the duration of the disease by eliminating a 4-week or longer period of preparation. Nevertheless, I would not do it this way again. To me, it seems preferable to employ ATD preparation because of its more prompt control of the disease as well as its beneficial effects on the RAI.

Selected Current References for Case 2-23

1. Miller JM and Block MA: Functional autonomy in multinodular goiter. *JAMA* 214: 535–539, 1970

    Miller warns about the great frequency of autonomous function in multinodular goiter, of the gradual transition from the nontoxic to the toxic state, and of the dangers in treating the nontoxic patient with thyroid hormone.

2. Blum M, Weinberg U, Shenkman L, et al: Hyperthyroidism after iodinated contrast medium. *New Eng J Med* 291:24, 1974

This paper complements earlier observations (references are cited) indicating the dangers of administering iodides to patients with goiter, and emphasizes the sensitivity that may be present by showing that the iodide in a dose of contrast medium for a pyelogram was enough to precipitate hyperthyroidism.

CASE 2–24. GRAVES' OPHTHALMOPATHY

November, 1974. A 50 year old woman was referred for treatment of hyperthyroidism. In addition to the usual systemic features of thyrotoxicosis she complained bitterly of the change in the appearance of her eyes.

The exophthalmometric measurements were 15 mm right and 14 mm left, within normal limits. Treatment was planned.

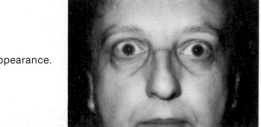

Figure 2–40. The patient's initial appearance.

With which of the following statements do you agree?

a. Thyroidectomy will most likely be followed by worsening of the eye problem.

b. Iodine-131 will most likely be followed by worsening of the eye problem.

c. ATD is the best treatment for patients with ophthalmopathy.

d. After restoration of the euthyroid state, the eyes will improve.

e. After restoration of the euthyroid state, the eyes may not improve.

f. After restoration of the euthyroid state, the proptosis will probably increase.

g. After restoration of the euthyroid state, the patient's appearance may improve, even though the proptosis is greater as determined by exophthalmometric measurements.

h. Without recession of the levators of the upper lids, these lids will not come down.

i. The patient will require tarsorrhaphy.

j. Orbital decompression is the only way to produce a satisfactory cosmetic result.

Case 2–24—Followup

The patient was treated with [131]I. Note the improvement in her appearance, even though her exophthalmometric measurements increased 1.5 mm bilaterally. Most patients have a slight increase in proptosis after correction of hyperthyroidism. Usually it is not apparent. The improved appearance, of course, is the result of a drop in the previously retracted upper eyelids.

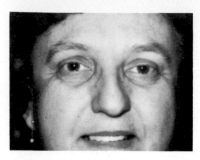

Figure 2–41. The patient when euthyroid.

Hyperthyroidism per se can produce retraction of the upper lids, and this is one of the characteristic features of the disease. As long as there is no fixed contracture of the levators, the eyelids will come down after correction of the hyperthyroidism. However, one cannot be certain in advance, and it is not safe to make promises.

There are reports in the literature that suggest that one or another method of treating hyperthyroidism is better for the eyes. No informed thyroidologist still believes this. The eye problem follows a course that is independent of the thyroid aspect of the problem.

Selected Current References for Case 2–24

1. Hamburger JI and Sugar HS: What the internist should know about the ophthalmopathy of Graves' disease. *Arch Intern Med* 129:131–139, 1972

   This review article is worth careful reading by all who deal with Graves' ophthalmopathy. Diagnostic principles and medical and surgical management are discussed and illustrated photographically.

2. Donaldson SS, Bagshaw MA and Kriss JP: Supervoltage orbital radiotherapy for Graves' ophthalmopathy. *J Clin Endocrinol Metab* 37:276–285, 1973

   This article summarizes Kriss' studies of radiotherapy for Graves' disease. His results are not overly impressive and do not seem much better than those achieved with steroids. Nevertheless, this treatment, if available, deserves consideration. The morbidity must be less than that for steroids. Also, some patients who failed to respond to steroids did improve with radiotherapy. Best results were obtained with patients demonstrating recent active progression, and worst results occurred with those who had late-stage severe asymmetrical extra-ocular paralysis.

3. Ravin JG, Sisson JC and Knapp WT: Orbital radiation for the ocular changes of Graves' disease. *Am J Ophthal* 79:285–288, 1975

   These authors again emphasize the advantage of radiotherapy — i.e., no serious complications when done properly. Best results were obtained with patients with optic neuropathy.

4. Day RA and Carroll FD: Corticosteroids in the treatment of optic nerve involvement associated with thyroid dysfunction. *Arch Ophthal* 79:279–282, 1968

   These physicians report favorable results with adrenal steroids in patients with optic neuropathy.

5. Gorman CA, DeSanto LW, MacCarty CS, et al: Optic neuropathy of Graves' disease. *New Eng J Med* 290:70–75, 1974

   These workers employed orbital decompression for optic neuropathy. So there you are. Radiation, steroids, or orbital decompression — all seem to work some of the time. The choice depends as much upon the availability of local talent as on any inherent superiority of method. Fortunately, the problem is rare. Transantral decompression is accomplished with less morbidity than the transfrontal approach.

CASE 2–25. GRAVES' OPHTHALMOPATHY

March, 1976. A 64 year old man was treated with ^{131}I in 1966 for TDG. Since 1974 he had been troubled with protrusion of the eyes, excessive lacrimation,

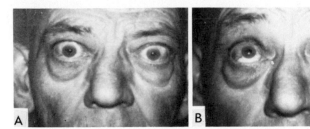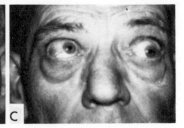

Figure 2–42. *A,* The patient looking straight ahead. *B,* The patient looking up. *C,* The patient looking to the left.

photophobia, a foreign body sensation, and diplopia in the upward and left lateral fields of gaze. The patient had never taken thyroid hormone following the ^{131}I treatment. He complained of occasional paresthesias and dry skin.

Examination revealed obvious proptosis. Exophthalmometric measurements were 20 mm bilaterally (normal measurements are between 18 and 20 mm). There was bilateral upper eyelid retraction, moderate chemosis, limited ability to elevate the globes bilaterally (worse on the left), and reduced ability to rotate the left eye laterally. There was no lagophthalmos. Visual acuity and visual fields were reported to be intact by his ophthalmologist.

The skin was dry and coarse, the heart rate 60, and the voice rather deep. The reflexes appeared normal.

The FTI was 1.6, the TSH(RIA) 30 μU/ml, and the T$_3$(RIA) 120 ng per 100 ml.

With which of the following statements do you agree?

a. If the patient had been treated with ATD this eye problem would not have developed.

b. The patient is hypothyroid.

c. The patient should take thyroid hormone, but do not expect that to do much for the eyes.

d. The patient has weakness of the superior recti and the left lateral rectus.

e. The patient has contractures of the inferior recti and the left medial rectus.

f. The patient needs an orbital decompression.

g. The patient will probably benefit from high doses of prednisone.

h. If prisms fail to control the diplopia, surgical correction may be needed.

i. This patient may fail to close his eyes during sleep.

j. Dark glasses outdoors, elevation of the head during sleep, avoidance of smoking and smoky environments, and covering the eyes at night with clear plastic after introducing a bland ointment are all helpful measures for patients with this problem.

Comment—Case 2–25

The ophthalmopathy of Graves' disease is one of the more difficult problems with which the thyroidologist must deal. There is no easy solution to the various aspects of this problem. First, let us deal with the mundane matters relative to his thyroid status.

Whether he has hypothyroidism or not is a semantic problem. His clinical features are minimal. The FTI was at the lower level of normal, and the TSH(RIA) value was elevated. The question is whether the elevated TSH concentration served to maintain normal hormonal secretion with some shift to T_3 secretion in preference to T_4 secretion, or whether the elevated TSH concentration per se means that the patient has hypothyroidism. This point can be argued persuasively either way. However, when the arguments are over, the proper thing to do is to give thyroid hormone in a supplemental dose adequate to suppress the elevated TSH level. In this instance, 0.1 mg of levothyroxine daily was ordered. One should be careful not to prescribe full doses of thyroid hormone because the residual thyroid function will very often be nonsuppressible.

The thyroid hormone will not do very much for the eyes. More marked hypothyroidism may increase orbital and periorbital fluid content, but this does not appear to be a major problem in this patient.

There have been claims that one or another of the treatments for hyperthyroidism is more or less likely to be followed by ophthalmopathy. These claims have no sound scientific basis. Graves' ophthalmopathy should be viewed as a phenomenon associated with the thyroidal component of Graves' disease but with a course that is independent of thyroid functional status. The ophthalmopathy may become evident before, during, or after the hyperthyroidism. Sometimes the eye problem is quite severe and hyperthyroidism never develops. Other patients develop the eye problem many years after the correction of the hyperthyroidism, even though they have remained euthyroid. Proper treatment of the ophthalmopathy demands careful analysis of the disability.

The disease may be considered under three major headings—vision, appearance, and conjunctival irritative phenomena.

1. Vision. Deterioration of vision is the most important problem. Depending upon the precise site of involvement, the patient might have diminishing visual acuity, reduced visual fields, or expansion of the physiologic blind spot. These types of impairment of vision are exceedingly rare in patients with Graves' ophthalmopathy and constitute the prime indications for orbital decompression.

Another cause of loss of vision is exposure keratitis. This is the result of neglect. Long before this situation develops something should have been done to protect the globes, either an operation to permit the upper lids to drop or an orbital decompression.

Diplopia is the most common visual disturbance. This is caused by muscular contracture. The inferior recti usually are the first muscles to be involved, and limited elevation of the globes is the result. Often this is misinterpreted as a weakness of the opposing muscles. This error is easily avoided if one remembers that the disease tends to produce a contracture of the involved muscles. The next most commonly involved muscles are the medial recti; limitation of the lateral gaze results. If the involvement is asymmetrical, the patient will experience diplopia when attempting to move the globes in a direction opposite to the pull of the involved muscle.

Prisms may correct the problem if it is not too severe. Otherwise, the correction requires a recession of the involved muscle. One should not attempt any surgical correction until the condition has been stable for at least 1 year. Nothing is more disconcerting than to undergo an operation that provides only a temporary benefit. While waiting for stability, the unpleasantness of diplopia may be avoided by patching one eye.

Adrenal steroids will seldom be of value for muscular involvement, unless the process seems to be quite acute. In this case the muscles may be swollen with fluid and inflammatory cells. High doses of steroids (e.g., prednisone, 100 to 150 mg daily) may produce rather prompt improvement. The presence of increasing periorbital edema and chemosis suggests a trial of steroids.

2. Appearance. The appearance of the patient may be the major complaint.

Severe proptosis can be disfiguring. There are two weapons the physician may employ for this problem — steroids and decompression surgery. Occasionally the proptosis is not very marked, but the fixed upper eyelid retraction (resulting from shortening of the levators of the upper lids) creates the illusion of severe proptosis. This can be corrected by freeing the levators from the tarsal plates, permitting the lids to drop.

3. Conjunctival Irritative Phenomena. Chemosis (edema and injection of the conjunctiva) results from obstruction of the venous return and the irritative effects of dryness of the conjunctivae because the lids fail to cover the globes. This is particularly likely to occur during sleep. Thus the patient may be unaware of what is happening, other than knowing that the eyes are especially irritated and dry in the morning. Someone should observe the patient while asleep to assess this point. Patients with this problem typically complain of excessive lacrimation, photophobia, foreign body sensation, and the bloodshot appearance of the eyes. Nocturnal eye care is essential. A bland ointment followed by taping a piece of clear plastic wrap (Saran Wrap) over each eye will produce considerable relief. Sleeping with the head elevated, wearing dark glasses outdoors, and avoiding the added irritation of smoke are additional beneficial measures.

Treatment of the ophthalmopathy of Graves' disease requires not only a careful assessment of the various elements of the disease but also an appraisal of the patient's attitudes and needs. What one patient might consider an unacceptable cosmetic defect, another might completely ignore. Some patients are severely incapacitated by diplopia, whereas others with similar muscular involvement accommodate very quickly by unconsciously suppressing one image.

Selected Current Reference for Case 2–25

1. Sterling K, Brenner MA, Newman ES, et al: Significance of triiodothyronine (T₃) in maintenance of euthyroid status after treatment of hyperthyroidism. *J Clin Endocrinol* 33:729–731, 1971

Sterling and associates describe nine patients with subnormal T_4 values and elevated serum TSH concentrations but normal serum T_3 concentrations. There were no clear clinical signs of hypothyroidism. However, they admit that borderline hypothyroidism is hard to exclude. They conclude that the elevated TSH levels were sustaining the euthyroid state by augmenting the T_3 output. This is a nice analysis, but clinicians (as opposed to scientists) will treat these patients with thyroid hormone. One of their patients became frankly hypothyroid later. They plan followup studies to see how many of the others follow suit. I wonder if they have informed consent for this experiment. Will they promise to correct any vascular disease that long-term mild hypothyroidism may promote?

CASE 2–26. GRAVES' OPHTHALMOPATHY

August, 1975. A 47 year old man had received ¹³¹I therapy for TDG in February of 1974. Three months later he noted the onset of increasing proptosis. He had been taking levothyroxine, 0.15 mg daily, since June of 1974 to control post-¹³¹I hypothyroidism. He was very upset about both his appearance and excessive lacrimation. A trial of adrenal steroids was advised, but he balked at having to take 20 pills daily (of prednisone, 5 mg each). He was then advised that orbital decompression was needed. He had been considering this advice but elected to seek another opinion.

Examination revealed a small thyroid gland and no clinical evidence of thyroid dysfunction; the rest of the significant findings were related to the eyes. There was bilateral upper lid retraction, extensive periorbital edema, 2 mm lagophthalmos bilaterally, striking bilateral chemosis, limitation of upward and

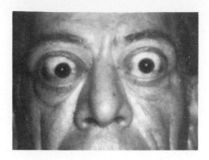

Figure 2–43. The patient's initial appearance.

lateral movements bilaterally, and obvious proptosis with exophthalmometric measurements of 33 mm right and 32 mm left.

While taking levothyroxine, 0.15 mg daily, the FTI was 3.0, the TSH(RIA) less than 2 μU/ml, and the RAI 17 per cent. A gamma camera image revealed a normal amount of normally functioning thyroid tissue.

A chest x-ray was negative, and an OT skin test was also negative. All parameters of vision were normal.

The patient was informed that there were only two therapeutic options available for consideration to improve his appearance — adrenal steroids and surgical decompression. When he was told that he could be treated with only three tablets daily (prednisone, 50 mg each), he agreed to a trial of adrenal steroids, and the treatment was begun. In addition, he was asked to cover the eyes at night with plastic wrap taped at the margins, after applying a bland ophthalmic ointment. He was also asked to sleep with his head elevated, to stop smoking, and to wear dark glasses outdoors.

September, 1975. After 2 weeks of treatment with prednisone, 150 mg daily, the patient was asked to take the medication every other day. The Hertel measurements had dropped to 31 mm right and 26 mm left. The excessive lacrimation was greatly reduced. Over the next 6 months, prednisone was gradually withdrawn.

March, 1976. The eyes were almost as bad as they had been originally. They measured 33 mm right and 30 mm left.

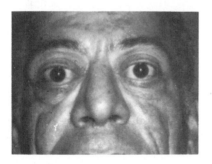

Figure 2–44. The patient after 1 month's treatment with prednisone.

With which of the following statements do you agree?

    a. Resume high doses of prednisone, and treat for a longer period of time.

    b. Advise orbital decompression.

    c. In the absence of any visual impairment there is no indication for orbital decompression.

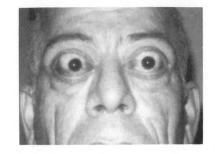

Figure 2-45. The patient after withdrawal of prednisone.

    d. Immediate tarsorrhaphy is indicated.

    e. Ablate the residual nonsuppressible function, and the eyes will improve.

    f. Advise patience; the natural course of this illness is one of gradual improvement if one allows enough time. There is no urgency in view of the normal vision.

Case 2-26—Followup

An orbital decompression was performed with a very satisfactory result. Note that the shortened right medial rectus muscle produced deviation of the right eye inward after the operation. Remarkably, the patient experienced no diplopia, apparently spontaneously suppressing one image. He was greatly pleased with the improved appearance.

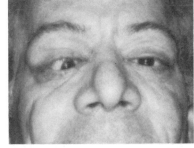

Figure 2-46. The patient after orbital decompression.

Cosmetic considerations are a valid indication for this type of operation. To require that a patient go through life with the gross proptosis this patient demonstrated because there is no visual impairment is unreasonable.

A further trial of prednisone held little prospect for success. It seemed more likely to produce iatrogenic Cushing's syndrome than adequate permanent regression of the eye problem.

Catz's claim that total ablation of the thyroid will produce regression of proptosis has not been supported by others. If one wished to try it, there would be no harm in it other than further delay in resolution of the problem if the treatment proved unsuccessful.

The natural course of this illness may include gradual eventual improvement, but this does not always happen. In view of the severity of the abnormality and the magnitude of the current disfigurement, it was our opinion that the patient should not be forced to live with this problem with only a small hope that some improvement might occur after an indefinite but long period of time.

Tarsorrhaphy is the initial knee-jerk response of many physicians (ophthalmologists) to an abnormal appearance from Graves' ophthalmopathy. It should be appreciated that this operation will reduce the widened lateral palpebral fissure and tend to elevate the lower lid somewhat in the process, but it will not bring the upper lid down and of course will do nothing for the proptosis. In fact. this procedure may make matters worse by calling attention to the eyes because of the obviously abnormal lid relationships produced. A tarsorrhaphy in conjunction with an upper lid procedure that frees the levator from the tarsal plate may improve the coverage of the globes by the lids but will still be inadequate to control the markedly abnormal appearance when there is extreme proptosis.

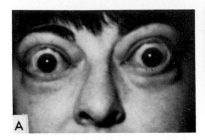 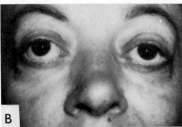

Figure 2–47. *A,* An inappropriate tarsorrhaphy. The patient looks worse than before the operation. Nothing was done to bring the upper lids down. *B,* A tarsorrhaphy and a freeing of the levators from the tarsal plates produced this gratifying result in a different patient.

CHAPTER 3

HYPOTHYROIDISM

PART I.   PATHOPHYSIOLOGY

Hypothyroidism is a complex clinical syndrome resulting from a deficiency of thyroid hormone. There are only a limited number of pathophysiologic mechanisms which produce hypothyroidism, and they are outlined in Table 3–1. Some are too obvious to require further discussion, but others do require some elaboration. Since thyroid hormone influences all organ systems, the manifestations of hypothyroidism are multiple and diverse.

In my referral patients hypothyroidism is suspected about twice as often as hyperthyroidism. However, confirmed diagnoses of these conditions are encountered with roughly equal frequency.

HASHIMOTO'S DISEASE

Hashimoto's disease is perhaps the most common noniatrogenic cause of hypothyroidism. This disease appears in two locations in Table 3–1, reflecting the different presentations of the disease depending upon the stage. Early in the course of this illness, there may be impairment of hormonal synthesis with compensatory hypertrophy and hyperplasia in response to increased stimulation by TSH. At this point there will be goiter. Late in the course of Hashimoto's disease, there is progressive fibrous atrophy leading to a more profound degree of hypothyroidism, even to the point of virtual athyreosis.

SUBACUTE THYROIDITIS (SAT)

As SAT progresses from the acute phase to recovery, there is often a period during which there is impaired capacity for hormonal synthesis in conjunction with depleted hormone stores (as a result of the discharge of preformed hormone during the acute inflammatory phase). This period is relatively brief, usually only a few weeks, and may easily pass unrecognized by either patient or physician unless the patient happens to be re-evaluated at just the right time. Well over 90 per cent of

TABLE 3-1. PATHOPHYSIOLOGIC MECHANISMS THAT CAUSE HYPOTHYROIDISM

I. **INADEQUATE MASS OF FUNCTIONING THYROID TISSUE**
   A. Congenital — athyreotic cretin
   B. Acquired
      1. Iatrogenic
         a. After thyroidectomy
         b. After ^{131}I therapy
         c. After x-ray therapy to the thyroid gland or other structures in the neck (e.g., for lymphoma)
      2. End stage of inflammatory disease
         a. Hashimoto's disease (common)
         b. SAT
            (1) Transient (common)
            (2) Permanent (rare)
II. **INTRINSIC DEFECT IN SYNTHESIS OF THYROID HORMONE**
   A. Congenital — goitrous hypothyroidism, dyshormonogenesis
   B. Acquired — Hashimoto's disease
III. **SUPPRESSION OF THYROID HORMONE SYNTHESIS BY EXTRINSIC AGENTS**
   A. In the treatment of hyperthyroidism
      1. PTU
      2. Methimazole
      3. Perchlorate or thiocyanate (rarely if ever used in the United States)
   B. In the treatment of other diseases
      1. Iodide (common)
      2. Lithium (occasional)
      3. Miscellaneous — PAS, cobalt, phenylbutazone, tolbutamide, chlorpropamide, and isoniazide (rarely important)
IV. **LACK OF THYROIDAL STIMULATION BY TSH**
   A. Secondary (pituitary) hypothyroidism
   B. Tertiary (hypothalamic) hypothyroidism
V. **DEFICIENCY OF PRECURSORS FOR THE SYNTHESIS OF THYROID HORMONE**
   A. Iodide
      1. Reduced intake (rare now because of iodized salt)
      2. Reduced availability (soybean diets)
   B. Lack of protein precursors (of theoretical significance only)

patients with SAT recover completely. Only a very small proportion have permanent impairment of function.

DYSHORMONOGENESIS

Dyshormonogenesis is a term that covers a number of discrete defects in thyroid hormone synthesis or secretion. In each case the problem is a deficiency of an essential enzyme needed for efficient thyroid function. If the deficiency is only partial, compensatory hypertrophy and hyperplasia may be effective in restoring hormonal output to normal — at the expense, however, of a diffuse goiter.

It is possible to determine the precise site of defective thyroid function by a combination of more or less sophisticated tests. However, this is not necessary for clinical purposes. It is enough to demonstrate that the patient has goitrous hypothyroidism and then institute treatment with thyroid hormone.

DRUG-INDUCED HYPOTHYROIDISM

The outline initiating this chapter includes a partial listing of the drugs that have been incriminated as potential causes of hypothyroidism. These drugs are generally not the sole cause of the problem but often merely enhance some pre-existing defect (e.g., Hashimoto's disease or compensated mild dyshormonogenesis), so that the goitrous hypothyroidism that ensues is the result of a combination of effects.

By far the most common culprit is iodide. The widespread use of lithium salts in the treatment of depression has produced a small number of cases of goitrous hypothyroidism. The other drugs are only rarely associated with this complication. If it is necessary to continue the drug (of whatever kind), supplemental thyroid hormone will control both the goiter and the hypothyroidism.

IODIDE DEFICIENCY

Although iodide deficiency is a rare cause of goitrous hypothyroidism in the United States, it is perhaps the foremost cause of this condition worldwide; goiter is still prevalent in undeveloped areas of the world where lack of iodide is endemic. In the United States, it is much more common to see thyroid problems resulting from the excessive intake of iodide (either goitrous hypothyroidism when iodide is given to patients with Hashimoto's disease, or hyperthyroidism due to the jodbasedow's phenomenon).

No Goiter — No Hypothyroidism

In previous publications I have suggested that the concept of no goiter — no hypothyroidism had clinical utility if applied with discretion. The exceptions include:
1. Iatrogenic hypothyroidism.
2. Endstage Hashimoto's disease, or rarely after SAT.
3. Congenital athyreotic cretinism
4. Secondary and tertiary hypothyroidism.

These exceptions are not troublesome, since it is obvious that in most instances the hypothyroidism in the first three on the list will be severe and thus not a diagnostic problem. It is possible for hypothyroidism to be relatively mild after ^{131}I therapy without goiter, and this may present a problem if the history is unclear. After thyroidectomy hypothyroidism is only mild if there is enough thyroid tissue remaining to maintain some hormonal secretion. Since that tissue will be under high TSH stimulation, it will tend to undergo hypertrophy and hyperplasia, often producing a nodular remnant.

Secondary hypothyroidism is uncommon and is associated with other target organ difficulties (except in very rare instances) that should alert one to the nature of the disease. Tertiary hypothyroidism is too rare to constitute a serious objection to the utility of the concept.

Having mentioned the exceptions it is now appropriate to emphasize the usefulness of the concept. I have proposed this concept for application to that large portion of the population whose thyroid glands have not been subjected to prior destructive therapy and who do not present the full-blown picture of myxedema, but for whom one or more clinical features raise the consideration of hypothyroidism. By definition these patients will have mild to moderately severe hypothyroidism, if they have it at all. Therefore, also by definition, these patients will necessarily have some functioning thyroid tissue producing the thyroid hormone which, although inadequate to prevent mild hypothyroidism, still serves to prevent the obvious severe hypothyroidism which can be diagnosed almost at a glance. This remaining thyroid tissue will be under increased TSH stimulation and thus should undergo hypertrophy and hyperplasia to produce goiter.

Note that this analysis leads to the inevitable conclusion that the milder the hypothyroidism, the more likely it is that goiter will be present. Since the milder the hypothyroidism, the more difficult the diagnosis will be from the clinical standpoint, it is fortunate that for just these patients the concept of no goiter — no hypothyroidism has greatest relevance.

When this hypothesis was tested in 265 consecutive hypothyroid patients, it held for 75 per cent of patients overall, 70 per cent of patients over 40 years of age, 82 per cent of patients between 20 and 40 years, and 88 per cent of patients less than 20 years old. Therefore, it is a concept which is far from absolute. Nevertheless, it is a simple and useful tool, particularly in young people. The point to remember is that most hypothyroid patients have goiter. If you suspect hypothyroidism and there is no goiter and the patient does not have obvious myxedema, you are betting against the odds. Therefore, you should take pains to insure that a diagnosis of a specific form of nongoitrous hypothyroidism is verified by appropriate laboratory data before committing the patient to life-long treatment. Failure to adhere to this rule will subject the physician to the risk of having his diagnosis destroyed by the new doctor in town who empirically discontinues thyroid hormone for all patients for whom there is no prior ironclad diagnosis.

References

1. Pittman JA, Jr, Haigler ED, Jr, Hershman JM and Pittman CS: Hypothalamic hypothyroidism. *New Eng J Med* 285:844–845, 1971
2. Lawrence AM, Wilber JF and Hagen TC: The pituitary and primary hypothyroidism. *Arch Intern Med* 132:327–333, 1973

PART II.   CLINICAL DIAGNOSIS OF HYPOTHYROIDISM

When hypothyroidism is overt, the diagnosis is usually obvious. When it is mild it may be overlooked quite easily. Two brief case reports will illustrate these extremes.

SEVERE HYPOTHYROIDISM

A 50 year old woman was referred for gradual onset of hoarseness, muscle cramps, paresthesias, hair loss, cold intolerance, and dry skin of 6 months' duration (Fig. 3–1A). There was marked facial edema, coarse skin, delayed reflexes, no palpable thyroid tissue, and a heart rate of 60.

Laboratory Data.   The FTI was 0.2, the TSH(RIA) 110 μU/ml.

Treatment.   Graded daily doses of LT$_4$ from 0.05 mg to 0.15 mg restored the euthyroid state within 2 months. Figure 3–1B shows the patient's final appearance. The FTI value was 2.4, and the TSH(RIA) value was 5.5 μU/ml. Note the change from flat to upright T waves on the EKG.

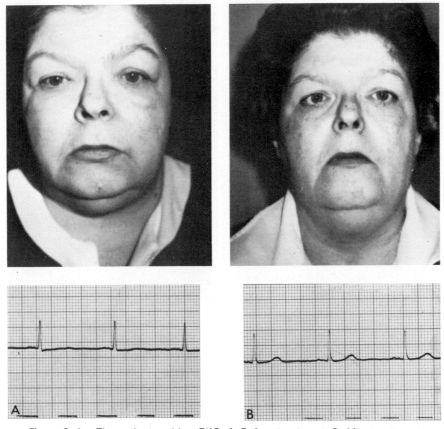

Figure 3–1. *The patient and her EKG. A,* Before treatment. *B,* After treatment.

CLINICALLY MILD HYPOTHYROIDISM

A 41 year old woman was referred for evaluation of thyroid function. Her complaints were fatigue and headaches. The skin and reflexes were normal. The heart rate was 78, the blood pressure 130/80. The thyroid gland was slightly firm and minimally prominent on palpation. Figure 3–2 shows her appearance. The FTI was 0.4, the T_3(RIA) 25 ng per 100 ml, the TSH(RIA) 128 μU/ml, and the RAI 6 per cent with no response to TSH stimulation testing.

Because of these grossly abnormal laboratory values the patient was requestioned and reexamined. She acknowledged occasional paresthesias and a slight increase in constipation and thought that her face was more puffy lately, especially in the morning. I could not convince myself of any additional physical findings suggestive of hypothyroidism.

She was treated with LT_4, 0.15 mg daily, and in 1 month she was euthyroid. Figure 3–2B shows the dramatic changes in her appearance.

This case shows that the diagnosis of hypothyroidism may be quite difficult on clinical evaluation, even when laboratory data are strikingly abnormal.

The clinical presentation of hypothyroidism is often much less overt than that of hyperthyroidism. Even a relatively severe deficiency may be difficult to recognize if the physician is not alert. The cardinal clinical features that suggest a working diagnosis of hypothyroidism include (1) facial edema, (2) goiter, (3) husky voice, (4) coarse, dry, flaky skin, (5) muscular cramps, (6) paresthesias, (7) delayed return phase of deep tendon reflexes, and (8) a surgical scar on the neck.

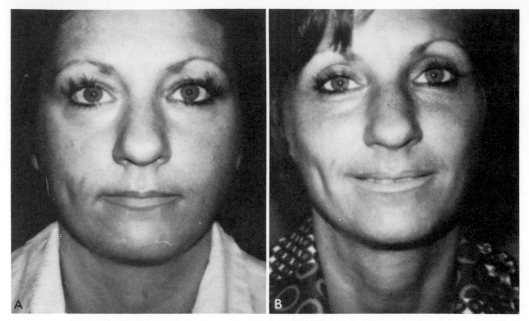

Figure 3-2. *The patient. A,* Before treatment. *B,* After treatment.

These easily documented findings indicate the need to search for further corroboration by history and physical examination of each of the systems likely to be involved.

A. CUTANEOUS SYSTEM

History. Facial puffiness and dry coarse skin are the primary cutaneous complaints of the hypothyroid patient.

Physical Findings. Facial edema is particularly pronounced in the infraorbital area. The skin often has a slightly yellowish cast, reflecting the carotenemia so commonly present. The skin of the forearm, easily accessible for examination, reveals the characteristic thickening and dry flakiness. The subcutaneous tissues are also less supple than normal, and the underlying muscles feel as if they are in a constant state of semicontraction. The hair is coarse and brittle and may be extracted easily.

B. VOICE CHANGES

The voice becomes increasingly husky as hypothyroidism progresses, eventually resulting in the characteristic croaking, slurred speech of severe myxedema.

C. THYROID GLAND

History. A scar may disclose the fact that the patient has undergone thyroidectomy. A history of radioiodine therapy may be more difficult to obtain. Some patients do not realize the significance of the treatment or believe that they have received therapy when only tracer studies were performed.

Physical Findings. Barring those patients who have had thyroidectomy or radioiodine therapy and the athyreotic cretin, most patients with primary hypothyroidism have goiter as already discussed. Consideration of the possible pathophysiologic mechanisms that are capable of producing hypothyroidism makes it obvious why this is so.

D. NERVOUS SYSTEM

History. The more the patient depends upon mental acuity in his daily activities, the more likely he is to complain of forgetfulness and loss of intellectual facility. Occasionally a history of psychotic behavior is obtained from the family; paranoid ideas are particularly common. As hypothyroidism is prolonged and becomes increasingly severe, a progression from somnolence to confusion, semistupor, and finally coma may be observed. The impairment of cerebral function may result from cerebral edema as part of the consequences of inappropriate antidiuretic hormone secretion. Seizures may also be observed. Less striking but more common neurologic manifestations are paresthesias, particularly those located in the hands in the distribution of the median nerve—a consequence of a reversible form of carpal tunnel syndrome. Impaired hearing is also common.

Reference

1. Frymoyer JW and Bland J: Carpal-tunnel syndrome in patients with myxedematous arthropathy. *J Bone Joint Surg* 55-A:78–82, Jan, 1973

E. MUSCULAR CHANGES

History. Muscular cramping is a particularly common complaint in hypothyroidism.

Physical Findings. Muscular myotonia accounts for the palpatory findings that suggest that the muscles are continuously in a state of semicontraction. This loss of normal ability to relax the muscles accounts for the characteristic delay in the return phase of the deep tendon reflexes ("hung up" reflexes).

F. CARDIOVASCULAR SYSTEM

History. It is important to detect the occasional association of angina with myxedema because this complicates management.

Physical Findings. Apparent cardiomegaly may reflect only pericardial effusion. However, there may be cardiac enlargement as well. The heart rate is slow, and hypertension is common. The electrocardiogram reveals low voltage and flattened to inverted ST segments and T waves.

G. GASTROINTESTINAL SYSTEM

History. Constipation and obstipation are common.

Physical Findings. Fecal impaction may result in intestinal obstruction. Flabby intestinal musculature may lead to ileus.

Laboratory Findings. The levels of serum enzymes such as SGOT, LDH, and CPK are often elevated in hypothyroidism. This is more troublesome now because panel testing is increasingly used for screening purposes. The unwary physician may be misled into considering a diagnosis of liver disease (or even heart disease). These laboratory abnormalities disappear with treatment.

H. METABOLIC CHANGES

History. Hypothyroidism in childhood leads to physical and mental retardation. Cold intolerance is common.

Physical Findings. In advanced cases the skin is cool and the temperature may fall to below 90° F. A falling temperature is a sign of impending myxedematous coma.

I. REPRODUCTIVE SYSTEM

The most common finding is menorrhagia.

PART III. LABORATORY CONFIRMATION OF A DIAGNOSIS OF HYPOTHYROIDISM

The flowsheet provides an approach to the use of modern thyroid function tests for the confirmation of a clinical diagnosis of hypothyroidism. The selection of tests depends upon whether the patient is or is not taking thyroid hormone in full replacement doses.

A. THE PATIENT IS NOT TAKING THYROID HORMONE

The laboratory confirmation of a diagnosis of *primary* hypothyroidism usually is simple if the patient is not taking thyroid hormone. Both the FTI value and the baseline TSH(RIA) value will be elevated. The response to TRH (which is not really necessary) will be augmented. Lack of an elevation in the baseline TSH(RIA) value and a blunted response to TRH suggest secondary hypothyroidism. A positive response to a TSH stimulation test provides support for that diagnosis.

If the FTI is only marginally depressed or is at the lower level of normal, the TRH test is of particular value. An augmented response indicates impaired thyroid function, a normal response excludes this diagnosis, and a blunted response suggests secondary hypothyroidism. In the past a TSH stimulation test was employed to evaluate these patients further, but the TRH test is simpler and more sensitive. Also, recent iodide ingestion from any source may invalidate the TSH stimulation test, and occasionally it will be impossible to exclude this consideration. Thus the TRH test, a

FLOWSHEET FOR CONFIRMATION OF WORKING DIAGNOSIS OF HYPOTHYROIDISM

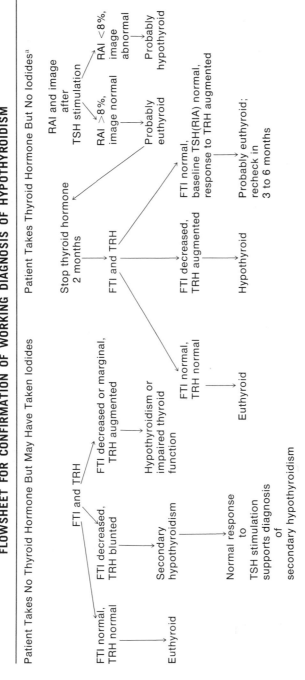

[a]If the patient has taken thyroid hormone and iodides, wait 3 weeks and then proceed with TSH testing.

test not altered by iodide ingestion, offers distinct advantages over the TSH stimulation test for patients whose baseline TSH(RIA) values are not clearly elevated.

B. THE PATIENT IS TAKING FULL REPLACEMENT DOSES OF THYROID HORMONE

The patient who has been taking full doses of thyroid hormone for some time and for whom a definite diagnosis of hypothyroidism had not been established initially is a common problem. The patient wants to know whether or not to continue the medication. One could stop thyroid hormone for 2 months and then proceed with testing as if thyroid hormone had not been given. Some normal patients will have normal FTI and baseline TSH(RIA) values at this point but will still have an augmented response to TRH, an abnormality that may take several additional months to correct.

Patients often object to stopping thyroid hormone without some assurance that they will not become severely hypothyroid. TSH stimulation testing may provide this assurance if a normal RAI and thyroid image are obtained. Nevertheless, it is still important to check the FTI and TRH response after stopping thyroid hormone, for there may be a discrepancy between the capacity to concentrate iodide and the ability to synthesize and secrete thyroid hormone (this is particularly common in Hashimoto's disease and after ^{131}I therapy for hyperthyroidism). Naturally a positive TSH response does not exclude secondary hypothyroidism. However, in the absence of other clinical features of pituitary disease, secondary hypothyroidism is unlikely and could be recognized by a subnormal FTI with a normal TSH(RIA) value which is not responsive to TRH after withdrawal of thyroid hormone.

Although a grossly subnormal response to the TSH stimulation test provides reasonably clear support for a diagnosis of primary hypothyroidism, the more nearly normal the response, the more one must consider that an unknown source of iodide might be the cause of the low value. If there is doubt, withdrawal from thyroid hormone and subsequent assay of the FTI and the TSH(RIA) response to TRH will be definitive (see CAUTION at bottom of page 15.

If a fluorescent scanning device is available, it provides an alternative method of solving this problem. If a normal image is obtained, one can infer that the iodide stores are intact and the patient almost certainly has a normal thyroid gland. Deficiency of iodide stores is a finding compatible with hypothyroidism but does not preclude the capacity for normal thyroid function. The TSH stimulation test would then be useful to indicate what action should be taken.

Patients frequently take less than full replacement doses of thyroid hormone. In these patients a depressed FTI value and an elevated TSH(RIA) value signify both that the patient has hypothyroidism and that the dose of thyroid hormone is insufficient. Some patients will have FTI values at the lower end of the normal range and a TSH(RIA) value at the upper range of normal. Here again TRH testing will be helpful.

A depressed FTI value with a suppressed TSH(RIA) value means that the patient is taking a product with a disproportionately high T_3 component. Obviously the FTI value alone could be misinterpreted. In these patients and also in those with normal FTI values and suppressed TSH(RIA) values, either the euthyroid state is maintained because of the effect of the supplemental exogenous thyroid hormone added to a subnormal endogenous output, or there is normal thyroid function. One must proceed with the workup as if the patient were taking a full replacement dose of thyroid hormone.

PART IV. TREATMENT OF HYPOTHYROIDISM

The treatment of hypothyroidism is administration of thyroid hormone. The preparation of choice is levothyroxine (LT_4). A proper dose of LT_4 will consistently and reliably supply both of the natural thyroid hormones T_4 and T_3 (the latter by deiodination of T_4). Whether T_4 acts only as a prohormone for the release of T_3, as some maintain, has no clinical significance, since abundant experience indicates that pure LT_4-containing products are efficient in the correction of hypothyroidism in athyreotic patients. The cost of LT_4 for most hypothyroid patients is only about 10 dollars per year. A solution of LT_4 suitable for intravenous administration is available. This product also may be given by tube to patients unable to swallow whole food.

DISADVANTAGES OF OTHER FORMS OF THYROID HORMONE

Desiccated Thyroid Hormone and Thyroglobulin

The continued use of these archaic and unreliable products cannot be condemned too strongly. One can be certain about neither the hormonal content in any given batch nor the consistency of the hormonal content from batch to batch. Frequently these products contain an inappropriate excess of T_3 over T_4. FTI values will thus be low even though the patient is not hypothyroid. The TSH(RIA) will not be elevated. The undesirability of these forms of thyroid hormone has received repeated emphasis in the literature. There is no economic advantage in their use. Nevertheless, we still see patients who have been treated with desiccated thyroid hormone without improvement; they have changed physicians convinced either that the diagnosis of hypothyroidism was in error or that their previous physician did not know how to treat the disease. Other patients report having had to take desiccated thyroid hormone in doses of 6 to 8 grains or more to feel well. In spite of these "high" doses, values for the FTI and T_3(RIA) tests were normal and occasionally subnormal with elevated TSH(RIA) values. On the other hand, other patients who had taken similar doses were intoxicated. It seems to me that the practice of medicine is difficult enough without needlessly complicating and confusing such a simple matter as replacement therapy for hypothyroidism.

Some practitioners tell me that they have been using desiccated thyroid hormone exclusively for years and never had any problem. Of them I inquire how often have they bothered to check the serum TSH concentration in their patients. Others have informed me not only that their patients do well on desiccated thyroid hormone but that their PBI values are "normal," ignoring the fact that the PBI measures iodinated protein whether metabolically active or not. This discussion always reminds me of a young girl who was treated for hyperthyroidism with methimazole and 180 mg of desiccated thyroid hormone daily. She reported to her pediatric endocrinologist rather obvious symptoms of hypothyroidism. When the PBI was normal, her complaints were dismissed. However, her FTI was 0.5 and the TSH(RIA) was greater than 100 μU/ml.

References

1. Braverman LE, Ingbar SH and Sterling K: Conversion of thyroxine (T_4) to triiodothyronine (T_3) in athyreotic human subjects. *J Clin Invest* 49:855–864, 1970
2. Braverman LE and Ingbar SH: Anomalous effects of certain preparations of desiccated thyroid on serum protein-bound iodine. *New Eng J Med* 270:439–442, 1964
3. Mangieri CN and Lung MH: Potency of United States Pharmacopeia desiccated thyroid tablets as determined by the antigoitrogenic assay in rats. *J Clin Endocrinol Metab* 30:102–104, 1970
4. Macgregor AG: Why does anybody use thyroid B.P.? *Lancet* 1:329–332, 1961

T_3 (Cytomel)

The administration of T_3 produces a prompt elevation in the serum T_3 concentration to levels which are first higher than normal and then fall within a few hours to subnormal levels. Thus it is difficult to provide a sustained normal serum level of T_3 with this drug. These fluctuations in serum T_3 concentration seem at least theoretically undesirable. An additional disadvantage of the drug is its high cost. Finally, even toxic doses will fail to restore a subnormal FTI value to normal, since T_3 is not measured by this or any of the usual thyroid function tests that measure the serum T_4 concentration. In fact, if the patient had only a slightly depressed FTI to begin with, the value would become lower as the dose of T_3 was increased. I remember a phone call from a very concerned physician who described just such a sequence of events, concluding with: "What should I do, she's getting worse under my very eyes?" A less humorous situation involved the president of a local bank who developed angina and congestive heart failure while taking 200 μg of T_3 daily. T_3 had been given originally for fatigue and a borderline FTI value. To add insult to injury, without thyroid hormone the patient had had normal FTI and TSH(RIA) values.

T_3–T_4 Mixtures

These newer products have been introduced with the claim that they more nearly simulate the normal output of the thyroid gland and produce normal values for tests that measure the serum T_4 concentration (rather than the elevated values that may occur when LT_4 is given). Actually, these products may simulate normal physiology less closely than does LT_4, since the T_3 component has a short half-life in the serum and the T_4 component provides possibly the major amount of T_3 (by deiodination) necessary to fulfill body needs. In any event, these products cost more than LT_4 and offer no real advantage. Furthermore, the necessity to assure a constant mixture of two drugs increases the danger of compounding errors that could lead to inconsistency in composition. Finally, it is now clear that the elevated T_4 values observed in patients taking LT_4 probably indicate overdosage.

Dextrothyroxine (DT_4)

This product was introduced primarily to treat hypercholesterolemia. It has been claimed that it produces less stress on the cardiovascular system per unit of metabolic effect. It has the outstanding disadvantage of exceedingly high cost. In fact, for this single reason I consider it impractical. In the past, I employed DT_4 for patients with myxedema and angina, thinking that I might be able to achieve a more nearly complete correction of the hypothyroidism without aggravation of the angina. However, I have not had the opportunity to test this hypothesis with the TSH(RIA), since the elderly patients with severe hypothyroidism I have seen in the past few years have been managed satisfactorily with LT₄.

Reference

1. Stock JM, Surks MI and Oppenheimer JH: Replacement dosage of 1-thyroxine in hypothyroidism. *New Eng J Med* 290:529–533, 1974

METHOD OF TREATMENT WITH THYROID HORMONE

In the usual patient with primary hypothyroidism in whom there is no concern for heart disease, particularly if the hypothyroidism is not of long duration, replacement therapy may be instituted with the full dosage of the drug chosen. I generally give LT₄, 0.15 mg daily, and recheck the TSH(RIA) level in 2 months to see if suppression has been achieved. If so, the patient may be seen annually. If the TSH(RIA) remains elevated, the dosage may be increased to 0.2 mg daily and the TSH(RIA) again checked in 2 months. Rarely will more than 0.2 mg daily be required. The fine titration of dosage recently suggested is seldom necessary.

If the patient is uncomfortable but otherwise young and healthy, I do not hesitate to start with 0.45 mg of LT₄ for the first 4 days and then reduce the dose to 0.15 mg daily. This produces a more rapid resolution of the clinical manifestations of hypothyroidism.

The cautious introduction of thyroid hormone accompanied by repeated clinical and laboratory assessments that has been so emphasized in the literature, unnecessarily prolongs the illness and increases the cost and inconvenience for most patients. This cautious approach may be necessary only for older patients (i.e., those over 40) and those with coexistent heart disease.

Before proceeding it should be emphasized that one cannot assess the adequacy of replacement therapy with the FTI. A value within normal limits does not assure that the TSH(RIA) value is suppressed. The proper study is the TSH(RIA).

SPECIAL SITUATIONS

Impaired Thyroid Reserve

The term "low thyroid reserve" was introduced by Jeffries to apply to patients who failed to respond normally to parenteral TSH by an increment in the RAI above baseline values. These patients had normal levels in tests that estimated the serum concentration of thyroid hormone. Of course, serum TSH assays were not available. It is now evident that some patients with decreased functional reserve also have elevated TSH(RIA) levels, whereas others do not, even though by definition the FTI is within normal limits. On the other hand, some patients with elevated TSH(RIA) values respond normally to TSH stimulation.

Whether these patients require treatment with thyroid hormone is arguable. If it were certain that all or even most of them would experience progressive deterioration of function to frank hypothyroidism within a reasonably short period of time, it would be clear that treatment is proper. However, there are no data on this point. Therefore, the physician's decision will be determined by whether he is more concerned about unnecessary thyroid hormone administration or the possibility of future unrecognized hypothyroidism. Most of these patients have goiter, and this strengthens the indication for treatment. Barring any special reluctance on the part of the patient, I generally advise thyroid hormone, usually LT_4, 0.15 mg daily. This simplifies the followup. Only a brief annual check is needed, and if all is well, it may not be necessary to perform any tests other than a TSH(RIA) every 2 or 3 years. The primary purpose of this test is to assure that the patient is faithfully taking the medication and only secondarily to be sure that the LT_4 dose is adequate and that there has been no profound deterioration in function.

Reference

1. Jeffries WM, Levy RP and Storanski MS: Use of the TSH test in the diagnosis of thyroid disorders. *Radiology* 73:341–344, 1959

Neonatal and Juvenile Hypothyroidism

Prompt treatment is essential if normal growth and physical and mental development are to be achieved. On the other hand, too vigorous treatment may give rise to psychotic behavior in children. In the first year of life the usual dose is between 25 and 75 μg of LT_4 daily. By 3 or 4 years of age, the usual adult dose of 150 μg daily is employed.

Hypothyroidism in the Aged

Management of hypothyroidism in the elderly patient may be complicated by coexistent limitations in cardiac reserve, a reserve which is itself further impaired by the hypothyroid state. Hypothyroidism reduces myocardial contractility, produces pericardial effusion, and promotes coronary artery atherosclerosis. Although it is important to correct hypothyroidism and although the correction will ultimately improve the cardiac status, the treatment may be attended by aggravation of angina, the development of congestive heart failure, or a cardiac arrhythmia.

For these reasons it is imporant to assess the cardiovascular system carefully prior to beginning treatment with thyroid hormone. It is common for patients with myxedema to have EKG abnormalities, particularly flattening and depression of the ST segments and T waves, and low voltage. Chest radiographs usually reveal an enlarged cardiac shadow, part of which may be the result of pericardial effusion. As the treatment progresses, these abnormalities should regress or at least become no worse.

In these patients I generally start treatment with LT_4, 25 μg daily, for the first 2 weeks. If the patient is doing well clinically and the EKG is stable, I then progress to 50 μg daily, 75 μg daily, 100 μg daily, and finally 150 μg daily at 2-week intervals. If clinical evidence of deterioration in the cardiac status should become evident, particularly in the form of increased angina, it is necessary to reduce the dosage of thyroid hormone and to prolong the intervals between subsequent increments.

In some instances it may be necessary to accept less than an optimal level of replacement therapy because of the intractable cardiac limitation.

Myxedema and Angina Pectoris — Case Report

A 67 year old woman was seen for the first time in May of 1971 for management of myxedema associated with angina pectoris. In 1926 she had had a thyroidectomy for

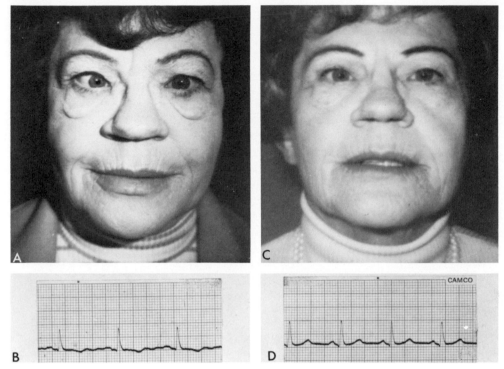

Figure 3-3. *Myxedema and angina pectoris. A* and *B,* Before treatment. *C* and *D,* After treatment.

TDG and subsequently was treated with thyroid hormone. She had been taking a combination of T_3, 25 μg daily, and desiccated thyroid hormone, 120 mg daily, up to 1 year prior to my first contact with her. Then thyroid hormone was discontinued because of increasing angina. She had tried LT_4 previously but was unable to tolerate as much as 0.1 mg daily without exacerbation of angina. The features of myxedema were pronounced (Fig. 3-3A). The T_4(D) value was 0.5 μg per 100 ml, and the serum cholesterol was 560 mg per 100 ml. The EKG is shown in Figure 3-3B.

Treatment was started with DT_4, 2 mg every other day. Gradual increments in dosage were made at 10-day intervals until a dose of 6 mg was reached in 1 month. At this point, the angina became worse and the dose of DT_4 was reduced to 4 mg daily. After 3 weeks, an increase in dose to 6 mg daily was tolerated. Three weeks later the dose of DT_4 was increased to 7 mg daily. One month later LT_4, 0.15 mg daily, was substituted for the DT_4. The serum cholesterol had fallen progressively to 255 mg per 100 ml, and there was striking improvement in the patient's appearance and EKG (Fig. 3-3C and D).

Successful management of these patients requires patience and very gradual dosage increments. Occasionally a temporary reduction in dosage is necessary. Although the patient previously had been unable to tolerate as much as 0.1 mg of LT_4 daily, after she had been on DT_4 for a while 0.15 mg was taken without difficulty.

Unfortunately, this patient was treated before the TSH(RIA) test was available. However, we were able to follow her satisfactorily with serial clinical evaluations, EKG's, and cholesterol determinations.

Hypothyroidism in the Intractable Patient

Over the years I have encountered several patients with rather severe hypothyroidism who maintained that they felt much worse when they took thyroid hormone than they did without it. They acknowledged the presence of the usual features of the hypothyroid syndrome and also that these features improved to some degree with treatment, but maintained nevertheless that they felt worse while taking thyroid hormone. An explanation of the potential serious consequences of untreated hypothyroidism was to no avail. These patients undoubtedly have some form of mental aberration.

For one such patient, I sent summaries of her records to five other physicians at her request. She was adamant that sooner or later she would find someone who would agree with her that thyroid hormone was not necessary. She had received psychiatric care for years in conjunction with attempted medical treatment, all without success. Recently, I learned that she has been hospitalized in a psychiatric hospital and now receives her thyroid hormone.

Myxedema Coma

Myxedema coma is a disease of neglect. It represents the endstage of failure to correct hypothyroidism for many months or years. The neglect may be the result of failure to diagnose the disease but may also represent a failure of the patient to take medication. The disease is rare and highly lethal and thus constitutes a true medical emergency. The usual treatment is intravenous LT_4 in an initial dose of 400 μg, and then 200 μg daily, in conjunction with adrenal steroids and supportive measures. Although the body temperature is usually subnormal, it is not necessary to take any vigorous action to warm the patient. Avoidance of heat loss by normal covering is adequate. Fecal impaction is a common problem and may cause intestinal obstruction. I treated one patient for this disease on three separate occasions over a period of several years. In each instance her myxedema coma resulted from failure to take her medication during a prolonged bout of alcoholism. The final episode was complicated by fractures, pneumonia, atrial fibrillation, and congestive heart failure to which she finally succumbed.

Secondary Hypothyroidism

Secondary hypothyroidism may be part of panhypopituitarism or, rarely, the result of an isolated deficiency of TSH. The availability of the TSH(RIA) determination simplifies the differential diagnosis of primary from secondary hypothyroidism, for values are high in the former but not in the latter. In patients with secondary hypothyroidism it is important to correct adrenal insufficiency in conjunction with the onset of thyroid hormone replacement. Spontaneous secondary hypothyroidism (as opposed to the surgically induced disease that follows hypophysectomy) is a rare cause of hypothyroidism. The deficiencies of other tropic hormones produce clinical features that are often more striking than those due to the TSH deficiency, and these features lead not only to the correct diagnosis but also to proper treatment.

Tertiary Hypothyroidism

The identification and synthesis of TRH, the hypothalamic-releasing hormone that participates in the regulation of TSH secretion by the pituitary, were followed by the recognition of a few patients who appeared to have hypothyroidism that was caused by TRH deficiency. The treatment of this disease is no different than that for primary hypothyroidism, as long as one can be certain that the process that gave rise to the TRH deficiency did not also involve, directly or indirectly, any other pituitary tropic hormone.

PART V.   SELF-ASSESSMENT

CASE 3–1. CHILDHOOD GOITROUS HYPOTHYROIDISM

March, 1974. A 5 year old girl was referred for evaluation of a goiter discovered on routine examination. Her height was 46 inches and her weight was 51 pounds, neither significantly deviating from the normal range. The skin and reflexes were normal. The heart rate was 92. The thyroid gland was twice the normal size and firm. The FTI was 0.8, the TSH(RIA) 58 μU/ml, and the T_3(RIA) 100 ng per 100 ml.

With which of the following statements do you agree?

   a.   The patient cannot be hypothyroid with a normal T_3(RIA) value.

   b.   The FTI reduction is balanced by the T_3(RIA) value; thus the patient is euthyroid.

   c.   The TSH(RIA) elevation is maintaining the euthyroid state by increasing the output of T_3.

   d.   Thyroid hormone is indicated. Start with levothyroxine, 0.05 mg daily, and gradually increase the dose to the amount needed to suppress the TSH(RIA) levels to normal.

   e.   Start with levothyroxine, 0.15 mg daily. There is no need to extend the treatment over several months.

   f.   The goiter will regress nearly completely in 2 months on levothyroxine, 0.15 mg daily.

Case 3–1—Followup

The patient was treated with levothyroxine, 0.15 mg daily. During the first year there was little change in goiter size; however, by the end of the second year the thyroid was only minimally enlarged.

The normal T_3(RIA) value represents an attempt by the thyroid gland to compensate for its inability to produce normal quantities of T_4. The compensation is inadequate, as evidenced by the considerably elevated TSH(RIA) value. Furthermore, the goiter is a reflection of a compensatory process in response to the continuing high TSH levels.

It is possible that a minor elevation in plasma TSH concentration may serve to restore the euthyroid state in a marginally functional thyroid gland at the expense of some degree of thyroid enlargement. In this instance the TSH(RIA) level was too high and the FTI level too low for one to accept this hypothesis. It is true that there were no obvious clinical signs of hypothyroidism, so perhaps the point is arguable. Nevertheless, it seemed prudent to put a halt to this pathophysiologic state if for no other reason than to prevent further thyroid enlargement.

In young people there is no need to introduce thyroid hormone gradually and slowly. This may be proper in the elderly when one must have respect for possible coronary artery disease. In the young, institution of the full dose at the beginning saves time and expense and reduces morbidity.

One cannot predict how rapidly these goiters will regress or indeed if they will regress at all. Some decrease in size rapidly, i.e., in a few months, some take several years, and some never completely regress.

The usual reason that some goiters regress less than expected is that the thyroid gland contains tissue that is largely nonfunctional—e.g., fibrotic or degenerated. The older the patient, the more likely that this will be the case.

There is another reason why some goiters do not regress in response to thyroid hormone—that's right, our old friend, nonsuppressible function. Whenever one elects to treat a goiter with thyroid hormone, this possibility should be kept in mind. If nonsuppressible function seems to be a realistic consideration, the simple expedient of performing an RAI while the patient is taking thyroid hormone will expose the abnormality.

The presence of diffuse nonsuppressible function is by definition equivalent to a diagnosis of Graves' disease. When there is no clinical evidence of hyperthyroidism and serum thyroid hormone concentrations are not yet elevated, the disease is in the euthyroid stage. In these patients the magnitude of the nonsuppressed RAI value is usually between 15 and 25 per cent. In my experience, the majority of these patients never progress to overt hyperthyroidism. Usually their condition remains stable over many years of followup. Occasionally, hypothyroidism is the end result.

Selected Current Reference for Case 3–1

1. Greenberg AH, Czernichow P, Hung W, et al: Juvenile chronic lymphocytic thyroiditis: Clinical, laboratory and histological correlations. *J Clin Endocrinol* 30:293–301, 1970

   This study of juvenile Hashimoto's disease reveals an inverse relationship between serum T_4 and TSH concentrations. A direct correlation was noted between the serum TSH concentration and antibody titers. These findings are, of course, what one would expect, but it is satisfying to see something work out as it should for a change.

CASE 3–2. BROTHERS WITH GOITERS

October, 1974. Two brothers aged 7 and 12 years were referred for evaluation of goiters. The younger boy's goiter had been observed for the first time 3 years earlier; the older boy had had a noticeable enlargement of the thyroid

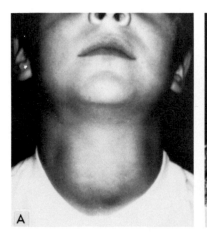
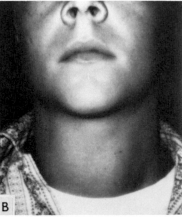

Figure 3–4. *Brothers with goiters. A,* The 7 year old. *B,* The 12 year old.

gland since birth, and the goiter had enlarged as the boy grew. Neither boy had obvious symptoms or signs of thyroid dysfunction. The only striking findings in both cases were diffusely enlarged, lobulated, slightly firm goiters.

RAI values were 47 and 51 per cent respectively. The FTI values were 1.0 and 1.1, and the TSH(RIA) values were elevated in both boys.

With which of the following statements do you agree?

    a. These are classic examples of juvenile Hashimoto's disease.

    b. These boys have Graves' disease in the euthyroid stage.

    c. These are dyshormonogenetic goiters.

    d. The elevated RAI values will prove readily suppressible in response to thyroid hormone.

    e. The elevated RAI values for these long-standing goiters may not be suppressible.

    f. The additional siblings and parents should be checked for goiter.

    g. The goiters result from pituitary TSH-producing tumors.

Case 3–2—Followup

These boys have goitrous hypothyroidism resulting from a defect in the synthesis of thyroid hormone at some stage after iodide is incorporated into thyroglobulin. The RAI is elevated in response to the increased stimulation of the thyroid by the pituitary (elevated serum TSH concentration), which is attempting unsuccessfully to increase hormonal secretion. The RAI, serum TSH concentration, and the goiter were all suppressed in response to treatment with thyroid hormone.

The boys had two sisters, both of whom had minimally enlarged thyroid glands and normal FTI and TSH(RIA) values. The mother and father were normal. Observation with an annual evaluation was advised for the girls, who presumably have a less overt defect.

It is possible by rather complex testing to pinpoint the location of the metabolic defect in patients of this type. However, this has no clinical significance because the treatment is thyroid hormone in any event.

Rare examples of pituitary TSH-secreting tumors have been reported, but they are not associated with subnormal FTI values and to suggest that two brothers have the same exceedingly rare disease is unrealistic.

CASE 3–3. HYPOTHYROIDISM AND GALACTORRHEA

June, 1975. A 17 year old girl was referred for evaluation of "combined hyperthyroidism and hypothyroidism." Because of goiter she had been referred for thyroid function tests. Serum T_4 concentrations were low, but the RAI was elevated. In addition, the patient reported galactorrhea of 2 months' duration.

Examination revealed a goiter that was two and a half times the normal size and normal in consistency. Milk was easily expressible from both breasts. The skin was slightly dry, and the pulse rate was 70.

The FTI was 1.2, the TSH(RIA) 40 μU/ml, and the RAI 46 per cent.

With which of the following statements do you agree?

    a. The patient has a pituitary tumor producing TSH and prolactin.

    b. The patient has goitrous hypothyroidism on the basis of dyshormonogenesis.

    c.   The patient has the overlap syndrome.

    d.   Thyroid hormone will increase the galactorrhea by increasing the general metabolism.

    e.   Goiter and galactorrhea will both regress with administration of thyroid hormone.

    f.   Although the patient does not have hyperthyroidism now, the high RAI means that she may soon develop hyperthyroidism and that thyroid hormone may be poorly tolerated.

Case 3–3—Followup

The overlap syndrome described by Grumbach a number of years ago is a condition in which provocation of pituitary TSH release by hypothyroidism may trigger simultaneous release of other pituitary tropic hormones, particularly gonadotropins, with the development of premature menarche. Thyroid hormone both corrects the hypothyroidism and leads to cessation of menses until the physiologic menarche occurs. In this case, it is probable that prolactin secretion was promoted by the hypothyroidism. This patient's situation is similar to the overlap syndrome but not precisely the same. Hypothyroidism will lead to increased release of the hypothalamic-releasing hormone (TRH), which stimulates TSH release from the pituitary. TRH also happens to have a prolactin-releasing effect —hence, this is not really an overlap phenomenon. Nevertheless, thyroid-hormone in this case did correct galactorrhea, hypothyroidism, and also the goiter.

The elevated RAI value in conjunction with a subnormal FTI value and an elevated TSH(RIA) value defines an abnormality of intrathyroidal physiology whereby the processes necessary to synthesize thyroid hormone are inadequate in spite of avid intake of iodine. The high RAI value reflects a compensatory response of the thyroid gland to increased TSH stimulation. The subnormal FTI and elevated serum TSH concentration indicate that the compensatory mechanism is ineffective.

One should not seriously think of a TSH-producing tumor in a patient with a subnormal FTI unless he is planning to make two diagnoses. Incidentally, long-standing hypothyroidism may be associated with enlargement of the sella turcica. Hence, one must be very careful to avoid misinterpretation of this finding in such a patient. The proof of the diagnosis is the patient's response to thyroid hormone.

Selected Current References for Case 3–3

1. Lawrence AM, Wilber JF and Hagen TC: The pituitary and primary hypothyroidism. *Arch Intern Med* 132:327–333, 1973

    This report notes the association of pituitary enlargement and hypothyroidism and warns against inappropriate treatment for a pituitary neoplasm.

2. Bayliss PFC and Van't Hoff W: Amenorrhoea and galactorrhoea associated with hypothyroidism. *Lancet* 2:1399–1400, 1969

    These authors suggest prolactin as the cause of the galactorrhea.

CASE 3–4. IODIDE-INDUCED GOITER

October, 1975.   A 45 year old woman was referred for the evaluation of a goiter discovered on routine examination. She was a chronic asthmatic who was taking adrenal steroids and Quadrinal tablets four times daily. She complained of fatigue, facial swelling, muscle cramps, and cold intolerance. The thyroid gland was two and a half times normal size and firm. The FTI was 0.8, and the TSH(RIA) 38 μU/ml.

With which of the following statements do you agree?

a. The iodine content of the Quadrinal precludes any imaging of this thyroid gland.

b. Iodide must be discontinued promptly.

c. Since many thousands of patients take this amount of iodide with no thyroid problems, the iodide did not contribute to the goiter or the hypothyroidism.

d. This amount of iodide, if taken chronically, will cause goiter in 75 per cent of people.

e. People who develop goiter while taking iodide do so because of some special sensitivity to the suppressant effect of the iodide.

f. If thyroid hormone is given, this goiter will regress even if the iodide is continued.

Case 3–4—Followup

Although the iodide did preclude the use of conventional scanning techniques, this was an ideal candidate for the fluorescent scanner. This instrument contains an americium-241 source that can cause the iodide within the thyroid gland to become temporarily radioactive, permitting a scan to be performed. The scan revealed uniform iodide stores in a thyroid gland which was diffusely enlarged as the physical examination had suggested.

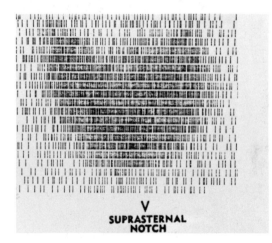

Figure 3-5. The initial fluorescent scan.

We encounter iodide-induced goiters about five to ten times each year. Since so many people tolerate similar quantities of iodide without developing either goiter or hypothyroidism, it seems reasonable to conclude that those who have trouble are particularly sensitive to the suppressant effects of the iodide.

Goiters of this type result from compensatory hyperplasia in response to high pituitary TSH levels secondary to inadequate thyroid hormone secretion. By giving thyroid hormone, regression in the goiter can be obtained even if iodide is continued. Many patients seem to require iodide for their pulmonary problems, and there is no need to discontinue the medication.

This patient was treated with levothyroxine, 0.15 mg daily.

April, 1976. The patient was free of symptoms of hypothyroidism. The FTI and TSH(RIA) were normal. The thyroid gland was normal in size, and this was confirmed by a normal fluorescent scan.

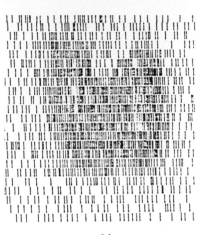

Figure 3–6. The fluorescent scan, April, 1976.

V
**SUPRASTERNAL
NOTCH**

Selected Current References for Case 3–4

1. Oppenheimer JH and McPherson HT: The syndrome of iodide-induced goiter and myxedema. *Am J Med* 34:281–288, 1961
2. Wolff J: Iodide goiter and the pharmacologic effects of excess iodide. *Am J Med* 47:101–124, 1969

   Although neither of the above articles are very current, they are the classics on the subject. Wolff's article has an encyclopedic bibliography of 280 papers. The authors of both articles appreciate that iodide goiter can be treated with thyroid hormone if iodide cannot conveniently be discontinued.

3. Braverman LE, Ingbar SH, Vagenakis AG, et al: Enhanced susceptibility to iodide myxedema in patients with Hashimoto's disease. *J Clin Endocrinol* 32:515–521, 1971

   Increased susceptibility to iodide myxedema was demonstrated in six patients with Hashimoto's disease. Since most people who take large quantities of iodide do not develop either goiter or myxedema, it is reasonable to assume that those who do have some basic defect rendering them particularly susceptible to the effects of iodide. The same may be said for lithium-induced goiter, as we shall see later.

4. Carswell F, Kerr MM and Hutchison JH: Congenital goiter and hypothyroidism produced by maternal ingestion of iodides. *Lancet* 1:1241–1243, 1970

   Eight cases of congenital goiter and hypothyroidism resulting from maternal ingestion of iodide are reported. Iodides should not be given to pregnant women except occasionally (e.g., to the occasional hyperthyroid woman who develops toxic reactions to ATD and is prepared for thyroidectomy with iodides for 10 days).

5. Vagenakis AG, Wang C, Burger A, et al: Iodide-induced thyrotoxicosis in Boston. *New Eng J Med* 287:523–527, 1972

   To complete the story, iodide also may induce hyperthyroidism. It is becoming ever more clear that iodide is not a good long-term medicine for most patients with goiter. It may produce hypothyroidism or hyperthyroidism, and it is not very often of any real benefit.

CASE 3–5. SUSPECTED LITHIUM-INDUCED HYPOTHYROIDISM

December, 1974. A 53 year old woman had been taking lithium for depression for 6 months. Her psychiatrist noted that she had facial edema and a hoarse voice and sent her for a thyroid evaluation.

Physical examination revealed marked facial edema, coarse dry skin, re-

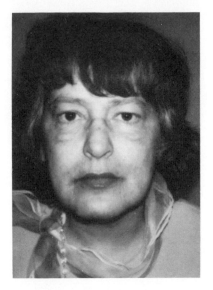

Figure 3-7. The patient.

flexes delayed in the return phase, a pulse rate of 68, hoarse voice, and an impalpable thyroid gland.

The FTI was 0.5, the TSH(RIA) 128 μU/ml, and the RAI 2 per cent.

With which of the following statements do you agree?

a. The patient has lithium-induced hypothyroidism.

b. Lithium must be discontinued promptly.

c. Lithium may be continued, but thyroid hormone is also needed.

d. Expect antithyroid antibodies to be strongly positive.

e. Review the past medical history to exclude the possibility of her having received ^{131}I therapy.

f. The infraorbital edema is too extensive for hypothyroidism alone; she may have nephrotic syndrome.

Comment—Case 3-5

This patient had primary hypothyroidism, and the lithium was incidental. Antithyroid antibodies were strongly positive, suggesting that Hashimoto's disease was the underlying pathophysiologic process. How could we have inferred that this was the nature of the problem?

In the first place, lithium exerts an antithyroid effect by blocking release of thyroid hormone. This will lead to a fall in the thyroid hormone levels in the blood, activating TSH release from the pituitary. TSH levels were high in this patient; therefore, if all this was the result of the lithium, why was there no hyperplastic response on the part of the thyroid gland? Lithium-induced hypothyroidism is goitrous hypothyroidism. No goiter, no lithium-induced hypothyroidism. Furthermore, in lithium-induced hypothyroidism, one would not expect an RAI of only 2 per cent. It might be normal or even high. Finally, so many people are taking lithium and so few develop thyroid problems that it might reasonably be suspected that those who do have some intrinsic thyroid defect that is only compounded by the lithium.

Incidentally, the facial edema is characteristic of myxedema; hence, there is no need to look for renal disease. The suggestion that the patient might have received ^{131}I therapy is at least worth considering once it is clear that lithium is not the culprit. However, the positive antithyroid antibodies suggest that Hashimoto's disease was the cause.

Of course, thyroid hormone was given, and the psychiatrist was advised that lithium could be continued. He could have continued the lithium even if this had been lithium-induced hypothyroidism as long as thyroid hormone had been given too. This is similar to the situation with iodide-induced goitrous hypothyroidism.

Selected Current References for Case 3–5

1. Burrow GN, Burke WR, Himmelhoch JM, et al: Effect of lithium on thyroid function. *J Clin Endocrinol* 32:647–652, 1971
2. Luby ED, Schwartz D and Rosenbaum H: Lithium-carbonate-induced myxedema. *JAMA* 218:1298–1299, 1971

    The above papers describe the syndrome of lithium-induced goitrous myxedema. The fact that lithium blocks thyroid hormone release was not yet fully appreciated.

3. Shopsin B, Shenkman L, Blum M, et al: Iodine and lithium-induced hypothyroidism: Documentation of synergism. *Am J Med* 55:695–699, 1973

    If either is bad, both are worse.

4. Temple R, Berman M, Robbins J, et al: The use of lithium in the treatment of thyrotoxicosis. *J Clin Invest* 51:2746–2756, 1972

    Sooner or later someone was bound to try this, even though the most casual perusal of the toxicity of this drug should lead one not to employ it whenever there are suitable alternatives (as there most certainly are for hyperthyroidism). In any event, the results were not impressive.

CASE 3–6. THE RECALCITRANT HYPOTHYROID

November, 1969. A 50 year old woman had undergone thyroidectomy 15 years earlier for Hashimoto's disease. Treatment with thyroid hormone was advised in May of 1969, but the patient did not take her medication regularly. No medicine had been taken for 1 month prior to her examination. There was clear-cut clinical evidence of hypothyroidism. The serum T_4 concentration was subnormal. Treatment with thyroid hormone (levothyroxine, 0.15 mg daily) was advised.

After taking three tablets the patient complained of severe palpitations. She was advised to have her symptoms checked by her physician but to continue taking the medication.

March, 1974. In the intervening period the patient had taken her medication only rarely, complaining that whenever she took it she had headaches. Once again, the evidence for hypothyroidism was unequivocal. The FTI was 0.6, the TSH(RIA) 58 μU/ml. The patient was advised that thyroid hormone was essential for her health.

October, 1974. The patient wrote a letter of complaint that the medication ordered was useless and that "At the price you charge you certainly should be such an expert that you would be able to recommend the proper thyroid pill."

With which of the following statements do you agree?

a. Better notify your malpractice carrier.

b. This patient has hypersensitivity to exogenous thyroid hormone. Do not dismiss her complaints lightly.

c. She should have been started on a smaller dose of levothyroxine with very gradual increments.

d. This may be only one aspect of a more serious emotional disorder.

Comment — Case 3-6

Needless to say, I have no further followup data to offer. This patient is an example of a problem I encounter every few years — i.e., the hypothyroid patient who refuses to take replacement medication. No amount of explanation, threats, or pleadings will convince these patients that they should take the thyroid hormone. Invariably they maintain that the thyroid hormone causes this or that symptom; often the symptoms are those of hypothyroidism, but the patient insists that the medication makes her worse rather than better.

The most striking example of this phenomenon in my experience was a woman who had shopped from doctor to doctor and from endocrinologist to endocrinologist until she had essentially exhausted the medical resources of the Northern Metropolitan Detroit area, all in search of a physician who would agree with her that thyroid hormone was not needed for her obviously severe myxedema. Her psychiatric disorder finally reached such a stage of decompensation that she was institutionalized.

Although this type of patient is a medical oddity, lesser degrees of unfaithfulness are far more common. In years past I checked hypothyroid patients taking replacement medication annually, relying upon my clinical evaluation to assess the adequacy of their treatment. In the last few years I have been routinely obtaining a serum TSH assay as a check on the reliability of self-administration and the adequacy of the dosage and a double check on my clinical acumen. I must say that the TSH assay has been a much more sensitive indicator of patient dereliction than my clinical examination. Armed with the laboratory data I have been able to obtain admission of lack of regular ingestion of medication, whereas upon the initial questioning the same had been denied.

Selected Current Reference for Case 3-6

1. Gorman CA, Wahner HW and Tauxe WN: Metabolic malingerers. *Am J Med* 48:708–714, 1970

This is the classic reference for the malingering or recalcitrant thyroid patient.

CASE 3-7. A 51 YEAR OLD WOMAN WITH HYPOTHYROIDISM

June, 1973. A 51 year old woman with classical features of myxedema was referred for management. Her symptoms had become progressively more promi-

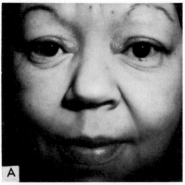
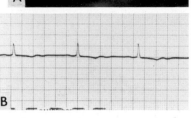

Figure 3-8. *A*, The patient. *B*, Her EKG.

nent over the previous 6 months. There was no history of prior thyroid surgery or radioiodine therapy. Otherwise, she had enjoyed good health in the past.

Examination revealed coarse skin, reflexes that were sluggish in the return phase, a heart rate of 90, no palpable thyroid tissue, and rather striking facial edema.

The FTI was 0.4, and the TSH(RIA) was 200 μU/ml. The EKG revealed ST segment depression and T-wave inversion in the left ventricular leads.

A chest radiograph revealed generalized enlargement of the cardiac shadow.

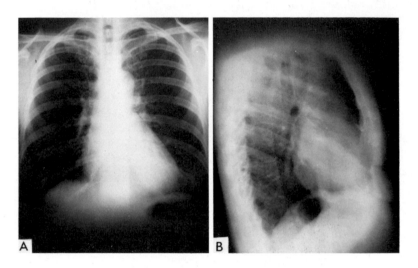

Figure 3-9. The initial chest x-ray. *A*, PA view. *B*, Lateral view.

With which of the following statements do you agree?

a. The EKG suggests that this patient may be having a myocardial infarction.

b. The EKG is not compatible with myxedema.

c. With an EKG like this, the administration of thyroid hormone would be hazardous.

d. One should administer levothyroxine, 0.025 mg daily, initially.

e. One should administer levothyroxine, 0.15 mg daily, initially.

f. One should increase the dose of levothyroxine at 10- to 14-day intervals.

g. One should increase the dose of levothyroxine every other day until a full dose is achieved.

h. The final dose required to restore a balanced pituitary thyroid axis will probably be 0.1 to 0.15 mg of levothyroxine daily.

i. The final dose required to restore a balanced pituitary thyroid axis will probably be 0.2 to 0.3 mg of levothyroxine daily.

j. The EKG abnormality may worsen in response to treatment with levothyroxine.

k. The EKG abnormality may improve in response to levothyroxine.

Case 3-7—Followup

The patient was treated with levothyroxine, beginning with 0.025 mg daily and increasing the dose at 2-week intervals until a final dose of 0.15 mg restored the FTI to

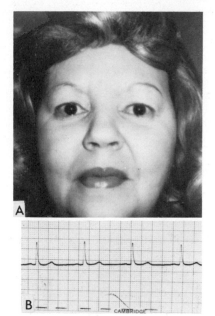

Figure 3–10. After restoration of the euthyroid state. *A*, The patient. *B*, Her EKG.

normal and suppressed the previously elevated TSH(RIA) value. Serial EKG's showed improvement. Her appearance and EKG after the hypothyroidism was corrected are shown.

A repeat chest radiograph showed reduction in the cardiac shadow.

The abnormal features of the EKG are characteristic of myxedema and, as in this patient, usually can be expected to improve with treatment. Enzymes such as SGOT, CPK, and LDH may be elevated, further confusing the issue. These also improve after treatment. If the introduction of thyroid hormone is too rapid and the coronary circulation has been compromised by atherosclerosis, one may induce myocardial ischemia, angina, and a deterioration in the EKG pattern. Therefore, older patients, especially those with long-standing hypothyroidism, should have EKG determinations serially prior to each dosage increment. Any deterioration in the EKG, especially if accompanied by angina, is an indication for a reduction in the dose of levothyroxine rather than an increment. The lower dose should be maintained for a longer period of time before another attempt is made to increase the dose.

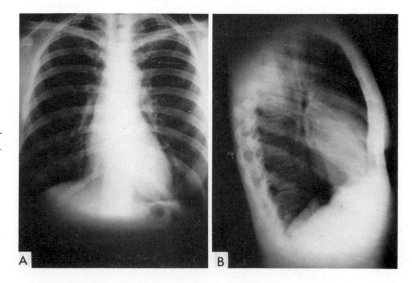

Figure 3–11. The chest x-ray after restoration of the euthyroid state.

In some instances one must accept a compromise between full restoration of normal thyroid pituitary balance and intolerable angina.

Most hypothyroid patients can be successfully treated with a dose of levothyroxine ranging from 0.15 to 0.2 mg daily. For those over 50 years of age, a dose of between 0.1 and 0.15 mg frequently proves adequate, and one should not give more than the dose needed to restore an elevated TSH(RIA) value to a suppressed level (e.g., to less than 10 μU/ml).

Selected Current References for Case 3–7

1. Mangieri CN and Lung MH: Potency of United States Pharmacopeia desiccated thyroid tablets as determined by the antigoitrogenic assay in rats. *J Clin Endocrinol* 30:102–104, 1970

   Again, the lesson that desiccated thyroid hormone is an unreliable source of thyroid hormone.

2. Evered D, Young ET, Ormston BJ, et al: Treatment of hypothyroidism: A reappraisal of thyroxine therapy. *Brit Med J* 3:131–134, 1973
3. Stock JM, Surks MI and Oppenheimer JH: Replacement dosage of L-thyroxine in hypothyroidism. *New Eng J Med* 290:529–533, 1974

   These two papers call attention to the fact that most hypothyroid patients require between 0.1 and 0.2 mg daily of levothyroxine for restoration of the euthyroid state. Larger doses are unnecessary and potentially harmful. However, there is a catch. The dose required is determined on the basis of the amount needed to suppress an elevated serum TSH level to within normal limits. In patients who are hypothyroid but not athyreotic a smaller dose of thyroid hormone will be needed to suppress serum TSH levels because of the contribution of hormone of endogenous origin. If this smaller dose is given it must be remembered that endogenous secretory activity may further decline in time, so that an initially adequate dose of thyroid hormone may no longer prove to be enough.

   Since 0.15 mg of levothyroxine daily is an adequate replacement dose for most patients with athyreosis and is seldom excessive, it is simpler to employ this dose, thinking in terms of total replacement rather than supplementation. This will work well most of the time, since any residual functional capacity will be suppressed. On the other hand, in patients for whom nonsuppressible functional remnants must be anticipated (e.g., in treated hyperthyroid patients), it may be better to employ supplemental rather than total replacement doses of thyroid hormone.

4. Bernstein RS and Robbins J: Intermittent therapy with L-thyroxine. *New Eng J Med* 281:1444–1448, 1969

   This is a technique that may be useful to expose malingering patients who claim that thyroid hormone fails to improve their myxedema when the truth is that they are not taking their medication. A single oral dose of 2.5 mg of levothyroxine given in the presence of the physician will produce striking improvement in laboratory indices of thyroid function.

5. Braverman LE, Ingbar SH and Sterling K: Conversion of thyroxine (T_4) to triiodothyronine (T_3) in athyreotic human subjects. *J Clin Invest* 49:855–864, 1970

   This is the classic article showing that T_4 is converted to T_3. Thus, there is no need to employ the more expensive replacement products containing mixtures of T_4 and T_3. Furthermore, they are probably not truly physiologic, for the T_3 component may have a more transient period of availability than is the case with T_3 derived from T_4.

6. Bastenie PA, Vanhaelst L, Bonnyns M, et al: Preclinical hypothyroidism: A risk factor for coronary heart disease. *Lancet* 1:203–204, 1971
7. Vanhaelst L, Neve P, Chailly P, et al: Coronary-artery disease in hypothyroidism. *Lancet* 2:800–802, 1967

   The authors of the above two papers emphasize the fact that mild hypothyroidism predisposes to coronary artery disease.

8. Newmark SR, Himathongkam T and Shane JM: Myxedema coma. *JAMA* 230:884–885, 1974

   There is no other place to cite this concise summary of the principles of management of myxedema coma, since I have not seen a case for several years. Therefore, I have arbitrarily placed it here.

CHAPTER 4

SIMPLE GOITER

PART I. PATHOPHYSIOLOGY

Simple goiter is the term I apply to a conglomerate of pathologic entities having in common generalized thyroid enlargement with neither a deficient nor an excessive secretion of thyroid hormone and no suggestion of thyroid cancer. For these patients further precision in the diagnosis in terms of either histology or pathophysiology will not materially influence the treatment. Usually these goiters are the result of a combination of chronic inflammatory disease (Hashimoto's disease), degeneration, and dyshormonogenesis.

Simple goiter is an extremely common cause of referral for thyroid evaluation. The goiter may be long-standing, or it may be discovered for the first time on a routine physical examination. The pathophysiologic mechanisms that may give rise to goiter are listed in Table 4–1.

TABLE 4-1. PATHOPHYSIOLOGIC MECHANISMS THAT CAUSE GOITER

I. **COMPENSATORY HYPERTROPHY–HYPERPLASIA**
   A. Iodine deficiency
   B. Iodine excess
   C. Dyshormonogenesis
   D. Goitrogens
      1. Drugs (propylthiouracil, methimazole, lithium carbonate, phenylbutazone, isoniazide, cobalt, tolbutamide, chlorpropamide, etc.)
      2. Food (rare in the United States)
II. **INFLAMMATION**
   A. Acute suppurative thyroiditis
   B. Subacute thyroiditis
   C. Hashimoto's disease
   D. Riedel's struma
III. **DEGENERATION**
IV. **HYPERFUNCTION**
   A. Toxic diffuse goiter (Graves' disease)
   B. Toxic autonomous goiter
      1. Toxic multinodular goiter
      2. Solitary toxic autonomously functioning adenoma
V. **PRIMARY NEOPLASIA**
   A. Benign
   B. Malignant
VI. **INFILTRATION (UNCOMMON)**
   A. Lymphoma
   B. Metastatic carcinoma to the thyroid
   C. Amyloid goiter

The first three of these mechanisms are responsible for simple goiters. Similar pathophysiologic processes are associated with goitrous hypothyroidism. Indeed, it is proper to consider simple goiter as an early stage in the development of goitrous hypothyroidism, a stage during which the TSH-induced hypertrophy–hyperplasia has proved successful in compensating for some impairment of thyroid synthesis or secretory capacity. Goiter is the price for the maintenance of the euthyroid state.

It is critical and fundamental that thyroid dysfunction be excluded prior to assigning a diagnosis of simple goiter, because this diagnosis carries with it therapeutic implications, the most obvious of which is the understanding that treatment for correction of thyroid dysfunction is not necessary. Therefore, the physician may concern himself with other clinical considerations that determine what treatment, if any, is employed. These are related to the size of the goiter and include:

1. The cosmetic implications of the goiter, and
2. The presence of obstructive phenomena.

References

1. Wiener JD: Lithium carbonate-induced myxedema. *JAMA* 220:587, 1972
2. Shapiro ST, Kohut RI and Potter JM: Amyloid goiter. *Arch Otolaryngol* 93:203–208, 1971

PART II.   CLINICAL EVALUATION OF SIMPLE GOITER

Simple goiter is a diagnosis of exclusion. A euthyroid patient who has an enlarged thyroid gland without a nodule that may raise the possibility of thyroid cancer and for whom painless SAT can be ruled out has simple goiter. The diagnosis is not really a problem. The only test needed is one that excludes thyroid dysfunction. If the goiter is firm and there is any suggestion of tenderness, an ESR will be helpful to exclude SAT. If titers of antithyroid antibodies are elevated, Hashimoto's disease is suggested as the underlying pathologic process, but this is not a critical consideration in the planning of treatment.

PART III.   TREATMENT OF SIMPLE GOITER

Size is the most important factor to be considered in planning treatment. Obviously these goiters can vary from a just perceptible enlargement to a massive increase in size. Although there is some tendency for larger goiters to be seen in older patients, this is far from invariable. A more consistent observation is the correlation between nodularity and size. Most large goiters appear nodular, while smaller goiters generally have smoother surfaces. Indications for treatment of simple goiter include:

1. Obstruction of either respiration or deglutition.
2. Cosmetic considerations.
3. Prevention of hyperthyroidism.
4. Prevention of further enlargement.
5. Prevention of hypothyroidism.

Thyroidectomy is the most effective method of eliminating a sizeable goiter. The operation should be bilateral and extensive to assure removal of all diseased tissue. Postoperatively, permanent administration of thyroid hormone is necessary both to assure normal supplies of thyroid hormone and to prevent recurrent goiter. If thyroidectomy is contraindicated or refused a trial of ^{131}I therapy might be considered if scanning indicates that the goiter has substantial uptake of the tracer. An effort should be made to improve the tracer uptake to 30 per cent or greater before ^{131}I is given. TSH stimulation, 5 units daily for 3 days, may be sufficient. If not, treatment may be tried with PTU, 300 mg four times a day for 1 month; then the

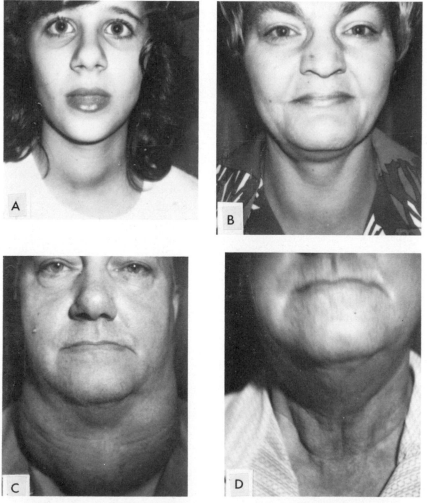

Figure 4-1. *Simple goiter. A,* A small goiter in a 12 year old girl. *B,* A larger goiter in a 48 year old woman. *C,* A massive goiter in a 62 year old man. *D,* Same patient as in *C,* after thyroidectomy.

rebound increase in uptake should be assessed 48 hours after stopping PTU. Another method of increasing the uptake of ^{131}I by the goiter is diuretic-induced iodide depletion.

Enthusiasm for prophylactic thyroidectomy to prevent hyperthyroidism has declined markedly in recent years. Fear of future toxicity has lessened as the means of dealing with this complication have been improved and simplified. The demonstration of nonsuppressible function in an elderly patient (for whom thyroid hormone had been given to control the goiter) might be an indication for prophylactic ^{131}I therapy, particularly if the FTI or T$_3$(RIA) values are at high normal levels.

Thyroid hormone is given frequently to goiter patients on the assumption that goiter is an expression of compensatory hyperplasia secondary to impaired secretory activity and that the underlying process will progress inexorably without treatment. Also, there is the expectation that thyroid hormone will shrink the existing goiter. Neither of these expectations will be realized consistently. I have followed many patients with small goiters for years and have noticed no real change in size or function. By contrast, I have treated many goiter patients with thyroid hormone, and not all regressed. Furthermore, routine administration of thyroid hormone to goiter patients is not entirely safe. Many goiters, particularly the long-standing multi-nodular variety, have nonsuppressible tissue. Hence, endogenous secretion will continue in spite of the administration of full doses of thyroid hormone. This can lead to iatrogenic thyrotoxicosis. The elderly patient is particularly prone to this complication. Because of these experiences I employ the following criteria for the treatment of simple goiter:

1. If the goiter is no larger than twice the normal size of the thyroid gland, I advise annual observation, looking for further enlargement or the development of thyroid dysfunction. An exception is the patient with a long, slim neck, which makes even a small goiter cosmetically unacceptable. I would treat such a patient with thyroid hormone.

2. For patients less than 40 years of age with diffuse goiters that are larger than twice normal size I prescribe LT$_4$, 0.15 mg daily. I routinely check the RAI in 2 months to exclude nonsuppressible function. If suppression has been achieved (the RAI will be less than 5 per cent), I continue the medication and check the patient annually.

3. If the patient is more than 50 years old, I seldom administer thyroid hormone unless there is hypothyroidism or an obstructive problem. (For a large goiter I might order a small dose of thyroid hormone to prevent further enlargement.)

a. For hypothyroidism I employ supplemental doses of thyroid hormone, beginning with LT$_4$, 0.05 mg daily (less if hypothyroidism is severe), and progressing with 0.05 mg increments at 2-week intervals until the TSH(RIA) value is suppressed. I have seldom found it necessary to exceed a daily dose of 0.15 mg of LT$_4$.

b. In patients with an obstruction for whom thyroidectomy is contraindicated or refused, a trial of thyroid hormone may be considered if the obstruction is not severe (for severe obstruction, of course, operation is mandatory). I would use LT$_4$, 0.15 mg every other day for 2 weeks and then daily if it is well tolerated and if the RAI suppresses normally in response to the treatment.

4. I advise against the recommendation of thyroidectomy for subjective complaints of compression. There is a very poor correlation between goiter size and complaints of compression. Many patients with large goiters have no complaints, whereas some with small goiters complain bitterly. If the latter are subjected to thyroidectomy, their complaints may increase rather than decrease, since they are usually neurotic in origin. The surgical scar merely increases their concern with the neck.

PART IV. SELF-ASSESSMENT

CASE 4–1. A CHILD WITH SUBMENTAL THYROID

November, 1974. A 9 year old child had a midline mass which had been enlarging for several years. It was firm, about 2.5 cm in diameter. The skin was dry, and the reflexes were somewhat sluggish in the return phase. The heart rate was 84.

A fluorescent scan revealed no activity in the normal thyroid location, and the submental mass had normal iodine content.

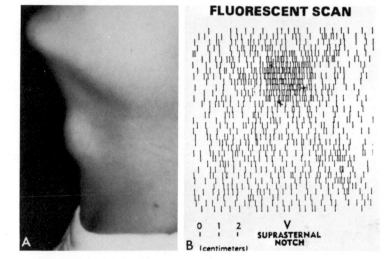

Figure 4–2. *A,* The patient. *B,* Her fluorescent scan.

With which of the following statements do you agree?

    a. This papillary cancer should be removed.

    b. Expect the FTI value to be low and the TSH(RIA) value to be high.

    c. Expect the FTI value to be high and the TSH(RIA) value to be low.

    d. The FTI and TSH(RIA) values may be normal, but the T_3(RIA) value will be high.

    e. This is an AFTA arising in the pyramidal lobe, suppressing the function of the normal thyroid. A scan after TSH stimulation will make the diagnosis.

    f. Thyroid hormone will cause this lesion to regress without surgical intervention.

    g. This is an example of the common prepubertal goiter. There is no need to worry; in a few years it will go away.

Case 4–1 — Followup

The FTI was 1.0, and the TSH(RIA) 128 μU/ml. This is a classic case of maldescent of the thyroid. Most of these thyroid glands are not only ectopic in location but also incapable of

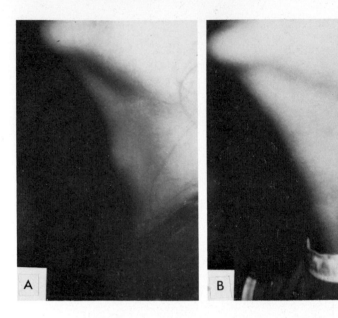

Figure 4-3. *A,* After treatment with thyroid hormone for 3 months. *B,* After treatment for 9 months.

normal thyroid secretory activity. Hence, the tissue undergoes compensatory hyperplasia. Failure to understand the underlying pathophysiology has led to inappropriate removal of masses of this type, producing permanent athyreosis. Several law suits have resulted from this error. It is of interest that this child has the same last name as a rather prominent consumer advocate who has made a career of suing incompetent people and the firms they represent.

In this case, the patient was treated with thyroid hormone, and there was complete regression of the mass over an 8-month period. Of course, thyroid hormone will be needed for life.

Selected Current References for Case 4-1

1. Katz AD and Zager WJ: The lingual thyroid. *Arch Surg* 102:582–585, 1971
2. Neinas FW, Gorman CA, Devine KD, et al: Lingual thyroid: Clinical characteristics of 15 cases. *Ann Intern Med* 79:205–210, 1973

   These two papers deal with lingual thyroid, a less common condition than maldescent of the thyroid, in which the aberrant tissue is located in the region of the hyoid. The authors emphasize that these lesions can be treated successfully with thyroid hormone and do not require excision. They found hypothyroidism in only 10 per cent and 33 per cent of cases respectively, whereas all of our patients were either hypothyroid or at least had elevated TSH(RIA) values.

3. Strickland AL, Macfie JA, Van Wyk JJ, et al: Ectopic thyroid glands simulating thyroglossal duct cysts. *JAMA* 208:307–310, 1969

   This report deals with ectopic thyroid glands located in the midline of the neck. All of their patients were hypothyroid. The lesions were excised because they failed to appreciate the nature of the tissue. These errors are avoidable simply by routine preoperative scanning. For this purpose the fluorescent scan is ideal. No tracer need be given. The radiation delivered to the neck is negligible compared to that resulting from any of the available tracers, and no radiation is given to the rest of the body.

CASE 4-2. SIMPLE GOITER IN A YOUNG WOMAN

November, 1974. A 20 year old woman gives a history of a goiter which has been present for the past 3 years. She had taken thyroid hormone initially for a few months, during which the goiter seemed to regress. However, when she stopped the medication, it recurred.

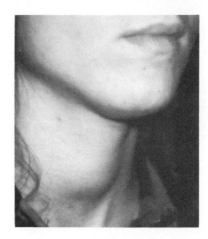

Figure 4-4. The patient.

The thyroid gland was twice the normal size on palpation and only moderately firm. The patient was clinically euthyroid, and the FTI and TSH(RIA) values were normal. Titers of antithyroid antibodies were not elevated.

With which of the following statements do you agree?

a. The duration of her original treatment was too short. If thyroid hormone had been given for 2 years, regression would have been sustained, even after withdrawal of thyroid hormone.

b. Thyroid hormone will not produce a permanent cure; only thyroidectomy will do the job.

c. Why not leave her alone, since the goiter is not that large and she has normal thyroid secretory capability?

d. Lifelong thyroid hormone will be needed.

e. Radioactive iodine therapy followed by thyroid hormone will simply and decisively eliminate this problem.

Case 4-2 — Followup

The patient was given levothyroxine, 0.2 mg daily. In 6 months the goiter had regressed markedly.

These goiters usually arise because of inefficient thyroid hormone synthesis and/or secretion. The defects are usually permanent. If treatment is not maintained indefinitely, any regression obtained will be lost as the process reactivates.

Thyroidectomy and ^{131}I offer no advantages over thyroid hormone, and indeed, thyroid hormone would be needed after either of these treatments. Hence, thyroid hormone alone is all that is indicated.

It is proper to ask whether any treatment is mandatory in a euthyroid patient who has only a small goiter. In most instances, I choose to observe patients with goiters smaller than two and a half times normal size. Most of these goiters do not progressively enlarge. In patients with smaller goiters the decision is based largely upon whether the goiter constitutes a cosmetic defect. This is determined as much by the individual neck structure as by the size of the goiter. For patients with long slim necks, such as this young lady, a relatively minor enlargement of the goiter can become unsightly. She was very pleased with the cosmetic result. It was important to explain to her that the goiter would recur unless she continued to take the medication indefinitely.

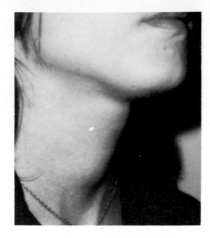

Figure 4-5. The patient after treatment for 6 months.

CASE 4-3. LONG-TERM FOLLOWUP OF A SMALL GOITER

July, 1972. A 33 year old woman was referred for evaluation of an enlarged thyroid gland, discovered on a routine examination. The thyroid was twice normal size, firm and lobulated. There were no clinical features of hypothyroidism.

The FTI was 2.2, the TSH(RIA) 20 μU/ml, and the RAI 16 per cent; after TSH stimulation the RAI increased only to 20 per cent, a subnormal response compatible with impaired functional reserve. The scan revealed a patchy and irregular distribution of the tracer.

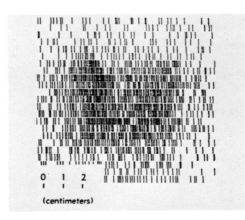

Figure 4-6. The initial scan.

With which of the following statements do you agree?

a. Treatment with thyroid hormone is indicated because of the reduced functional reserve. The treatment is primarily prophylactic.

b. The thyroid gland will probably undergo gradual progressive deterioration of endogenous secretory capacity. Treatment with thyroid hormone now will prevent both hypothyroidism and further thyroid enlargement.

c. If elevated titers of antithyroid antibodies were demonstrated the indication for treatment with thyroid hormone would be strengthened.

d. Whenever thyroid hormone is given to a patient with a small diffuse goiter the possibility that function will be nonsuppressible should be anticipated.

e. If thyroid hormone is well tolerated for 1 year, there is no need for further concern for nonsuppressible function.

Case 4–3 — Followup

I prescribed levothyroxine, 0.15 mg daily, even in the absence of clinical features of hypothyroidism. I was impressed by the combination of a mild elevation in serum TSH concentration, the subnormal response of the RAI to TSH stimulation, and the very patchy function demonstrated by the scan. I am not sure that high antibody titers in a euthyroid patient mean that hypothyroidism necessarily will occur in the near future. I am studying this point, but I suspect it will take a long time to find the answer.

The possibility of nonsuppressible function is a real consideration whenever one orders thyroid hormone for control of goiter. The older the goiter, the more likely it is that function will not be completely suppressible. Furthermore, there is no guarantee that because goiter function is suppressible at one point it will remain so in the future.

December, 1973. The patient was euthyroid clinically. The thyroid was no longer enlarged. The FTI was 3.2. Treatment with levothyroxine, 0.15 mg daily, was continued and annual evaluation advised.

September, 1974. The patient returned prematurely because of the onset of typical features of hyperthyroidism. The heart rate was 120. She had lost 10 pounds in the previous month. The thyroid gland had enlarged to two and a half times normal size.

The FTI was 6.4, and the RAI was 60 per cent, even though the patient was taking levothyroxine, 0.15 mg daily. The scan showed uniform tracer concentration in the diffuse goiter.

The patient was successfully treated with [131]I.

This patient demonstrates the unpredictable course of a goiter, even after an apparently satisfactory response to treatment with thyroid hormone. This is not a common occurrence if one considers the large number of patients who are treated in this fashion. However, the possibility must be kept in mind.

This patient also illustrates the diagnostic value of performing an RAI *without* discontinuation of thyroid hormone. This is a form of suppression test. A high value on a patient taking a reasonably full dose of a potent form of thyroid hormone is strong evidence for hyperthyroidism. (If the patient had been taking desiccated thyroid hormone, we would not be sure. The medication could have been impotent.) Discontinuing the thyroid hormone for a month or so prior to testing would only needlessly delay the diagnosis.

In patients with lesser degrees of nonsuppressible function it is possible that without supplemental thyroid hormone all studies could be normal. Therefore, unless the RAI is performed before thyroid hormone is stopped, it might not be evident that the hyperthyroidism was the result of the combined effect of the nonsuppressed endogenous hormonal

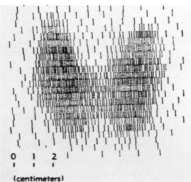

Figure 4–7. The scan, September, 1974.

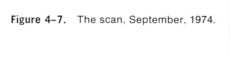

(centimeters)

secretion and the exogenous thyroid hormone. The physician might erroneously conclude that the problem was simply one of too high a dose of thyroid hormone. He might then order a lower dose, producing a recurrence of the hyperthyroidism. This error is easily avoided if one remembers to check the RAI value while the patient is still taking thyroid hormone.

The necessity for such a test is suggested even in the absence of overt hyperthyroidism in the following clinical situations:

1. An unexpectedly high FTI value for the dose of thyroid hormone given.

2. Failure of a diffuse goiter to regress in spite of treatment with a full replacement dose of thyroid hormone for more than 1 year.

3. Regression of part of an enlarged thyroid gland with a persistent nodular remnant. This may prove to be an autonomously functioning thyroid adenoma.

It is important to know what RAI values to expect in patients taking full doses of thyroid hormone (e.g., levothyroxine, 0.15 to 0.2 mg daily). A normal RAI response to such treatment is a value of less than 5 per cent. A higher value is abnormally high. Occasionally small nodules may be shown to function autonomously on scanning even when the RAI value on thyroid hormone is as low as 3 to 5 per cent.

CASE 4–4. LONG-TERM FOLLOWUP OF A SMALL GOITER

September, 1972. A 25 year old woman was referred for evaluation of a small goiter discovered on a routine physical examination. She was clinically euthyroid. The thyroid gland was firm and somewhat lobulated. The FTI was 2.2, and the TSH(RIA) 3.0 μU/ml. The RAI was 22 per cent. The scan was normal in appearance. Observation was advised.

October, 1974. The patient was returned for recheck because of muscle cramps, coarsening of the skin, paresthesias, and further enlargement of the thyroid gland. The thyroid was now about twice the normal size and distinctly firm. The FTI was 1.3, and the TSH(RIA) was 22 μU/ml. The RAI was 18 per cent, and there was no increase in response to TSH stimulation.

With which of the following statements do you agree?

a. Ignore the slight elevation in TSH(RIA). This patient has only a small goiter of no clinical significance.

b. If she had been treated with thyroid hormone in the first place, this further clinical deterioration could have been avoided.

c. Observation is all that is necessary. This condition may be reversible.

d. This sequence of events will happen to more than 50 per cent of patients with small goiters who are not treated with thyroid hormone.

e. Decline in thyroid function of this magnitude is unlikely to occur within 10 years in more than 10 per cent of patients.

Case 4–4 — Followup

The condition of most patients with small goiters remains stable for many years. This is the exception. Previously we have seen a patient who became hyperthyroid within 2 years (Case 4–3). Now we have one who became hypothyroid. The point is that there is no alternative to observation and reevaluation of these patients.

Our experience has been that the conditions of most young patients with small diffuse goiters remains relatively stable for many years. Hence, we do not insist that they be treated with thyroid hormone unless one of the following criteria is present:

1. The patient has laboratory data establishing impaired thyroid function.

2. The goiter is two and a half times normal size or larger. At this point it seems logical to try to prevent further enlargement by giving thyroid hormone, unless the patient is elderly (see p 182).

3. The goiter presents a visible cosmetic defect. This may relate not only to the size of the goiter but also to the structure of the neck. A long slender neck exposes the thyroid to a greater degree than does a short neck (see Case 4–2).

Admittedly, the second and third of these criteria are arbitrary and somewhat subjective. In the past I gave thyroid hormone to all patients with enlargement of the thyroid gland, hoping to prevent further growth. My patients taught me that this may not be the best idea for two reasons:

1. I see literally thousands of patients with small goiters every year. To ask them all to take thyroid hormone for life is a vast undertaking.

2. Many of those for whom I had made this recommendation failed to follow my advice but returned 1 to 10 years later no worse off without taking the thyroid hormone than they were at first.

Selected Current Reference For Case 4–4

1. Cassidy CE and Eddy RL: Hypothyroidism in patients with goiter. *Metabolism* 19:751–759, 1970

   These authors attribute the development of goiter in most instances (excluding hyperthyroidism) to impaired synthesis of thyroid hormone, leading to compensatory hypertrophy and hyperplasia. They reported a high incidence of hypothyroidism in their patients. However, their methods were crude, and perhaps some of their diagnoses were incorrect.

CASE 4–5. RECURRENT GOITER AFTER THYROIDECTOMY

October, 1974. A 26 year old woman had undergone thyroidectomy 4 years earlier for hyperthyroidism. No thyroid hormone was given after the operation. A recurrent mass was detected on the right side of the neck.

She was clinically euthyroid. The FTI was 1.5, the TSH(RIA) 4.5 μU/ml, and the T_3(RIA) 125 ng per 100 ml. The RAI was 58 per cent. The scan showed that the mass contained essentially all of the tracer concentrated in the neck area. The patient was primarily concerned about the cosmetic aspects of the problem.

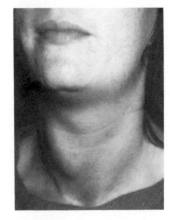

Figure 4–8. The patient.

With which of the following statements do you agree?

a. Treatment with thyroid hormone would produce a regression in the mass.

b. ^{131}I is the most appropriate treatment.

c. Before deciding which of the above two treatments might be better, an additional test is essential.

d. Thyroidectomy should be simple and effective.

e. Lugol's solution will cause this goiter to regress. The high RAI in conjunction with an FTI toward the lower level of the normal range means that this enlargement is the result of iodine deficiency.

f. If the patient had been treated with ^{131}I in the first place, this would not have happened.

g. If the patient had been given thyroid hormone after the original operation, this would not have happened.

Case 4–5 — Followup

This enlargement is clearly functioning tissue. The question is whether the recurrent thyroid tissue is the result of TSH-dependent compensatory hyperplasia, or is independent of TSH for its growth and function and has developed because of continuing activity of the mechanism that produced hyperthyroidism in the first place. The differential diagnosis is important. In the first instance treatment with thyroid hormone would be indicated and would be likely to produce regression of the mass. However, if the second diagnosis were correct, then thyroid hormone not only would be contraindicated (for it would probably lead to recurrent hyperthyroidism) but would surely be futile.

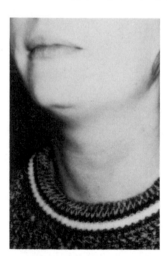

Figure 4–9.   The patient after ^{131}I therapy.

Therefore, an additional study is essential—you guessed it—a suppression test. After 1 week of treatment with T_3, 50 μg twice daily, the RAI remained nonsuppressible at 52 per cent. Therefore, it was concluded that treatment with thyroid hormone would be useless and also would not have prevented this recurrence. Iodine-131 therapy was given both to improve the patient's appearance and to prevent a recurrence of hyperthyroidism, a distinct possibility if the condition were permitted to progress untreated.

Clearly this would not have occurred had ^{131}I therapy been given initially. This is not the elevated RAI of iodine deficiency, because this form of elevation is readily suppressible in response to T_3. A repeat operation is more hazardous than the initial procedure and is unnecessary.

CASE 4–6. HASHIMOTO'S DISEASE

March, 1967.   A 37 year old euthyroid woman was referred for evaluation of a firm lobulated goiter twice the normal size. The FTI was 2.5, and the RAI 39 per cent.

Antithyroid antibodies were strongly positive, suggesting a diagnosis of Hashimoto's disease. The patient was treated with LT_4, 0.2 mg daily.

June, 1967. The goiter was unchanged. The RAI, while the patient was taking LT_4, was 7 per cent. Treatment with LT_4 was continued. Annual reevaluation was advised.

July, 1968. The goiter had not regressed. The patient remained clinically euthyroid. She had been taking her LT_4 faithfully; however, the RAI had increased to 33 per cent. Discontinuation of LT_4 was advised because of concern for future hyperthyroidism. Annual observation was continued.

May, 1969. She had been taking LT_4, 0.2 mg daily, for 6 months on the advice of another physician. The goiter was unchanged. She was euthyroid. The FTI was 3.8, the RAI 28 per cent. A scan showed diffuse function. Again we suggested discontinuation of LT_4 and annual reevaluation.

With which of the following statements do you agree?

a. She has Hashimoto's disease and Graves' disease. She will soon be hyperthyroid.

b. The strongly positive antibodies suggest that hypothyroidism will become evident within 5 years.

c. Prophylactic treatment with ^{131}I is proper.

d. Lugol's solution will control this goiter simply and safely.

e. Lugol's solution may precipitate jodbasedow's phenomenon.

f. Since she is euthyroid on LT_4, continue it to prevent further goiter enlargement.

g. If LT_4 is discontinued, she may be hypothyroid, even though she has nonsuppressible function.

Case 4–6 — Followup

Thyroid hormone was discontinued and the patient reevaluated on six subsequent occasions, at 12- to 18-month intervals through March of 1976. She remained euthyroid. The goiter remained stable. Her most recent FTI was 2.3; the TSH(RIA) was 4.4 $\mu U/ml$. Antibodies to thyroglobulin were positive at 1 to 250, and microsomal antibodies were positive at 1 to 25,600.

We conclude that the patient did have the combination of Hashimoto's disease and Graves' disease called euthyroid Hashitoxicosis (if you enjoy medical jargon). The Hashimoto's component limits the secretory capacity of the thyroid gland, thus preventing the development of hyperthyroidism even though there is diffuse nonsuppressible function.

This patient shows that positive antibodies do not necessarily indicate that hypothyroidism will soon develop. It does seem prudent to continue her regular followup examinations, because eventually I would assume that hypothyroidism will be her fate.

There was no need to give ^{131}I. Most patients with euthyroid Graves' disease, in my experience, do not rapidly become hyperthyroid. Lugol's solution may induce hypothyroidism. Patients with Hashimoto's disease are especially sensitive to the suppressant effects of iodine. This is not the usual type of goiter that will exhibit the jodbasedow phenomenon. More often it is the long-standing multinodular goiter that reacts in this fashion.

Continued treatment with thyroid hormone to prevent the development of hypothyroid manifestations might have been considered. However, this patient remained euthyroid for 9 years and may remain so for many more. Why should she take thyroid hormone unnecessarily for all that time? Obviously the small goiter was not an indication for thyroid hormone, and the known nonsuppressible function made it unlikely that thyroid hormone would have altered the course of the goiter itself.

CASE 4–7. GOITER IN MIDDLE AGE

January, 1975. A 44 year old woman reported that a goiter had been discovered on routine examination 2 weeks earlier. She had noted lack of pep, fatigue, facial puffiness, hoarseness, muscle cramps, and paresthesias in the previous 3 to 6 months. There was no history of heart disease. On examination the skin was coarse and dry, the heart rate was 72, and the blood pressure was 130/80. The reflexes were depressed in the return phase, there was moderate facial edema, and the thyroid gland was twice the normal size and firm.

The FTI was 0.6, the TSH(RIA) 100 μU/ml, and the RAI 15 per cent before and 14 per cent after TSH stimulation. Antithyroid antibodies were strongly positive. The EKG was normal.

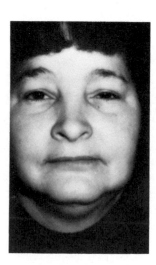

Figure 4-10. The patient.

With which of the following statements do you agree?

    a.   This patient has Hashimoto's disease.

    b.   This patient has hypothyroidism.

    c.   The normal RAI value is inconsistent with the diagnosis of hypothyroidism.

    d.   The treatment is levothyroxine, 0.15 mg daily.

    e.   The treatment is levothyroxine, 0.05 mg daily initially, with phased increments to full replacement doses over a period of 6 weeks.

Case 4-7 — Followup

This patient is relatively young and has only moderately severe hypothyroidism; hence, she was given levothyroxine, 0.15 mg daily. In 2 months she was rechecked and was found to be euthyroid. The goiter had regressed about 25 per cent. Her improved appearance is evident in Figure 4–11.

There is no need for gradual introduction of thyroid hormone for a patient like this. It will only prolong her morbidity.

This is a typical case of Hashimoto's disease in middle age that produces goiter and hypothyroidism. The normal RAI value is commonly seen at this point in the course of Hashimoto's disease. This disease should be viewed as a continuum beginning with the triggering of an autoimmune process that leads to impairment of thyroidal cellular function. As the secretory activity of the thyroid gland falls, pituitary TSH release is increased,

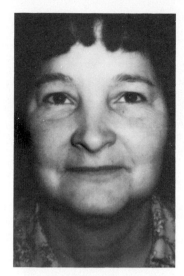

Figure 4–11. The patient when euthyroid.

promoting goiter on the basis of compensatory hyperplasia. The inflammatory reaction also plays a role in the goiter.

Hence, early in the course of the disease, there may be a picture of goiter, an elevated serum TSH concentration (often of modest degree), and elevated titers of antithyroid antibodies. The microsomal antibodies are more often positive, and positive in higher titers than the antithyroglobulin antibodies. The elevated TSH concentration may be lacking if compensatory hyperplasia restores thyroid hormone output to normal. The RAI is usually normal at this point; it may even respond normally to TSH stimulation if there is still some functional reserve intact.

A later stage reflects the progressive nature of the disease, with further deterioration in thyroidal secretory activity leading to hypothyroidism. At the same time, the intrathyroidal disease advances with increasing fibrosis. Antibody levels rise to higher titers. The RAI may still be within normal limits but does not respond to TSH stimulation. The normal RAI value only means that the thyroid gland still has functional tissue capable of incorporating iodine into thyroglobulin. However, the necessary additional function needed for the production of metabolically active thyroid hormone is inadequate to permit the maintenance of the euthyroid state.

By the end stage of the disease the patient has severe myxedema with very low levels of thyroid hormone in the plasma. TSH concentrations reach the highest possible levels. Similarly, the antibody titer becomes exceedingly high. The thyroid gland has undergone extensive fibrous atrophy and is barely enlarged, if enlarged at all; it varies in texture from firm and irregular to finely nodular. By this time the RAI value is essentially zero.

CASE 4–8. THE MULTINODULAR GOITER

November, 1966. A 42 year old woman was referred for evaluation of a large multinodular goiter, discovered on routine examination. She was clinically euthyroid. The thyroid gland was three times the normal size, firm, and multinodular.

The FTI value was 2.2 and the RAI 19 per cent. The scan showed gross patchiness and irregularity of function. This is characteristic of a multinodular goiter which has undergone degeneration, possibly in conjunction with chronic inflammatory disease (i.e., Hashimoto's disease).

Treatment with thyroid hormone was advised. The patient was given levothyroxine, 0.3 mg daily (by another physician). This medication was continued through January of 1975.

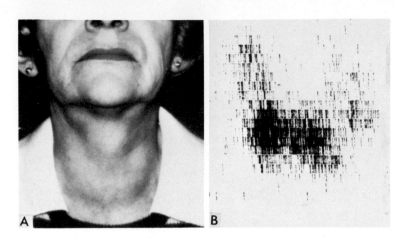

Figure 4-12. *A*, The patient. *B*, Her scan.

January, 1975. The patient was referred for reevaluation because of tachycardia and nervousness. The heart rate was 112. The thyroid gland was still enlarged to three times the normal size and was still multinodular.

With which of the following statements do you agree?

a. The patient has been taking an overdose of thyroid hormone.

b. The RAI value will be less than 5 per cent.

c. The RAI value will be greater than 5 per cent.

d. It may be hazardous to treat elderly people with multinodular goiters with thyroid hormone.

Case 4–8 — Followup

This patient was given too large a dose of levothyroxine. Almost all patients are adequately treated with 0.15 to 0.2 mg of levothyroxine daily. I never use more than 0.15 mg daily unless there is evidence of an incompletely suppressed serum TSH concentration. The elderly patient with a long-standing multinodular goiter is particularly likely to be intolerant of thyroid hormone because there is a tendency for the goiter to have nonsuppressible function. The normal response of the RAI to a full dose of levothyroxine is a drop to levels of less than 5 per cent. In this patient the value was 9 per cent. This was a drop from the original 19 per cent, indicating that some of the tissue of this goiter was responding to suppression of TSH by thyroid hormone, but some tissue was at least partially independent of TSH for its continued function.

Therefore, the patient developed hyperthyroidism because of the combined effects of an overdose of levothyroxine and continued nonsuppressed endogenous secretory activity.

What should be done, if anything, in addition to stopping the thyroid hormone? In this instance, after thyroid hormone was discontinued, the patient was euthyroid. We, therefore, suggested observation with retesting annually to rule out the possibility of future development of spontaneous hyperthyroidism. Of course, we cannot exclude the possibility of eventual hypothyroidism either.

CASE 4–9. AN ELDERLY WOMAN WITH A LARGE, ENLARGING GOITER

March, 1975. A 76 year old woman was referred for an enlarging goiter. She had undergone a partial thyroidectomy in 1941 but was not advised to take thyroid

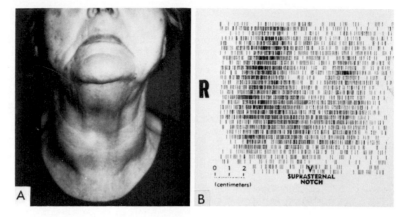

Figure 4-13. *A,* The patient. *B,* Her scan.

hormone subsequently. The recurrent goiter was first noted 10 to 15 years ago and had been gradually increasing in size. She had no obstructive complaints. She was clinically euthyroid. On palpation the thyroid gland was multinodular and about five times the normal size.

The FTI was 2.4, the T_3(RIA) 110 ng per 100 ml, and the TSH(RIA) 2.4 μU/ml. Antibodies to thyroid microsomes were strongly positive.

The scan revealed patchy and irregular function throughout this large multinodular goiter.

A chest radiograph with special attention to the thoracic inlet revealed deviation of the trachea to the left but no tracheal narrowing.

With which of the following statements do you agree?

a. Thyroidectomy is essential to prevent progressive asphyxiation as this goiter inexorably enlarges.

b. If thyroid hormone had been given after the initial operation, this problem might have been prevented.

c. Levothyroxine, 0.3 mg daily, should be given now.

d. Levothyroxine, 0.2 mg daily, should be given now.

e. Thyroid hormone may be hazardous because these goiters often have significant nonsuppressible function.

f. If the patient lives long enough, hypothyroidism is inevitable in view of the strongly positive antibody titer.

g. If the patient lives long enough, hyperthyroidism is likely to ensue.

h. Treatment with ^{131}I will prevent future toxicity and eliminate or at least greatly reduce the goiter mass.

i. The safest thing to do is to leave well enough alone — observation only is indicated.

Case 4–9 — Followup

This was a difficult problem, primarily because of the history of recent gradual enlargement. Although there was no evidence of significant obstruction, the possibility of obstruction if no action were taken seemed at least worthy of serious consideration. For a patient of this age, elective thyroidectomy for prophylactic purposes was not a very attractive prospect. Therapy with ^{131}I probably would not be very effective because a large portion of the goiter was not functional tissue—the end result of years of degeneration. Furthermore, these long-standing multinodular goiters are notoriously resistant to ^{131}I because of the nonuniform uptake of the radionuclide throughout a thyroid gland composed of tissue with variable functional activity.

These long-standing multinodular goiters often have significant nonsuppressible function. Hence, full replacement doses of thyroid hormone may add to the endogenous secretory activity to produce iatrogenic toxicity. If thyroid hormone is given, it should be given cautiously, no more than 0.1 mg of levothyroxine daily initially. This is actually what was done. It was well tolerated, and 1 year later the goiter was slightly smaller.

It is reasonable to assume that had thyroid hormone been given after the initial operation, this recurrent goiter might have been prevented. It is disheartening to see so many patients like this, most of whom have been told by their surgeons that enough thyroid tissue was left to produce all the hormone they will need. This statement represents a rather poor understanding of the pathophysiology underlying most nontoxic goiters. The thyroid enlarged in the first place because of compensatory hyperplasia in response to inefficient synthesis and secretion of thyroid hormone. If a substantial mass of thyroid tissue is removed, one of two things will eventually happen (and both are bad). Either the remaining thyroid tissue will be unable to produce adequate quantities of thyroid hormone, and hypothyroidism will occur; or the remaining thyroid tissue will again undergo compensatory hyperplasia, resulting in a recurrent goiter (with or without hypothyroidism). The simple expedient of administering thyroid hormone postoperatively (e.g., levothyroxine, 0.15 mg daily) will prevent these complications.

What the future holds for this patient is unclear. The high antibody titer suggests that Hashimoto's disease is present and that the end result may be hypothyroidism. However, these goiters have a definite propensity to produce thyrotoxicosis, even after many years of quiescence. One must be alert to either possibility.

CASE 4–10. SUDDEN ONSET OF THYROID ENLARGEMENT IN A MIDDLE AGED WOMAN

November, 1974. A 55 year old woman was referred for evaluation of a massive swelling in the neck that had been enlarging during the previous 2 months. It had not been painful or tender at any time. There was no fever. Her voice had become husky in the past month. Her past health had been excellent, and there was no evidence of heart disease.

The patient had minimal facial edema, a heart rate of 100, a normal temperature, and a massive, firm lobulated goiter. The FTI was 0.5, the T_3(RIA) 65 ng per 100 ml, the TSH(RIA) 64 μU/ml, and the RAI 5 percent. The ESR was 17 mm/hour. The scan revealed patchy and irregular function throughout this massive goiter.

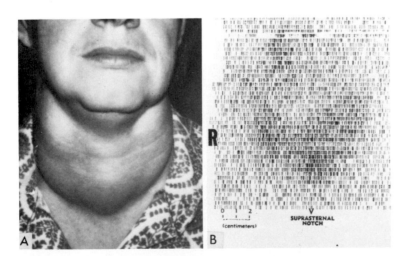

Figure 4–14. *A,* The patient. *B,* Her scan.

With which of the following statements do you agree?

a. This patient has an anaplastic thyroid cancer. The husky voice means there has been involvement of the recurrent nerve. The prognosis is hopeless.

b. This could be occult subacute thyroiditis in a resolving stage. The husky voice may reflect only the hypothyroidism.

c. A biopsy is necessary.

d. Thyroid hormone should be given promptly. Start with levothyroxine, 0.15 mg daily.

e. Same as d, but start with levothyroxine, 0.05 mg daily, and gradually progress to 0.15 mg daily over a period of 2 months.

f. This is an acute presentation of Hashimoto's disease.

g. Don't forget lymphoma.

h. Needle biopsy may be considered.

i. Open biopsy is better; almost certainly a decompression procedure will be needed.

j. The combination of thyroid hormone and adrenal steroids will produce prompt regression of this goiter.

Case 4–10 — Followup

This was a very worrisome situation. The possibility of lymphoma or anaplastic cancer was prominent in our thinking. However, neither of these diseases is likely to cause hypothyroidism. Thus, it would be necessary to make two diagnoses or else discard consideration of lymphoma and anaplastic cancer. Hashimoto's disease was a possible diagnosis, but I have never seen such an acute presentation of Hashimoto's disease. A diagnosis of subacute thyroiditis is possible and is perhaps the most attractive diagnosis. True enough, there was no pain or fever by history. However, the relatively rapid thyroid enlargement is most consistent with that diagnosis. Hypothyroidism often occurs in the later stages of resolution of this disease. At that point there is no longer any elevation in the sedimentation rate. In any event, we were most concerned about missing a diagnosis of malignancy, and the attending physician (a surgeon) was most concerned about potential obstruction.

Therefore, the patient was treated with levothyroxine, 0.15 mg daily, for 3 weeks to restore the euthyroid state. Note, this patient had relatively mild hypothyroidism of rather short duration. Her cardiac history was negative, there were no physical findings suggesting

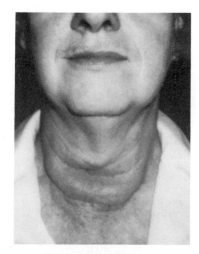

Figure 4–15. The patient after thyroidectomy.

heart disease, and an EKG was normal. Even though she was 55 years old, there was no need for a more gradual introduction of thyroid hormone. This would only have delayed the planned surgery. A subtotal thyroidectomy was performed, and the pathologist made a diagnosis of "chronic thyroiditis consistent with a fibrous variant of Hashimoto's disease."

However, the microscopic findings included extensive destruction of follicles, massive leukocyte infiltration including lymphocytes and plasma cells, no lymphoid follicles, multinucleated giant cells, extensive fibrosis, and microfollicles with only small amounts of colloid. In short, this is an excellent description of the histologic features of subacute thyroiditis. Unfortunately, pathologists do not have many opportunities to see examples of subacute thyroiditis. These patients come to surgery only when an incorrect diagnosis is made.

Had we been a bit more alert, we would have tried a course of adrenal steroids and thyroid hormone (goiter enlargement may have been promoted by the hypothyroidism with an elevated TSH concentration), and quite probably an unnecessary operation could have been avoided.

Needle biopsy of a goiter of this type might be very unsatisfactory. Since the pathologist was confused with a specimen consisting essentially of the entire thyroid gland, how could we have expected him to make a proper diagnosis with a small piece of tissue? If a very fortunate sample had been obtained, perhaps a very experienced pathologist might have been able to make a correct assessment, but it seemed to us unnecessary to put him under so much pressure. An open biopsy under local anesthesia would provide a much more generous sample of the tissue. The end result can be seen in Figure 4–15.

Recently I have seen an 80 year old woman who presented with an enlarging, somewhat tender goiter about eight times the size of the normal thyroid gland. She had an FTI of 1.0, a TSH(RIA) of 80 μU/ml and markedly elevated antithyroid antibody titers. The ESR was 24 mm/hour. A fine needle aspiration produced a specimen that was cytologically consistent with Hashimoto's disease. A needle biopsy specimen was inadequate for histologic diagnosis. Treatment with thyroid hormone was instituted. However, the goiter continued to enlarge. Treatment with adrenal steroids was considered because of the possibility that this might represent a more acute stage in the development of Hashimoto's disease with considerable infiltration of inflammatory cells. We rejected this treatment because she had a history of a bleeding duodenal ulcer 10 years earlier. Within 2 months from the time we first saw her the goiter had grown so large that swallowing was very difficult. An open biopsy was performed under local anesthesia, and it was found that, to be sure, the patient had Hashimoto's disease, but she also had a lymphoma of the thyroid. She improved in response to radiation therapy.

This is the second instance in which a fine needle aspiration failed to give us a clear picture of the underlying pathologic process in a patient with lymphoma. For the first patient a needle biopsy produced a satisfactory and diagnostic specimen.

Because of this experience we insisted upon obtaining a larger specimen for this patient, and the suspected diagnosis of lymphoma was established.

Thus, a diagnosis of Hashimoto's disease, even accompanied by hypothyroidism, does not preclude a second diagnosis of lymphoma, particularly in an elderly patient.

CHAPTER 5

THYROID NODULES AND THYROID CANCER

PART I. PATHOPHYSIOLOGIC MECHANISMS INVOLVED IN THE DEVELOPMENT OF THYROID NODULES

A thyroid nodule is simply a lump in the thyroid gland detected by palpation. A number of pathologic processes may give rise to nodular thyroid lesions. These are outlined in Table 5–1.

TABLE 5–1. PATHOLOGIC CONSIDERATIONS RELATIVE TO THYROID NODULES

I. **NON-NEOPLASTIC NODULES**
  A. Hyperplastic
    1. Spontaneous
    2. Compensatory after partial thyroidectomy
  B. Degenerative
  C. Inflammatory
    1. Hashimoto's disease
    2. SAT
II. **BENIGN NEOPLASMS**
  A. Nonfunctional
    1. Solid
    2. Cystic
  B. Autonomously functioning
III. **MALIGNANT NEOPLASMS**
  A. Primary
    1. Papillary
    2. Follicular
    3. Hürthle cell
    4. Medullary
    5. Anaplastic
  B. Lymphoma
  C. Metastatic cancer to the thyroid

HYPERPLASTIC NODULES

These nodules are thought to represent the consequences of successive phases of hyperplasia and involution, after which a portion or portions of the thyroid gland may remain enlarged, lobulated, or frankly nodular. These nodules are functional and remain dependent upon TSH for their function. The compensatory hyperplastic nodule that occurs after partial thyroidectomy is the result of essentially the same process, provoked in this instance by a nonphysiologic mechanism.

These nodules are benign and when necessary may be treated with thyroid hormone. Since hyperplastic nodules are TSH-dependent, one might expect that treatment with thyroid hormone in doses adequate to suppress pituitary release of TSH would regularly produce regression. This is not the case. Some regress while others do not. There are a number of reasons for this lack of regression in response to treatment, but I believe the most important is the extent of central degeneration. This leads us to the next section of this discussion.

DEGENERATIVE NODULES

Nodules generally derive their blood supply from the periphery. As the nodule enlarges, the more central portions may become ischemic, eventually undergo infarction, and thus degenerate. Hyperplastic nodules are prone to undergo degeneration as they age. Thus, what was originally a functional nodule may ultimately become functionless. This sequence of events has been demonstrated by serial imaging and ultrasound studies on nontoxic AFTA. Hence, central degeneration is a very common finding in large nodules, regardless of the pathologic process that produced the lesion.

INFLAMMATORY NODULES

Inflammatory processes that involve the thyroid usually do so in a uniform and diffuse fashion. However, on occasion a localized nodular lesion may occur. These lesions will have little or no functional activity and are easily confused with neoplastic nodules.

SAT commonly extends throughout the thyroid gland in a creeping fashion, beginning in one lobe and finally involving the opposite lobe over a period of a few weeks, more or less. If a patient with SAT is seen early in the course of the disease, a unilateral, firm, nodular lesion may be discovered. If the lesion is only minimally tender, as is often the case, it may not be easy to exclude a neoplastic process.

BENIGN NONFUNCTIONAL NEOPLASMS

These lesions are usually indistinguishable from their malignant counterparts until they are removed and examined histologically. Diagnostic ultrasound techniques permit the differentiation of purely cystic nodules from those that are solid or part solid and part cystic. The purely cystic lesions are almost certainly benign and probably represent the end stage of degeneration of a previously solid nodule.

Benign neoplasms may be classified on the basis of their histological appearance, but with one exception this has little or no clinical significance. Some of these nodules have papillary changes. If they lack other features of papillary cancer, they may be called papillary adenomas. Although they may appear to be benign from the pathologist's point of view, clinicians should be aware that they have a pronounced tendency to recur locally. Some pathologists prefer to consider them papillary carcinomas.

AUTONOMOUSLY FUNCTIONING THYROID ADENOMAS

The AFTA is a nodular lesion of the thyroid that functions independently of pituitary regulation. AFTA are regularly benign but may be associated with cancer elsewhere in the thyroid more often than dictated by chance alone. However, this association seems not to be great enough to constitute a mandate for thyroidectomy unless one happens to find another nodule that fulfills criteria for a possible cancer.

Macroscopically, AFTA are usually solitary. However, a high proportion of patients with apparently solitary macroscopic AFTA may be shown to have autonomously functioning micronodules. Why one lesion grows to a large size while others do not is unknown. There are occasional instances in which two or three grossly palpable AFTA may coexist in the same thyroid gland, but these are the exceptions. Suppression scanning may reveal tiny areas of autonomous function in addition to the palpable AFTA. These small lesions are usually not palpable as discrete nodules.

There is only one reported case (with which I am familiar) of a recurrent toxic AFTA after removal of a prior toxic AFTA.

As already noted, AFTA tend to undergo spontaneous degeneration. Over a number of years an initially functional solid lesion may be converted into a largely functionless predominantly cystic mass. This process is a major limiting factor in the progression of nontoxic AFTA to the toxic stage.

Most nontoxic AFTA remain nontoxic and stable in size for many years. A smaller number enlarge somewhat but remain nontoxic. It is the exceptional AFTA that progresses from the nontoxic to the toxic state within a 10-year period.

It has been claimed that AFTA may become TSH-dependent. This claim was not substantiated by the data presented and has not been confirmed. The evidence better supports the contention that AFTA are TSH-independent from the earliest recognizable stage and remain so throughout their life history (see reference 3). Of course, if the lesion becomes completely degenerated so that no functional tissue remains, then obviously there will be no further functional autonomy.

References

1. Hamburger JI: Solitary autonomously functioning thyroid lesions. *Am J Med* 58:740–748, 1975
2. Wiener JD: A systematic approach to the diagnosis of Plummer's disease (autonomous goitre), with a review of 224 cases. *Neth J Med* 18:218–233, 1975
3. Hamburger, JI: *Hyperthyroidism, Concept and Controversy.* Springfield, Illinois, Charles C Thomas, 1972, pp. 50–53.

PRIMARY MALIGNANT NEOPLASMS OF THE THYROID

This histologic diagnosis of malignant neoplasms carries with it certain useful clinical implications. However, overlap between histologic categories is common, and it is difficult, impractical, and indeed often impossible to study completely the histologic pattern throughout the primary and metastatic lesions. Nevertheless, the following generalizations are reasonably sound rules of thumb.

Papillary cancer usually is poorly encapsulated, locally invasive, and often multifocal; it spreads predominantly to the regional lymph nodes and progresses slowly, often requiring 10 to 20 years before producing metastases.

Follicular cancer is usually well encapsulated and less likely to be locally invasive. It usually presents as a solitary thyroid lesion. It metastasizes primarily via the blood stream and is somewhat less predictable in terms of malignancy.

The Hürthle cell variant of follicular carcinoma is more aggressive.

Medullary cancer is similar in presentation to papillary and follicular lesions. It metastasizes initially to the lymph nodes but also via the blood stream to distant sites and has a poorer prognosis.

Anaplastic cancer is almost invariably rapidly fatal.

Lymphoma of the thyroid is rare and carries a poor prognosis, but it may respond to radiation therapy, occasionally with an apparent cure.

DIFFERENTIATED THYROID CANCER (PAPILLARY AND FOLLICULAR)

There are many exceptions to the generalizations just listed, particularly within the differentiated group. The presence of follicular elements in a papillary cancer does not alter the probability that the cancer will behave like a papillary lesion. Hence, papillary and mixed papillary and follicular lesions may be considered a single entity. Furthermore, if one confines a diagnosis of follicular cancer to those tumors that are purely follicular, both in the primary and the metastatic lesions, this becomes a rather uncommon type of thyroid cancer. Since it is practically impossible to determine the purity of a follicular cancer in the clinical setting in time to influence the surgical management, this diagnosis is primarily of retrospective significance. Hence, it may be reasonable to accept Winship's suggestion that papillary, follicular, and mixed papillary and follicular cancers of the thyroid can all be treated alike as differentiated tumors.

The occult sclerosing papillary cancer perhaps may be considered a distinct variant of differentiated cancer, worthy of subclassification by virtue of its regularly benign course. These tumors by definition are less than 1.5 cm in diameter, are clinically unsuspected, and are often found in the course of thyroidectomy for another reason. There is general agreement that the prognosis is excellent. However, one cannot conclude from these observations that all small papillary cancers are entirely unimportant, since many patients presenting with overt evidence of metastasis from papillary cancer have tiny primary lesions. In actuality, the concept of the benign occult sclerosing papillary cancer is purely retrospective. When such a lesion is discovered incidental to thyroidectomy for another reason, obviously grossly evident disease has not yet occurred. Under these circumstances the prognosis is good. By contrast, the tiny papillary cancer that is likely to produce bulky metastases before the primary lesion is detectable by palpation obviously can be uncovered only in the course of a search for the primary lesion after grossly evident metastases have developed. It seems doubtful that these clinical distinctions define fundamentally different pathologic entities. Perhaps they reflect only differences in the age of the lesion. Nevertheless, extensive experience with the benign nature of a thyroid cancer that fulfills the criteria for an occult sclerosing papillary lesion seems to justify attitudes of conservatism and optimism.

About 70 to 80 per cent of cancers of the thyroid are differentiated. The most common mode of presentation is the discrete thyroid nodule. Less often, the presenting manifestations may be related to metastases. These may involve the cervical lymph nodes (palpable and even visible neck masses); the lungs (radiographic defects); or bone (lytic lesions with or without pathologic fractures). Even if the primary lesion appears solitary, experience indicates quite clearly that multifocal involvement or intraglandular dissemination is very common, if not the rule. Furthermore, occult cervical lymph node involvement is about equally frequent. Hence, one can conclude that by the time a primary differentiated thyroid cancer becomes detectable by palpation, the probability of additional tumor elsewhere in the gland or in the cervical nodes is very great.

Those cancers that seem to arise because of prior radiation therapy to the thymus or the general area of the neck are particularly likely to be multifocal.

The prognosis for differentiated thyroid cancer is generally good. The overall 10-year survival rate is similar to that for the population at large. However, there are important factors in addition to histology that appear to have a critical influence upon survival. Of greatest importance is the age of the patient when the cancer is discovered. If the patient is less than 40 years old the prognosis is excellent. In older patients the outlook may be somewhat poorer. Although women have thyroid cancer three times as often as men, the prognosis for men is not as good. The presence of distant metastases also makes the prognosis worse. However, cervical node involvement, even if extensive (as often occurs in children), does not appear to influence the chances for survival materially. Thus, a young woman with differentiated thyroid cancer, whether cervical node metastases are present or not, is likely to survive as long as a comparable woman without thyroid disease selected from the population at large.

Recently it has been suggested that differentiated tumors of the thyroid may dedifferentiate after many years into the anaplastic variety. The evidence offered to support this sequence of events includes the coexistence of foci of differentiated tumor in a high proportion of anaplastic cancer specimens. Furthermore, biopsies of recurrences of differentiated carcinomas at times demonstrate a progressively less well differentiated pattern that may ultimately become frankly anaplastic. Of course, it is impossible to provide direct proof of a progression from differentiated to anaplastic cancer, and the existing evidence can also be interpreted as indicating only the association of both types of cancer in the same patient. Nevertheless, the possibility of anaplastic transformation must be given consideration. This may account for the poor prognosis for some older patients whose cancers appear to be of the differentiated type.

Reference

1. Sampson RJ, Oka H, Key CR and Iijima S: Metastases from occult thyroid cancer. *Cancer* 25:803–811, 1970

HÜRTHLE CELL CANCER

Hürthle cell tumors are generally considered to be a variety of follicular cancer. Whether they should be classified as a separate entity is a matter of dispute. Those who argue to the contrary observe quite correctly that Hürthle cells can be seen in every type of thyroid cancer, in benign neoplasms, and in every other kind of thyroid gland whether goitrous or not. Therefore, the mere presence of Hürthle cells has no fundamental significance. However, this is not the point. Some tumors are composed predominantly if not entirely of Hürthle cells. They tend to be bulky and invasive. They metastasize widely and prove lethal in a high proportion of patients.

MEDULLARY CANCER

Medullary thyroid cancer has been recognized as a separate entity only in the past 20 years. Within the past 10 years it has become clear that this tumor arises from nests of parafollicular cells, or "C cells." These cells are of neural crest origin and travel with the ultimobranchial body into the thyroid gland. The similarity in origin of these cells to those of the adrenal medulla may explain the association of medullary cancer with pheochromocytoma. Microscopically, there are sheets of cells with a characteristic deposition of amyloid. It is frequently a familial disorder, inherited as an autosomal dominant trait, and is associated with pheochromocytoma, hyper-parathyroidism, and multiple mucosal neuromas involving the eyelids, lips, tongue, and buccal mucosa. Medullary thyroid cancer may produce hormonal substances, including calcitonin, 5-hydroxytryptamine, histaminase, and prostaglandins. The latter three substances may be responsible for the flushing and diarrhea sometimes observed. In addition, these tumors rarely may produce an ACTH-like substance and induce a disorder resembling Cushing's disease. Association with carcinoid also has been observed. Radioimmunoassay of calcitonin is now available. This assay has been used to screen asymptomatic relatives of medullary cancer patients, and as a result the disease has been discovered even in the absence of palpable thyroid nodules. Assay of histaminase activity in serum and tissue is also of value in the diagnosis of metastatic medullary carcinoma.

Medullary thyroid cancer is intermediate in malignancy between the differentiated and anaplastic types. The primary lesion is likely to be bilateral in the familial form. In the absence of metastases, the prognosis is favorable. Unlike the situation with differentiated thyroid cancer, involvement of the cervical nodes significantly worsens the outlook for survival.

References

1. Paloyan E, Scann A, Straus FH, Pickelman JR and Paloyan D: Familial pheochromocytoma, medullary thyroid carcinoma and parathyroid adenomas. *JAMA* 214:1443–1447, 1970
2. Melvin KEW, Miller HH and Tashjian AH: Early diagnosis of medullary carcinoma of the thyroid gland by means of calcitonin assay. *New Eng J Med* 285:1115–1120, 1971
3. Block MA, Jackson CE and Tashjian AH: Medullary thyroid carcinoma detected by serum calcitonin assay. *Arch Surg* 104:579–586, 1971

ANAPLASTIC CANCER AND LYMPHOMA

Patients with anaplastic thyroid cancer comprise 10 to 15 per cent of most series. In my own series less than 3 per cent had anaplastic cancer, an unusually small proportion. This undoubtedly reflects the fact that my cases are culled exclusively from an outpatient population. By contrast, in the series of the Royal Marsden Hospital (a referral center for problem cancer patients) 25 per cent of patients had anaplastic cancer. Anaplastic cancer is almost exclusively confined to patients older than 40 years and is most common after 60. These tumors are uniformly fatal, usually within 1 year after the diagnosis has been made. The prognosis is so dismal that failure to succumb to the disease is grounds for reconsideration of the diagnosis. The cellular pattern may include giant cells, spindle cells, or small cells, but cell type has little clinical importance. However, the differentiation between small cell anaplastic thyroid cancer and lymphoma may be exceedingly difficult. Some authorities believe that there is no such entity as small cell anaplastic thyroid cancer and that all lesions of this type are actually lymphomas. Lymphomas may respond to radiation therapy. This may account for some relatively long-term survivals of patients who were thought to have anaplastic cancer. Surgical decompression is occasionally of value for palliation of anaplastic cancer, and some tumors may regress temporarily after radiation therapy.

References

1. Woolner LB, McConahey WM, Beahrs OH and Black BM: Primary lymphoma of the thyroid. *Am J Surg* 111:502–523, 1966
2. Rayfield EJ, Nishiyama RH and Sisson JC: Small cell tumors of the thyroid. *Cancer* 28:1023–1030, 1971

METASTATIC CANCER TO THE THYROID

Metastatic cancer to the thyroid is rare. The kidney and the breast are more common sites of primary lesions.

References

1. Wychulis AR, Beahrs OH and Woolner LB: Metastasis of carcinoma to the thyroid gland. *Ann Surg* 160:169–177, 1964
2. Burge JP and Blalock JB: Metastatic hypernephroma of the thyroid gland. *Am J Surg* 113:387–389, 1967

PART II. CLINICAL EVALUATION OF THYROID NODULES

The single overriding consideration in the evaluation of the patient with a thyroid nodule is the risk of cancer. A secondary problem that pertains only to functional nodules is the differentiation of those that function autonomously from those that arise on the basis of TSH-dependent compensatory hyperplasia.

The first step in such an evaluation is the determination that there are grounds for clinical concern for cancer. The major points to be assessed in the history and physical examination and the weight that might be assigned to each are summarized in Table 5–2.

HISTORY

Both benign and malignant nodules occur with greater frequency in older patients. However, the rate of increase for benign lesions is far greater than that for malignant. Hence, the younger the patient with a nodule, the greater the concern for cancer. Although thyroid cancers may remain dormant for many years, a nodule with a long history of lack of growth reduces somewhat the probability of cancer. Steady painless growth increases concern, whereas rapid enlargement, especially if accom-

TABLE 5–2. CLINICAL FEATURES THAT WEIGH FOR AND AGAINST THYROID CANCER IN A DISCRETE THYROID NODULE

	FOR CANCER	AGAINST CANCER
History		
Less than 20 years of age	+4	
More than 60 years of age		−2
Prior radiation therapy	+4	
Growth in spite of thyroid hormone treatment	+4	
"Complete regression" on thyroid hormone treatment (rare)		−2
Nodule present more than 20 years without change		−2
Rapid development		−2
Rapid development plus pain and tenderness		−3
Slow painless growth	+2	
Male sex	+1	
Positive family history	+1	
Positive family history of medullary cancer	+3	
Hoarseness	+1	
Physical Findings		
Freely movable	0	
Internally fixed	+3	
Rock-hard	+3	
Adjacent lymph nodes involved	+2 to +4	
Diffusely abnormal thyroid gland		−2

panied by pain and tenderness, is more likely to result from hemorrhage or subacute thyroiditis.

The association of radiation therapy 10 to 30 years before the subsequent development of thyroid cancer is well known. Most attention has been paid to thymic radiation; however, a history of radiation therapy to the tonsils, adenoids, skin, lungs, or virtually any tissue in the region of the thyroid should increase the index of suspicion.

The family history is of principal importance in patients with medullary cancer, for which calcitonin assay may demonstrate the presence of malignancy even before there is a palpable lesion.

Hoarseness is usually emphasized as an unfavorable sign. However, bulky benign goiters also may cause hoarseness, probably by compression of the laryngeal nerves. Finally, hoarseness may be caused by coincidental laryngeal disease.

I do not find much use for a trial of thyroid hormone for treatment of solid nodules that are hypofunctional on scanning. By definition, these lesions do not have normal TSH-dependent function. Therefore, suppression of pituitary TSH (which is all that thyroid hormone administration can accomplish) is not likely to be useful. When this type of nodule regresses during thyroid hormone administration, one can assume that the regression would probably have occurred without such treatment. For example, spontaneous regression may occur with localized subacute thyroiditis and hemorrhagic cystic nodules. Even nodules that seem to regress "completely" cannot be ignored, for there may well be a persistent nodule that is difficult to palpate, and the regression simply results from resorption of the bleeding which had caused a temporary expansion. Actually, the most important finding to be elicited from a trial of thyroid hormone is a history of further growth. This is almost certainly indicative of either autonomous function or neoplasia.

Figure 5–1 demonstrates the workup of a typical patient with thyroid cancer.

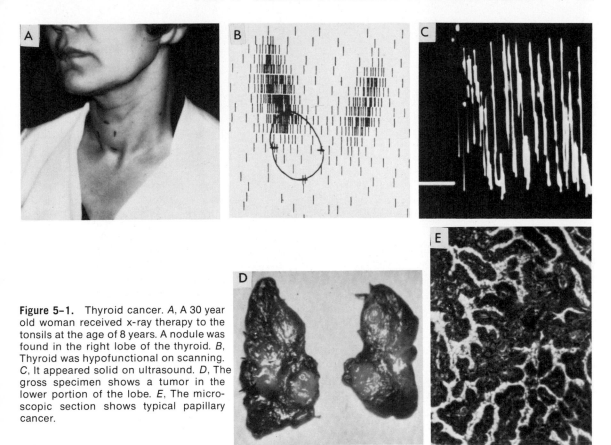

Figure 5-1. Thyroid cancer. *A,* A 30 year old woman received x-ray therapy to the tonsils at the age of 8 years. A nodule was found in the right lobe of the thyroid. *B,* Thyroid was hypofunctional on scanning. *C,* It appeared solid on ultrasound. *D,* The gross specimen shows a tumor in the lower portion of the lobe. *E,* The microscopic section shows typical papillary cancer.

TECHNIQUE FOR EXAMINATION OF THE THYROID GLAND

Experienced physicians sooner or later develop their own methods of examining the thyroid gland. There are those who favor the face to face approach and those who prefer to stand behind the patient. It is possible to use either method successfully, but it is more difficult to do a thorough job from behind where vision is obscured. Also, I am convinced that many physicians who examine from behind never actually palpate the thyroid gland completely. They are content with an appraisal of the anterior surface of the lobes and isthmus rather than actual palpation of the full thickness of the lobes between thumb and fingers. They will miss many small nodules, and the actual size of others will be incompletely assessed, to say nothing of an incomplete appreciation of the texture of the nodule. Since this book may be of interest to physicians with varying experience in the examination of the thyroid, I shall describe the technique I employ.

Initially, one should inspect the neck while the patient swallows. A nodule may be clearly visible, or one may see the slight protrusion of the lower third of the sternocleidomastoid muscle that signifies an underlying mass. The thyroid gland is examined one lobe at a time. With the opposite thumb, the larynx and thyroid should be displaced toward the side to be examined (Fig. 5-2 *A*).

Then the first two fingers of the examining hand should be inserted behind the sternocleidomastoid muscle and the lobe pushed forward into contact with the thumb. To facilitate this maneuver, one should have the patient tilt the head to the side being examined (Fig. 5-2 *B*). This will relax the sternocleidomastoid muscle. (Patients

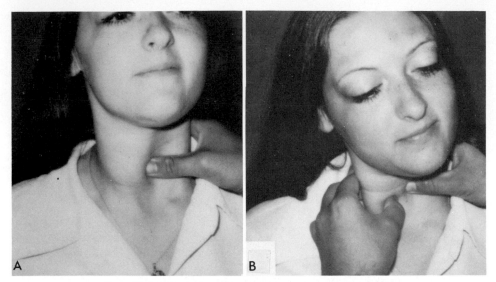

Figure 5-2. Technique for palpation of the thyroid gland.

apparently instinctively draw the head backward when a physician reaches for the neck. This makes adequate palpation virtually impossible.) The examiner then slides the fingers and thumb up toward the apex of the lobe and back down to the lower pole, judging the thickness, consistency, and nodularity as he proceeds.

For the patient who has a short neck or a low-lying thyroid it may be difficult to reach the lower poles. Having the patient swallow will be helpful. After both lobes have been examined, the isthmus may be palpated with the fingertips. Once the thyroid gland has been evaluated, one should examine the rest of the neck for enlarged lymph nodes or other palpable abnormalities. Special attention should be given to the area between the larynx and the sternocleidomastoid muscle, and the supraclavicular fossae. If the midline over the laryngeal cartilage is routinely examined, a cordlike structure extending from the thyroid up to the hyoid bone will occasionally be discovered; this is a thyroglossal duct. Cystic enlargement of this structure can present as a nodule and simulate a pathological lymph node. Carcinoma involving the thyroglossal duct does occur but is uncommon.

Reference

1. Bhagavan BS, Rao DRG and Weinberg T: Carcinoma of thyroglossal duct cyst: Case reports and review of the literature. *Surgery* 67:281–292, 1970

PHYSICAL FINDINGS

Physical findings of a rock-hard mass with multiple adjacent enlarged, rubbery, firm lymph nodes clearly mean thyroid cancer. In younger patients thyroid cancer may not be so hard, and in children these lesions may appear soft or cystic on examination. Advanced lesions tend to be internally fixed and relatively immovable. However, the usual early tumor is freely movable. If the thyroid gland is diffusely abnormal, it is more likely that a nodule is part of this diffuse process rather than a separate neoplastic entity. Of course, there may be exceptions to this guideline; therefore, any discrete thyroid nodule deserves careful evaluation.

PART III. LABORATORY EVALUATION OF THYROID NODULES

Once the balance of clinical findings suggests the necessity to consider a diagnosis of thyroid cancer, one should proceed with laboratory investigation. The primary function of laboratory study is to provide data that will reduce the clinical concern for cancer. The most useful data for this purpose is the demonstration of compensatory or autonomous function by imaging or a purely cystic lesion by ultrasound.

THE FUNCTIONAL NODULE

The Flowsheet presents the further steps necessary to evaluate nodules that appear functional ("hot") on a preliminary image. The objective is the differentiation of an AFTA from a nodule resulting from compensatory hyperplasia. AFTA are

FLOWSHEET FOR DIAGNOSIS OF FUNCTIONAL THYROID NODULES

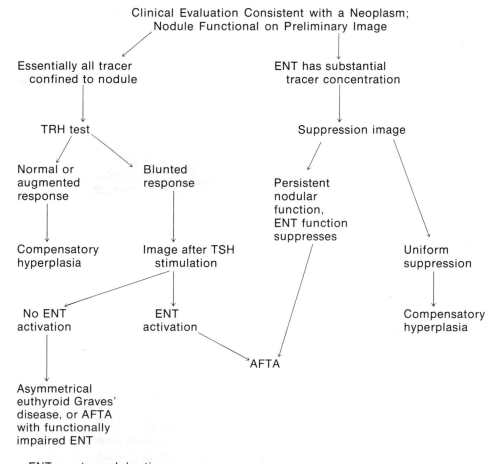

ENT = extranodular tissue
AFTA = autonomously functioning thyroid adenoma

nonsuppressible and suppress the function of extranodular tissue (ENT). Hyperplastic nodules readily suppress. For a nodule that concentrates virtually all of the tracer, a TRH test should be performed initially. If the response to this test is normal or augmented, compensatory hyperplasia is suggested as the diagnosis.

Most patients with blunted TRH responses have AFTA. An occasional patient will have asymmetrical Graves' disease, the result of either total or partial contralateral agenesis or atrophy. TSH stimulation will be helpful in the diagnosis. The ENT will respond to TSH if the patient has an AFTA (see Fig. 1–9). With asymmetrical Graves' disease there will be no activation of ENT function in response to TSH, since all tissue capable of function is already functioning. It is possible for a patient with an AFTA also to have nonfunctional ENT because of coincidental prior inflammatory disease or even a previous operation, but this is uncommon.

Note that a T_3 suppression test may be misleading if there is considerable tracer uptake by ENT. The RAI (which measures tracer uptake by the thyroid overall) may fall because of suppression of uptake by ENT while nodular uptake remains unchanged. A suppression image after 3 weeks' treatment with LT_4, 0.15 mg to 0.2 mg daily, will provide definitive data. If there is preferential suppression of ENT tracer uptake, a diagnosis of an AFTA is established (see Fig. 1–12).

Once a diagnosis of an AFTA has been confirmed, an ultrasound study may be useful. Evidence in favor of extensive cystic change suggests that the potential for toxicity is reduced. This is especially important if the AFTA is 3 cm in diameter or larger and has enough secretory activity to suppress ENT uptake relatively completely on a preliminary image.

FUNCTIONALLY NONDELINEATED NODULES

An imaging procedure may not satisfactorily define the functional activity of small nodules (smaller than 1 to 1.5 cm). If there is functioning tissue in front of or behind the nodule a functionless nodule may appear to be in an area of function. A suppression image may be helpful if the nodule has autonomous function, because the ENT will suppress while the nodule will continue to concentrate the tracer.

If there is no evidence of autonomous function, one might think that the nodule could still be a small area of compensatory hyperplasia. However, almost

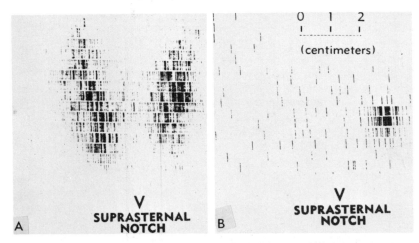

Figure 5–3. *Suppression scan of a nondelineated nodule.* A, The preliminary image. B, The suppression scan.

all small nodules that do not have autonomous function are hypofunctional. The inquisitive reader may ask how I know that this last statement is true. Hyperplastic nodules arise because of TSH stimulation. TSH does not selectively stimulate a small nodule; it stimulates all of the thyroid gland. It is increased when secretion of thyroid hormone is reduced. This occurs after partial thyroidectomy or partial destruction of thyroid tissue by chronic inflammatory disease. The remaining functional tissue undergoes hypertrophy and hyperplasia, and if the patient is euthyroid (a basic presumption when one is dealing with discrete nodules for which malignancy is a consideration), a sizeable hyperplastic nodule must be present, or else several smaller nodules. These nodules will almost always appear on a thyroid image as the tissue with best function. They will not, by definition, be small nodules obscured by better functioning tissue.

It may be asked how I can exclude a local area hypersensitive to TSH. When a well-documented study of such lesions is published, I will worry about it. Until then, I will assume that nonautonomous, functionally nondelineated nodules are hypofunctional.

THE HYPOFUNCTIONAL NODULE

Suspicious thyroid nodules that are hypofunctional on imaging and appear solid on ultrasound study usually should be removed. There is growing enthusiasm for the use of needle biopsy (Bx) (to obtain tissue for histologic evaluation) or fine needle aspiration (FNA) (to obtain material for cytologic evaluation) to assess further the probability of malignancy in thyroid nodules. I have been studying both procedures with Dr. J. Martin Miller since October of 1976. My preliminary impression is that FNA is the procedure of choice since it is much simpler, less traumatic, and less expensive. Also, the FNA procedure may be employed for nodules as small as 1 cm, whereas Bx is suitable only for nodules at least 2 cm in diameter and preferably larger. Of course, FNA does require an experienced cytologist.

With FNA or Bx it is possible with a relatively high degree of accuracy to separate non-neoplastic nodules (inflammatory, degenerative, and dysfunctional) from the neoplastic variety (benign and malignant). Although a diagnosis of cancer sometimes can be made with relative certainty, in many cases it is impossible to differentiate benign from malignant neoplasms. One should not expect otherwise, for it is well known that this may be a difficult job requiring multiple sections when the entire lesion has been removed. Therefore, I consider any findings that suggest a neoplastic lesion as evidence in favor of operation, and accept findings favoring a non-neoplastic lesion as support for observation.

The major limitation of these procedures is the potential for improper needle placement, which may produce a sampling error. Therefore, a negative finding should not reverse a strong clinical impression of malignancy. Actually, when the clinical picture is clear-cut there is no point to Bx or FNA. In doubtful situations when operation presents special risks, further study may be helpful.

Nodules that appear to be cystic by ultrasound study should be aspirated to confirm their cystic nature and reduce their size. If regression is complete or nearly complete, observation may be pursued, usually in conjunction with the administration of suppressive doses of thyroid hormone.

Whenever one elects to observe a patient with a thyroid nodule in preference to excision, he is committed to regular permanent followup. Should subsequent developments suggest that the lesion is behaving like cancer, operation may then be advised.

References

1. Miskin M, Rosen IB and Walfish PG: B-Mode ultrasonography in assessment of thyroid gland lesions. *Ann Intern Med* 79:505–510, 1973
2. Walfish PG, Miskin M, Rosen IB, et al: Application of special diagnostic techniques in the management of nodular goitre. *Can Med Assoc J* 115:35–40, 1976
3. Wang C, Vickery AL, Jr, and Maloof F: Needle biopsy of the thyroid. *Surg Gynecol Obstet* 143:365–368, 1976

PART IV.   TREATMENT OF THYROID NODULES

As already indicated, on the basis of clinical, imaging, and ultrasound data, those nodules for which there is increased concern for cancer can be separated from those that seem probably benign. Suspicious nodules are removed. Followup of cancer will be discussed below. If the nodule is benign, the patient is advised to take thyroid hormone in a dose adequate to suppress TSH (e.g., LT_4, 0.15 to 0.2 mg daily). This will prevent the development of a recurrent nodule in the remaining tissue on the basis of compensatory hyperplasia. Obviously, thyroid hormone must be taken permanently. All too often I see patients who have been advised that thyroid hormone is unnecessary after unilateral lobectomy because "enough thyroid tissue was left behind to provide all the thyroid hormone you need." This is both true (usually) and irrelevant (always). This advice may result some years later in a recurrent nodule, unnecessary concern on the part of the patient and physician, and needless expense for further testing to prove that the tissue is only an example of compensatory hyperplasia. The simple expedient of thyroid hormone administration will prevent these problems.

Nodules for which operation is not advised may be classified as follows:

1. Functional nodules that appear to be hyperplastic.
2. Purely cystic nodules.
3. Nontoxic AFTA.
4. Hypofunctional nodules that fail to fulfill the criteria for concern for malignancy, or those in patients for whom operation is contraindicated.

The treatment of these four categories of nodules varies and thus requires separate discussions.

THE FUNCTIONAL (HYPERPLASTIC) NODULE

These nodules usually arise in a thyroid gland that has suffered some insult leading to functional deterioration of part of the gland with compensatory hyperplasia of the rest, or of those portions that are least involved. The nodules appear to be functional on imaging and often seem to represent the best functioning tissue present. The differentiation from AFTA is made by a suppression study that will show that the nodular function is readily suppressible. Treatment may then be continued with LT_4, 0.15 to 0.2 mg daily; the larger dose is given to patients less than 40 years of age, whereas the smaller dose is given to older patients. For patients over 50 to 60 years (depending upon general health), I may elect simple observation unless there is evidence of hypothyroidism. Of course, any initial dose of thyroid hormone may require adjustment on the basis of subsequent evaluations. The purpose of treatment is twofold — first, to prevent further growth (this objective is usually achieved), and second, to bring about some regression of the nodule (more often than not success in this regard is only partial).

THE PURELY CYSTIC NODULE

A purely cystic lesion is usually the result of hemorrhagic degeneration of a preexisting hyperplastic or neoplastic (benign) nodule. As the lesion ages, blood is replaced by serous fluid. The principal indications for treatment are cosmetic, to allay concern by the patient, and to confirm the cystic nature of the entire lesion, thus excluding a partially cystic, partially solid nodule that might require more frequent further observation and possible future excision if there is growth. If the nodule is small, simple observation might be elected. If there is reason to do something, short of surgical excision, one might choose needle aspiration. In addition, I favor the use of thyroid hormone in younger patients to relieve the thyroid gland from further TSH stimulation, with the thought that further growth or recurrence of the nodules may be prevented. Suppression of TSH, of course, will have no direct effect upon the cystic nodule because the lesion has negligible if any TSH-dependent parenchyma. If a cystic nodule (on ultrasound examination) has arisen because of hemorrhage, a smaller, predominantly solid lesion may be left when the hemorrhage is reabsorbed. One might then advise excision, particularly if the patient is young and the nodule is hard and especially if the nodule enlarges in spite of treatment with thyroid hormone. Hence, even apparently purely cystic nodules require followup.

NONTOXIC AFTA

The autonomously functioning thyroid adenoma (AFTA) is a rather uncommon thyroid lesion. I have encountered only 234 patients with AFTA in 15 years. Of these, 32 had toxic AFTA, and 202 had nontoxic lesions. Diagnostic criteria for AFTA have been outlined earlier in this book and described in considerable detail in previous publications. It is clear that the toxic AFTA require treatment and thus have been discussed in Chapter 2. However, the majority of AFTA are nontoxic, and the treatment of these lesions deserves further discussion. Before outlining the therapeutic principles to which I adhere it will be worthwhile to discuss the potential risks of nontoxic AFTA, for this is a consideration that is basic to decisions on how aggressive one should be with treatment.

Natural History of Nontoxic AFTA

It is clear that toxic AFTA are derived from the nontoxic variety, and in effect represent the end stage of an evolutionary process that seems to begin with a lesion of microscopic dimensions. Thus, the first risk that must be considered when one makes the diagnosis of a nontoxic AFTA is that of future hyperthyroidism. That this is a potential risk is agreed, but the magnitude of the risk seems to be rather small. Several long-term studies of untreated nontoxic AFTA indi-

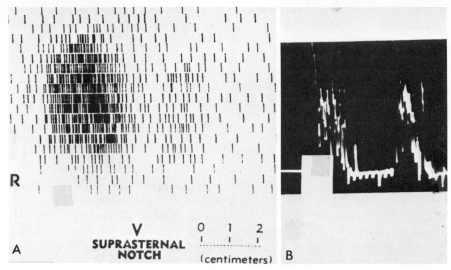

Figure 5-4. *A,* An autonomously functioning thyroid adenoma which appears solid on the scan. *B,* The ultrasound study reveals a cystic pattern.

cate that progression to toxicity is uncommon within 5 to 10 years. In fact, most untreated lesions do not seem to change very much at all. In addition, there is a second process (other than the evolutionary increase in function) that may involve a nontoxic AFTA and prevent the appreciation of its hyperfunctional potential. I refer, of course, to central degeneration. This probably results from outgrowth of blood supply with central hemorrhagic infarction and liquefaction of tissue, resulting in a functionless fluid-filled remnant. Evidence for degeneration may be provided by imaging, which reveals a central area of reduced function, or by ultrasound, which will reveal evidence of central cystic change (Fig. 5–4).

Thus, a nontoxic AFTA may follow one of three courses if left untreated:

1. No change for many years.
2. Spontaneous degeneration.
3. Progression to toxicity.

Since the first two seem much more common than the third, there is no urgent need to take definitive action for nontoxic AFTA. This holds unless the lesion appears to be in an advanced stage in the evolution toward toxicity and the patient is rather elderly, so that one might have reservations about the tolerance for any further increment in AFTA secretory activity (particularly from the cardiac standpoint). This presents a new problem. It is now necessary to establish criteria upon which to base a judgment as to how close a nontoxic AFTA is to producing toxicity.

Assessment of Secretory Activity of Nontoxic AFTA

Most toxic AFTA are 3 cm in diameter or larger; thus, the larger the lesion the greater the potential for hypersecretion. However, some large AFTA have already undergone degeneration; hence, size alone is not a reliable indicator of function. Obviously, the serum concentration of thyroid hormone gives some indication of the secretory activity of the AFTA. Since toxicity from AFTA may be of the T_3 toxicosis variety, it is necessary to have data from both the FTI and

T_3(RIA). The closer these levels are to the hyperthyroid range, the nearer the patient is to toxicity. Inspection of a baseline thyroid image provides another excellent indication of secretory activity. The more completely the function of extranodular tissue is suppressed, the closer the patient is to the toxic state.

Treatment of Nontoxic AFTA

Based upon the above observations, I have proposed the following approach to treatment of nontoxic AFTA:

1. For patients less than 40 years old, without coincidental illness that might increase the risk of hyperthyroidism (particularly heart disease) and for whom the AFTA does not fulfill criteria for imminent toxicity, I suggest observation with annual reevaluation.

2. If the AFTA is small (less than 2 cm in diameter) or if it exhibits prominent evidence of degeneration, I suggest observation at any age.

3. For patients over 40 years old who have larger lesions with enough secretory activity to suppress completely the function of the extranodular thyroid tissue, I suggest prophylactic ablative therapy, excision, or ^{131}I therapy. The final decision as to choice of therapy is usually made by the attending physician with consideration for the patient's preference. When ^{131}I is employed, an ablative dose should be given (15 to 20 mCi delivered to the AFTA) just as with toxic AFTA. After ablation of the AFTA has been achieved, permanent treatment with LT_4 is advised to prevent TSH stimulation of the inevitably irradiated extranodular tissue.

References

1. Hamburger JI and Meier DA: Cancer following treatment of an autonomously functioning thyroid nodule with sodium iodide I[131]. *Arch Surg* 103:762–764, 1971
2. Hamburger JI: Solitary autonomously functioning thyroid lesions. *Am J Med* 58:740–748, 1975

HYPOFUNCTIONAL NODULES THAT ARE PROBABLY NOT MALIGNANT

It is agreed by thoughtful and informed physicians that selective removal is the proper and practical approach for thyroid nodules. Selective removal implies the establishment of criteria upon which to base a decision about whether any given nodule is more or less likely to represent a neoplasm. If the physician accepts the principle of selective removal, he must realize that even though he achieves considerable success in patient selection he will not be infallible. Therefore, a decision against operation is not irrevocable. Far from it, the decision *against* prompt excision is equivalent to a decision *for* permanent regular observation. I hasten to add that this need not be an undue burden for the patient. My approach to the patient with a nodule I consider unlikely to be malignant consists of the following elements:

1. The patient is informed that my opinion, based upon the history, physical examination, and testing, and evaluated in the light of my personal experience, is that the nodule seems likely to be benign. Nevertheless, the only way to exclude thyroid cancer with absolute certainty is excision. However, surgical removal

also carries a small risk, and it is my judgment that the risk of the nodule might be less than the risk of the operation. Therefore, I believe that operation is not mandatory at this time and advise observation.

2. If the patient is unwilling to accept the risk of observation and prefers the risk of operation, I send him or her to the surgeon with my blessing.

3. If the patient is agreeable to observation, I then emphasize that the first principle of observation is that I reserve the right to change my mind if future events indicate that operation might be preferable to further observation. Similarly, I indicate that I also respect the right of the patient to change his or her mind on the matter.

4. Having cleared the air of the preliminaries, I then advise suppressive doses of LT_4 (e.g., 0.15 mg daily) to provide a controlled condition for observation. Since these are hypofunctional nodules by definition, I do not expect them to subside because thyroid hormone is given. On the other hand, I am not surprised if they do regress. Some have arisen on the basis of unappreciated inflammatory disease, either localized subacute thyroiditis or Hashimoto's disease. Others may represent hemorrhagic cysts. Thus, regression might have occurred even without the thyroid hormone. If such a fortunate turn of events should occur, everyone is pleased. Regardless of any regression, I continue the thyroid hormone for life on the presumption that TSH stimulation might have played a role in the genesis of the nodule, and TSH suppression may prevent a recurrence of this nodule or the development of others. I am satisfied as long as there is no growth of the nodule and no development of other nodules, either within the thyroid or in adjacent tissue (e.g., in lymph nodes). Growth in spite of TSH suppression by thyroid hormone is an unfavorable development that requires consideration of operation. If the patient is elderly (over 50 years old) or has a coexistent cardiac infirmity, I forgo thyroid hormone administration and simply observe.

5. The patient is advised to return initially in 3 months so that I can assess the tolerance to thyroid hormone and exclude the unlikely possibility that the nodule will enlarge rapidly. If all is well, I advise annual reevaluation.

PART V.   TREATMENT OF THYROID CANCER

ANAPLASTIC THYROID CANCER

There is no need to discuss the treatment of anaplastic cancer. These tumors are always rapidly fatal, and the course is uninfluenced by treatment. For more details on this oncologic disaster the interested reader is referred to a recent article.

Reference

1. Kyriakides G: Anaplastic carcinoma of thyroid. *Ann Surg* 179:295–299, 1974

MEDULLARY THYROID CANCER

Medullary thyroid cancer is also a relatively aggressive tumor which has the potential to kill. Timely and adequate surgical treatment can be curative. Current interest centers on the utlility of the serum calcitonin assay, both in the diagnosis of medullary cancer and in the evaluation of the adequacy of operative management.

Medullary cancer may be familial, and when this is the case elevated serum calcitonin levels will indicate the presence of the disease even in asymptomatic relatives without palpable abnormalities of the thyroid. Operation in such early cases offers an excellent chance for cure. As long as the disease is confined to the thyroid, thyroidectomy is as effective as it is with differentiated thyroid cancer. When medullary cancer extends beyond the thyroid, the prognosis becomes more ominous. Formal radical neck dissection is justified for these cancers if there are positive lymph nodes. The calcitonin assay may be of value in determining the adequacy of the operation and also (by selective venous catheter sampling) in determining the site of residual tumor when present.

Medullary cancer responds neither to ^{131}I nor to thyroid hormone. Since it is believed that the parafollicular cells that give rise to medullary cancer are of neuroectodermal origin and are not derived from the thyroid follicle, it is understandable that these tumors do not exhibit properties characteristic of thyroid follicular tissue.

References

1. Goltzman D, Potts JT, Jr, Ridgway EC and Maloof F: Calcitonin as a tumor marker. *New Eng J Med* 290:1035–1039, 1974
2. Hill CS, Jr, Ibanez ML, Samaan NA, Ahearn MJ and Clark RL: Medullary (solid) carcinoma of the thyroid gland: An analysis of the M.D. Anderson Hospital experience with patients with the tumor, its special features, and its histogenesis. *Medicine* 52:141–171, 1973

DIFFERENTIATED THYROID CANCER (PAPILLARY OR FOLLICULAR)

The differentiated thyroid cancers, papillary and follicular, constitute the vast majority of the lesions encountered in an unselected ambulatory practice. The natural history of differentiated thyroid cancer is protracted and is compatible with a long survival regardless of how the patient is treated. Yet everyone with experience has encountered the exceptional patient with differentiated cancer which for no obvious reason follows a more abbreviated and lethal course. This combination of a generally favorable prognosis, punctuated by uncommon but unpredictable exceptions, makes it difficult to assess the efficacy of any therapeutic regimen. Because of this uncertainty (or ignorance if you will), controversy abounds in the literature as to what constitutes optimal treatment for this disease.

This controversy involves all three major modalities of treatment — thyroidectomy, ^{131}I therapy, and thyroid hormone.

Table 5–3 outlines some of the issues generating the most heat.

Table 5–3 includes only the highlights of the current controversy. The details could easily fill a volume. In fact, I nearly succeeded in doing just that in

**TABLE 5-3. CONTROVERSIAL ASPECTS OF TREATMENT OF
DIFFERENTIATED THYROID CANCER**

I. CONTROVERSIES ON SURGICAL MANAGEMENT
   A. What is the proper primary operation?
      1. Operation unnecessary for most patients
      2. Lobectomy with or without isthmectomy
      3. Routine total thyroidectomy
   B. How should one deal with cervical node metastases?
      1. Prophylactic radical (modified) neck dissection
      2. Excision of grossly involved nodes, "berry-picking" as necessary

II. CONTROVERSIES ON ^{131}I THERAPY
   A. What are the indications?
      1. Rarely if ever is ^{131}I useful
      2. Only for known metastases concentrating ^{131}I
      3. For all postsurgical remnants concentrating ^{131}I
   B. How can one best promote ^{131}I uptake by the tumor?
      1. Administer exogenous TSH
      2. Permit hypothyroidism to promote endogenous TSH release
      3. Induce rebound after diuretic-induced stable iodide depletion
   C. What dose of ^{131}I should be given?
      1. An empirical dose given at arbitrary intervals until arbitrary and empirical criteria
         for ablation are fulfilled
      2. Variable doses depending upon the mass of the tumor and its ability to concen-
         trate ^{131}I

III. CONTROVERSIES ON THYROID ADMINISTRATION
   A. Thyroid hormone is the only treatment most patients require.
   B. Withhold thyroid hormone after operation to promote endogenous TSH stimulation
      of ^{131}I uptake by tumor.
   C. Do not withhold thyroid hormone after operation. Endogenous TSH stimulation
      may promote cancer growth and spread.

a recent book (74 pages) to which the reader may refer if he wishes further discussion and a bibliography on this subject.

In this book, which is concerned with the office management of thyroid disease and addressed primarily to the practicing physician, not the thyroidologist, an in-depth discussion of surgical or ^{131}I therapy technique is inappropriate. I shall limit myself to a brief listing of the principles of operation and ^{131}I therapy and then comment upon followup.

References

1. Hamburger JI: *Nontoxic Goiter — Concept and Controversy.* Springfield, Ill., Charles C Thomas, 1973, pp 125–199
2. Franssila KO: Is the differentiation between papillary and follicular thyroid carcinoma valid? *Cancer* 2:853–864, 1973

Surgical Principles

1. The high incidence of occult multifocal disease has prompted most surgeons to remove more than the ipsilateral lobe with the isthmus whenever a diagnosis of differentiated cancer is confirmed during the operation. If there is no gross involvement of the contralateral lobe, the decision to perform subtotal excision is largely a matter of preference. Of course, if gross bilateral involvement is evident, a total thyroidectomy is necessary.

2. Sometimes after lobectomy (including the isthmus) the frozen section suggests a benign lesion, but several days later a diagnosis of thyroid carcinoma is established. The physician must then decide whether additional surgical treatment is needed. If at the time of the initial operation careful palpation revealed neither positive ipsilateral cervical nodes nor contralateral thyroid nodularity, I would advise thyroid hormone and observation. This advice might be altered if the pathologist has reason to believe that the lesion is particularly aggressive.

3. In cases of cervical node involvement with differentiated thyroid cancer there is growing agreement that the less disfiguring, modified neck dissection is no less successful than the formal radical procedure.

4. In cases of recurrence after a limited excision, the thyroidectomy should be completed and modified neck dissection performed if the recurrence is in the cervical nodes. If a neck dissection has already been done, "berry-picking" may be satisfactory.

Principles of [131]I Therapy

I shall merely list the policies I currently advocate, with no claim that they are the only or even the best possible methods. I do not believe that any single physician can live long enough to follow enough patients for enough time to make that claim.

1. I no longer administer ^{131}I therapy for residual ^{131}I-concentrating tissue confined to the area occupied by the thyroid gland preoperatively, unless it seems probable that the tumor was incompletely excised and that further excision is not possible.

2. If there is palpable tumor tissue in the neck, I advise a repeat operation rather than therapy with ^{131}I, even if the tissue concentrates [131]I.

3. I reserve ^{131}I for impalpable, unexcisable, reasonably definite residual tumor in the neck and for distant metastases. Of course, ^{131}I is given only if there is evidence of adequate uptake of a tracer dose to suggest the possibility of a therapeutic effect.

4. Using these criteria, I am treating fewer patients with ^{131}I than in the past in the expectation that I shall not regret it at some future date.

Once thyroidectomy, with or without subsequent ^{131}I therapy, has been completed, treatment with thyroid hormone (usually LT_4 in full replacement dosage) is instituted for life.

References

1. Leeper RD: The effect of ^{131}I therapy on survival of patients with metastatic papillary or follicular thyroid carcinoma. *J Clin Endocrinol Metab* 36:1143–1152, 1973
2. Hamburger JI: Diuretic augmentation of ^{131}I uptake in inoperable thyroid cancer. *New Eng J Med* 280:1091–1094, 1969

Miscellaneous Measures Occasionally Employed For Thyroid Cancer

External Radiation

This treatment may be considered for palliation of anaplastic or other inoperable forms of thyroid cancer. With differentiated cancer it is important not to use x-ray therapy until every effort has been made to assess the possibility of employing ^{131}I, because ^{131}I has the potential to deliver far more radiation more safely than external radiation. Also, if external radiation therapy is given first it may impair uptake of ^{131}I by the tumor. Lymphoma, of course is another indication for external radiation therapy.

Chemotherapy

Chemotherapy for thyroid cancer continues to be studied. Data at this time indicate that no important benefit has been achieved.

Reference

1. Gottlieb JA and Hill CS, Jr: Chemotherapy of thyroid cancer with adriamycin. *New Eng J Med* 290:193–197, 1974

Followup Management of Thyroid Cancer Patients

All cancer patients are asked to return for annual examinations. I routinely examine the neck for any evidence of recurrence and obtain a chest radiograph, a serum calcium value (to rule out late onset hypoparathyroidism), and a blood count if ^{131}I therapy has been given. After I am satisfied that all necessary and possible treatment has been accomplished with excision and [131]I (if indicated), I do not repeat thyroid imaging on followup examinations unless there is clinical evidence of a recurrence, by either palpation of the neck or chest x-ray, or from a finding suggesting distant metastasis.

MANAGEMENT OF HYPOPARATHYROIDISM

I have chosen to discuss hypoparathyroidism at this point because it occurs rather commonly after the extensive surgical treatment that is often necessary for thyroid cancer patients.

Hypoparathyroidism Occurring Immediately After Operation (Possibly Transient)

1. Intravenous calcium gluconate will usually control tetany.
2. Calcium lactate, 2.4 gm, four times daily (one-half hour before meals and at bedtime without food) should be started immediately.
3. Parenteral parathyroid hormone may be used at bedtime if tetany is persistent, at least until calcium levels are restored to normal, with oral calcium in conjunction with vitamin D if necessary.

Permanent Hypoparathyroidism

1. Calcium lactate should be administered as described previously.
2. Vitamin D, 50,000 to 200,000 units, may be employed daily as necessary to maintain serum calcium levels between 8.5 and 9.5 mg per 100 ml. Higher

serum calcium levels, in the absence of parathyroid hormone, may produce hypercalciuria and nephrocalcinosis.

Problems in the Management of Hypoparathyroidism

1. Calcium lactate is the preferred oral calcium medication. It contains 18 per cent calcium by weight, twice as much as calcium gluconate. Since about 2 grams of calcium is needed daily, and the largest calcium lactate tablet contains 600 mg (about 110 mg of calcium), 16 tablets daily is the minimum dose. It should be taken in four divided doses (as already noted) about one-half hour before meals and at bedtime without food. It is essential to administer calcium in the interdigestive period. If calcium is given along with food the alkaline secretions of the gastrointestinal tract may block calcium absorption. Failure to appreciate this point is the cause of much of the difficulty physicians have in controlling hypoparathyroidism.

2. Dissolution of the calcium tablets may not be complete if they are swallowed whole. Chewing will solve this problem. If this is unpleasant, they may be ground and placed in capsules.

3. If the serum phosphorus value is elevated, it is almost always because the serum calcium is too low. One should check on the patient's timing of calcium ingestion, the type of calcium, and the dosage. If these are satisfactory, then a larger dose of vitamin D is necessary. Restricting the dietary phosphorus is usually not only unnecessary but also distracts the physician from searching for the actual cause of the elevated serum phosphorus level.

PART VI. EXPERIENCE WITH THE DIAGNOSIS OF THYROID NODULES AND THE TREATMENT OF THYROID CANCER

DIAGNOSIS OF THYROID NODULES

The age and sex distribution of 1094 patients with discrete thyroid nodules is given in Table 5–4.

In this table the patients have been segregated in three classes on the basis of relative concern for cancer, Class I being those for whom there is the most suspicion and Class III the least (including autonomous nodules that do not require separate classification for this purpose). Nodules were included in Class III whenever the risk to the patient from the nodule was thought to be less than the risk of thyroidectomy (considering the age of the patient and the presence of other illness). Note that almost 60 per cent of the patients with Class I nodules were less than 40 years old, whereas for Class II nodules the figure is 37 per cent and for Class III nodules it is 28 per cent. There is a somewhat greater proportion of males in Class I patients.

TABLE 5-4.   AGE AND SEX DISTRIBUTION OF 1094 PATIENTS WITH DISCRETE THYROID NODULES

AGE (YEARS)	CLASS I		CLASS II		CLASS III	
	M	F	M	F	M	F
<20	14	31	2	10	2	8
20–39	24	160	13	114	8	87
40–59	23	100	23	160	30	148
60+	6	17	8	33	4	69
Total	67	308	46	317	44	312

Histologic data were available for 336 Class I patients, and of these, 111 had cancer (33 per cent). Among Class II patients, 15 of 190 had malignancies (7.9 per cent). Only 3 of 59 Class III patients had cancer. Two of these patients were women in their 70's. Observation was quickly abandoned when it became clear that the lesions were rapidly growing. Both were anaplastic cancers and proved rapidly fatal. The third cancer was an 0.5 cm occult papillary lesion in the center of a 2.5 cm AFTA. The majority of patients with Class III nodules have been followed without operation, some for up to 15 years, with no important changes in the lesions.

This experience indicates that it is possible to classify patients with thyroid nodules on the basis of clinical and laboratory data so that those with a high risk of cancer may be advised to have operative treatment and those with less suspicious lesions may be treated with observation only. The advice given to patients with Class II lesions depends largely upon the patient's age and general health. For younger healthy patients I am more likely to recommend prompt surgical intervention.

Diagnostic ultrasonography has been helpful in avoiding unnecessary operations for patients with clinically suspicious nodules. A purely cystic pattern indicates a lower risk of cancer. Central hemorrhage may produce sudden enlargement of a nodule, and in such a case, an ultrasound study will reveal a cystic pattern. As the blood is absorbed, the ultrasound pattern may revert to that of a partially or predominantly solid lesion. Although most hemorrhagic nodules are benign, one cannot exclude the possibility of a focal malignancy. Therefore, cystic nodules require followup and may ultimately require excision if there is evidence of growth. More experience is needed with observation, aspiration, and excision of cystic nodules before the risk of these lesions can be defined properly. Therefore, although diagnostic ultrasound seems to be a valuable adjunct in the evaluation of thyroid nodules, the limits of its reliability in the diagnosis of cancer remain incompletely established. At this time I consider data from ultrasound to be simply one additional bit of information in the overall assessment of the patient.

Reference

1. Miskin M, Rosen IB and Walfish PG: B-mode ultrasonography in assessment of thyroid gland lesions. *Ann Intern Med* 79:505–510, 1973

TREATMENT OF THYROID CANCER

The data in my series of thyroid cancer patients (see Tables 5–5 through 5–11) are subject to several important limitations:

1. These patients were operated upon by many surgeons. Therefore, some variation in surgical approach can be expected. In addition, different pathologists classified tissue sections somewhat differently. For example, one pathologist's papillary cancer might be no different from another's mixed papillary and follicular carcinoma (or adenocarcinoma or even follicular carcinoma). Therefore, I have chosen to group these patients into the single category of differentiated thyroid cancer. Since the prognosis in this group of patients was uniformly good, subclassification does not seem to be essential for clinical purposes. In contrast, the poorer prognosis for patients with Hürthle cell lesions justifies a separate classification, in my opinion.

2. Six patients with lymphoma and one with metastatic cancer to the thyroid (from the lung) are not included. It is enough to say that the lymphomas were in older patients who experienced temporary improvement from x-ray therapy but ultimately died of their disease. The patient with metastatic lung cancer also died.

3. Not all patients were seen when the diagnosis was first established. Some were examined for the first time years later. This introduces a bias in favor of patients with a more favorable prognosis.

4. Followup has been incomplete. Some patients were referred only for diagnosis and others only for consultation at a single point during the course of the disease. These facts simply reflect the variable nature of the relationship between a large number of attending physicians and a consultant.

In spite of these limitations, I believe that this rather sizeable experience will serve to illustrate a number of clinically useful points.

Table 5–5 gives the age and sex distribution for 250 patients with thyroid cancer seen at Northland Thyroid Laboratory in the 13-year period ending July, 1974. In each case the age cited is the age at which cancer was first diagnosed.

Note that Hürthle cell and anaplastic lesions were seen only in women. The anaplastic cancers occurred predominantly in elderly patients, and Hürthle cell lesions also occurred more often in older patients. By contrast, 58 per cent of the patients with differentiated lesions were less than 40 years old.

Table 5–6 indicates that a consultant may see patients with thyroid cancer at varying stages in the disease and for a variety of reasons. The majority, of

TABLE 5–5. AGE AND SEX DISTRIBUTION FOR 250 PATIENTS WITH THYROID CANCER

AGE (YEARS)	DIFFERENTIATED		HÜRTHLE	ANAPLASTIC	MEDULLARY	
	M	F	F	F	M	F
<20	6	14	0	0	0	1
20–29	9	49	1	0	1	0
30–39	16	40	1	0	0	1
40–49	6	40	2	1	0	0
50–59	14	23	3	0	0	0
60–69	2	5	2	1	1	1
70+	1	6	0	3	0	0
Total	54	177	9	5	2	3

TABLE 5-6. MANNER OF PRESENTATION OF 250 THYROID CANCER PATIENTS

Discrete thyroid nodule		128
Class I	111	
Class II	15	
Class III	2	
Referral after diagnosis and initial operation elsewhere		97
Enlarged cervical lymph node		10
Pulmonary metastases noted on chest x-ray		1
Incidental to operation for another reason		14
Hyperthyroidism	5	
Obstruction	3	
Benign nodule	2	
Parathyroid adenoma	2	
AFTA	1	
Scalene node biopsy	1	

course, were seen initially for evaluation of a recently discovered nodule. Others were referred after the diagnosis had been made elsewhere, with a request for help with the postoperative management. In some cases, evidence of metastatic disease precipitated referral, whereas in others the discovery of cancer was incidental to thyroidectomy for another reason.

Total thyroidectomy was by far the predominant operation when feasible. In some instances only lobectomy was done because of a mistaken diagnosis of a benign tumor on frozen section. When it was later learned that the lesion was malignant, observation was preferred to immediate reoperation for reasons discussed earlier in this chapter.

In 113 patients thyroid hormone alone was the only treatment. Iodine-131 was given to 70 patients, some of whom were treated elsewhere and for whom I would not have advised this treatment. I must add that I would not now give ^{131}I to many of those that I chose to treat in this manner in years past. I no longer recommend ^{131}I for residual ^{131}I-concentrating tissue that may represent only residual normal tissue. The excellent survival record for my patients with differentiated thyroid cancer (no deaths yet from the cancer itself) suggests that these patients either are diagnosed very early or have less aggressive tumors than those reported by others. Hence, greater conservatism in the use of ^{131}I may be suitable. Avoidance of ^{131}I reduces the inconvenience and cost of the disease, to say nothing of the discomfort to the patient during repeated periods of hypothyroidism necessary for treatment and followup.

Note that 21 patients had a repeat operation for recurrent masses in the neck. In one of these the mass was benign tissue. An additional three patients had recurrent cancer that was considered inoperable. Of the 23 patients who had recurrent cancer, 12 had undergone total thyroidectomy as the primary procedure, while four patients had a less extensive operation; in seven patients the extent of the primary operation could not be determined. It appears that the extent of the primary operation was not a critical factor in the development of recurrent or persistent disease. It is probable that the extent of the disease at the time of diagnosis was more important. For example, it seems unlikely that those patients who had evidence of pulmonary spread prior to operation or soon afterward could have been cured regardless of the extent of the operation.

The data indicate the necessity for long-term followup before concluding that a cure has been achieved.

Table 5-10 gives the duration of followup for the 189 known survivors, of whom ten are known to have residual tumor.

TABLE 5-7. EXTENT OF PRIMARY OPERATION

Total thyroidectomy with or without cervical node dissection	145
Lobectomy	31
Limited resection or biopsy only	12
Bilateral subtotal thyroidectomy	9
Ipsilateral total lobectomy, contralateral subtotal lobectomy	5
Extent unknown	48
Total	250

TABLE 5-8. POSTOPERATIVE TREATMENT

LT_4 only	113
^{131}I, then LT_4	66
External radiation, then LT_4	10
^{131}I followed by external radiation, then LT_4	1
Repeat operation, then LT_4	16
Repeat operation followed by ^{131}I, then LT_4	3
Repeat operation, then external radiation	1
Repeat operation for benign disease	1
Treatment unknown	39
Total	250

TABLE 5-9. TIME LAPSE BETWEEN PRIMARY OPERATION AND CLINICAL EVIDENCE OF A RECURRENCE

TIME LAPSE (YEARS)	NUMBER OF PATIENTS
<1	5
1–2	9
3–5	1
5–10	6
18–20	2
Total	23

TABLE 5-10. DURATION OF FOLLOWUP FOR 189 LIVING THYROID CANCER PATIENTS

DURATION OF FOLLOWUP (YEARS)	NUMBER OF PATIENTS[a]
<5	92 (5)
5–10	74 (3)
11–20	19 (2)
>20	4
Total	189 (10)

[a]Numbers in parentheses indicate patients with known residual tumor.

TABLE 5-11. CAUSE OF DEATH FOR 19 THYROID CANCER PATIENTS

Anaplastic cancer		5
Hürthle cell cancer		3
Medullary cancer		1
Miscellaneous, not		9
due to thyroid cancer		
Stroke	3	
Cardiac causes	3	
Lung cancer	1	
Breast cancer	1	
Brain tumor	1	
Cause unknown		1
Total		19

No followup is available for 43 patients, and 19 patients are dead. The cause of death is given in Table 5-11.

None of the ten patients who had differentiated cancer and subsequently died are known to have died of thyroid cancer (although for one patient the cause of death could not be determined).

This experience permits the following conclusions:

1. Patients with anaplastic thyroid cancer can be expected to die from the disease within 1 year.

2. Patients with Hürthle cell lesions have a poorer prognosis than those with differentiated cancer. Three of nine such patients have died from this disease.

3. Patients with medullary cancer also may have a poor prognosis, although early and extensive surgical treatment may be curative.

4. Patients with papillary or follicular cancer generally can be expected to do well in terms of survival. The prognosis for recurrent or persistent disease seems to depend primarily upon the extent of the involvement at the time of diagnosis. The type of operation performed appears to be less important.

PART VII.   SELF-ASSESSMENT

CASE 5-1. INCIDENTAL THYROID CANCER

April, 1973. A 29 year old woman had a bilateral subtotal thyroidectomy for toxic diffuse goiter. The pathologist reported a papillary carcinoma 0.5 cm in diameter in the right lobe of the thyroid. Six weeks after the operation, a scan of the neck revealed bilateral uptake of ^{131}I in areas that were consistent with normal thyroid tissue deliberately left by the surgeon. The patient was clinically and biochemically euthyroid.

With which of the following statements do you agree?

a. Further surgical treatment is mandatory.

b. The residual thyroid tissue should be ablated with ^{131}I.

    c. A full replacement dose of thyroid hormone (e.g., 0.15 or 0.2 mg of levothyroxine daily) should be given.

    d. External radiation therapy should be given.

    e. Thyroid cancer is exceedingly uncommon in association with TDG.

    f. The prognosis for an occult lesion of this type is very good.

    g. The chance of a recurrence may be as great as 15 per cent.

    h. If ^{131}I therapy had been given, this dilemma could have been avoided.

Case 5–1 — Comment

Once or twice a year we receive a referral of this type. Our cancer group now includes 15 such patients. None have had any evidence of recurrent cancer. I have advised observation. Thyroid hormone is given only if the patient is hypothyroid. Occult tumors of this type may be found in a small proportion of the thyroid glands in the population at large, and they seem not to have significant biologic potential for malignant behavior. If this were not so, there would be many more patients with clinically evident thyroid cancer, and the mortality from this disease would be much higher.

Some authorities ablate all residual thyroid tissue with ^{131}I in patients who have thyroid cancer. I do not follow this policy. It is my opinion that this treatment is unnecessary for most of these patients, and that those few who do develop recurrences can as easily be treated at that time.

Since this patient was euthyroid, no treatment was given. In the subsequent 3 years, there has been no evidence of recurrent cancer.

Had she received ^{131}I therapy initially, to be sure, this problem would not have occurred. We would simply not have known about it. Since we know that as many as 1 or 2 per cent of patients harbor microcancers of this type, it is reasonable to assume that of the 2000 patients we have treated with ^{131}I, as many as 40 might have had coincidental cancer. To date, I have not detected a single cancer on followup examination of patients with TDG who were treated with [131]I. One patient with a toxic AFTA had clinically evident cancer 3 years and 9 months after ^{131}I therapy. This case was published because of the possibility that the treatment might have played a role in the development of the cancer. The conditions unique to AFTA that might justify such an inference have been discussed on page 79.

In any event, the discovery of only one cancer in so many patients suggests either that these microcancers are not biologically aggressive or that ^{131}I might have ablated those small lesions.

Selected Current References for Case 5–1

1. Shapiro SJ, Friedman NB, Perzik SL and Catz B: Incidence of thyroid carcinoma in Graves' disease. *Cancer* 26:1261–1270, 1970

   These authors found thyroid cancer in 9 per cent of 172 patients who had had a total thyroidectomy for Graves' disease, an extraordinary incidence. Most were grossly evident, but there were four microcancers, a figure in line with the expectation of 2 per cent in the population at large.

2. Simonowitz D, Thomsen S, Moossa AR, et al: The treatment of incidental thyroid cancer. *Arch Surg* 11:477–483, 1976

   This paper is primarily of interest because of the discussion in which the occult papillary cancer is considered. The high frequency with which such lesions can be found if a careful search is made is emphasized. A proper skepticism is maintained as to the biologic potential for malignant behavior of these lesions.

3. Sampson RJ, Key CR, Buncher CR, et al: Smallest forms of papillary carcinoma of the thyroid. *Arch Path* 91:334–339, 1971

   This provocative study of Japanese exposed to atomic bomb radiation suggests that these microscopic lesions may be initiated by radiation but require an additional provocative factor for them to grow and become invasive.

4. Hamburger JI and Meier DA: Cancer following treatment of autonomously functioning thyroid nodule with sodium iodide [131]I. *Arch Surg* 103:131–139, 1972

This paper reports our patient with a toxic AFTA who developed thyroid cancer after ^{131}I therapy. The reasons why we thought that the radiation therapy might have been causal in this special situation are presented.

CASE 5–2. PAPILLARY THYROID CANCER, MULTIFOCAL WITH CERVICAL NODE METASTASES

March, 1973. A 38 year old man had a thyroid nodule that was first discovered in 1970. He was treated with thyroid hormone for 3 years. On this treatment the nodule enlarged about 50 per cent. When first seen by me, the lesion was 2.5 cm in diameter, firm, and located lateral to the upper pole of the right lobe of the thyroid. It was functionless on thyroid scanning and solid on ultrasound examination.

April, 1973. A total thyroidectomy with bilateral cervical node excision revealed a multifocal papillary cancer with bilateral cervical lymph node metastases. Six weeks after the operation scanning of the neck and chest revealed no concentration of the tracer other than in a small midline focus suggestive of a pyramidal lobe. A 72-hour urine collection contained 92 per cent of the tracer.

With which of the following statements do you agree?

a. Bilateral cervical node metastases make the prognosis for more than a 10-year survival very poor.

b. The patient should have a bilateral radical neck dissection.

c. The patient should have a bilateral modified radical neck dissection (sparing the sternocleidomastoid muscles and internal jugular veins).

d. The patient should have a right modified radical neck dissection (the side of the primary).

e. The patient should have chemotherapy.

f. The patient should have ^{131}I therapy.

g. The patient should have external radiation therapy.

h. The patient should be given levothyroxine, 0.2 mg daily, and followed.

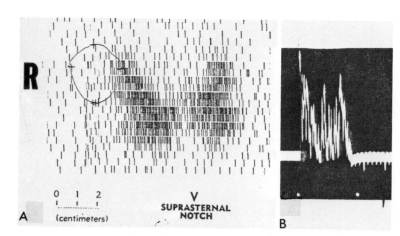

Figure 5–5. *A*, The scan. *B*, The ultrasound study.

i. If no additional excisional therapy is undertaken at this time, there is 50 per cent chance of a clinically evident recurrence.

j. Same as i, but a 10 per cent chance.

k. If a bilateral neck dissection is performed, the chance that additional foci of cancer will be found might be as high as 50 per cent.

l. Same as k, but no greater than 10 per cent.

Case 5–2 — Followup

The patient was given levothyroxine, 0.2 mg daily, and observed.

May, 1974. A 2.5-cm nodule was detected in the right side of the neck. A modified neck dissection was performed and proved that the nodule represented recurrent papillary cancer in a lymph node. No other positive nodes were found. Postoperatively, LT_4, 0.2 mg daily, was continued. In the 2 years that have passed, there has been no palpable evidence of recurrent tumor in the neck. Serial chest radiographs have been normal.

The presence of cervical node metastases from papillary cancer does not significantly alter the good prognosis for these lesions. It is very unlikely that such a patient will succumb to his thyroid cancer within even 20 years.

The argument in favor of prophylactic neck dissection (almost all surgeons favor the modified type) is the high frequency with which additional foci of cancer may be found in lymph nodes (50 per cent). The argument against prophylactic neck dissection is that clinical recurrences are seen in only about 10 per cent of these patients. Since these recurrences are likely to be just as amenable to excision when they become clinically evident as before, it seems unnecessary to subject all of these patients to further operative treatment to prevent recurrences in 10 per cent.

Chemotherapy has not been helpful in patients with papillary cancer. Perhaps the occasional patient who develops inoperable widespread metastases may be considered for such treatment if ^{131}I proves useless.

In this patient there is little likelihood that ^{131}I ablation of the pyramidal lobe activity (the only tissue concentrating the tracer) would have been beneficial.

There are a few enthusiasts for local external radiation therapy for patients with extensive thyroid cancer. I do not favor its use until it is certain that ^{131}I cannot be employed effectively. Since ^{131}I can deliver more radiation to the target tissue per unit of radiation to adjacent normal tissue, ^{131}I is the radiation therapy of choice. Premature use of external radiation may impair the ^{131}I concentrating capacity of the tissue. I restrict the use of external radiation therapy to patients with inoperable recurrent disease or those who have repeated recurrences in spite of extensive excision.

Selected Current References for Case 5–2

1. Franssila KO: Prognosis in thyroid carcinoma. *Cancer* 36:1138–1146, 1975
2. Richardson JE, Beaugie JM, Brown CL, et al: Thyroid cancer in young patients in Great Britain. *Brit J Surg* 61:85–89, 1974

   These two papers emphasize the good prognosis for differentiated thyroid cancer in the young.

3. Buckwalter JA and Thomas CG, Jr: Selection of surgical treatment for well differentiated thyroid carcinomas. *Ann Surg* 14:565–578, 1972

   This article contains a well-reasoned approach to the selection of an operative procedure for differentiated thyroid cancer, depending upon the extent of involvement and patient age. Emphasis is given to the necessity for long-term followup (more than 10 years) before differences in morbidity and mortality resulting from various operations become evident. A spirited discussion of the paper is included.

4. Crile G, Jr: Changing end results in patients with papillary carcinoma of the thyroid. *Surg Gynecol Obstet* 132:460–468, 1971

   This is a plea for conservative operations and thyroid feeding. Crile suggests that the increasing proportion of long-term survivals from papillary cancer may be related to the increased incidence of the disease resulting from the extensive use of radiation therapy to the upper body. Those tumors that seem to have occurred as a result of radiation therapy tend to be more readily curable than those of an earlier era.

5. Attie JN, Khafif RA and Steckler RM: Elective neck dissection in papillary carcinoma of the thyroid. *Am J Surg* 122:464–471, 1971
6. Noguchi S, Noguchi A and Murakami N: Papillary carcinoma of the thyroid. II. Value of prophylactic lymph node excision. *Cancer* 26:1061–1064, 1970
7. Block MA, Miller JM and Horn RC, Jr: Thyroid carcinoma with cervical lymph node metastasis. *Am J Surg* 122:458–463, 1971
8. Block MA, Miller JM and Horn RC, Jr: Significance of mediastinal lymph node metastases in carcinoma of the thyroid. *Am J Surg* 123:702–705, 1972

These four articles deal with the problem of lymph node metastases from differentiated thyroid cancer. Careful reading of these papers provides reassurance that these metastases are not really such an ominous finding.

CASE 5–3. PAPILLARY CANCER WITH PULMONARY METASTASES

September, 1973. A 35 year old woman had a 4-cm, firm mass in the left side of the neck that was hypofunctional on scanning. A total thyroidectomy was attempted. There were bilateral foci of papillary cancer with positive lymph nodes on the left side. A postoperative chest film revealed multiple nodules.

November, 1973. A scan of the neck and chest revealed that most of the right lobe was intact and there were multiple foci of tracer uptake in the left side

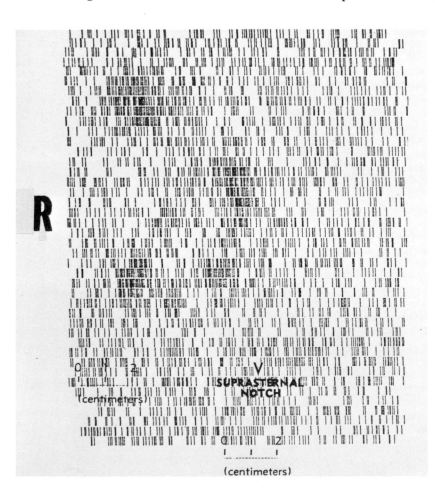

Figure 5–6. The neck scan reveals multiple foci of ^{131}I concentration.

of the neck. There was bilateral pulmonary uptake of ^{131}I. A further attempt at excision of the cervical thyroid tissue was advised.

January, 1974. Considerable additional normal tissue and a number of positive lymph nodes were removed.

March, 1974. Multiple foci of ^{131}I-concentrating tissue were seen in the neck (Fig. 5–6), and there were bilateral foci of tracer uptake in the lungs (Fig. 5–7).

The uptake of ^{131}I in the neck was 3 per cent. There was no increment in response to TSH stimulation, but after diuretic preparation, the uptake increased to 5 per cent. The 72-hour urine collection contained 80 per cent of the tracer. A dose of 200 mCi of ^{131}I was given.

With which of the following statements do you agree?

a. Pulmonary metastases from papillary cancer do not significantly alter the prognosis.

b. The chances of successful ablation of the multiple pulmonary metastases with ^{131}I are poor.

c. The chances for survival of this patient for 10 years are probably less than 25 per cent.

d. If necessary, the ^{131}I can be repeated every 3 to 6 months up to a total dose of 2 curies.

e. Fatal leukemia has been observed in patients who have received more than 1 curie of ^{131}I for thyroid cancer.

f. Although the ^{131}I therapy may successfully eliminate pulmonary concentration of ^{131}I, the gross pulmonary nodules visible on radiographs are unlikely to regress.

Case 5–3 — Followup

August, 1974. Scanning of the neck and chest revealed no significant tracer concentration above background. Chest radiographs revealed clearing of nodular infiltrates.

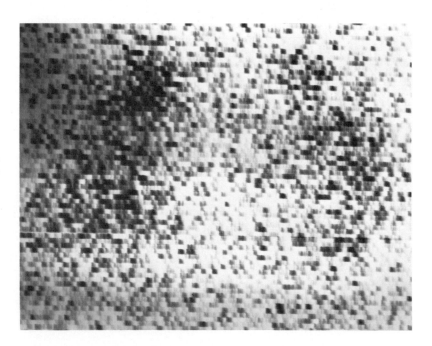

Figure 5–7. The lung scan reveals bilateral ^{131}I uptake in pulmonary metastases.

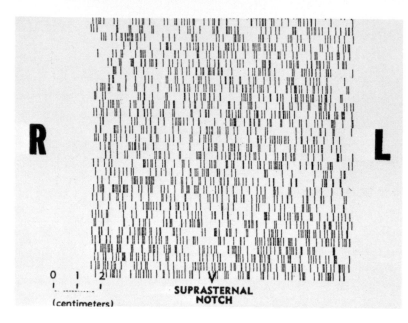

R   L

0 1 2

(centimeters)

SUPRASTERNAL
NOTCH

Figure 5–8. The neck scan after ^{131}I therapy shows only background activity.

Chest radiographs have remained clear through 1976.

Frankly, I was surprised and elated at this result. Pulmonary or osseous metastases, especially if widespread, do carry the implication of a poor prognosis. Nevertheless, a prolonged survival is the rule. More than 50 per cent of patients who have widespread disease that is discovered before they are 40 years old will survive for 20 years or more. My own experience with patients having differentiated thyroid cancer (papillary or follicular) with pulmonary metastases has been limited to six patients, three of whom have had successful ablation with ^{131}I. None has yet died of this disease. However, the duration of followup has been less than ten years for all of them.

Repeated doses of ^{131}I are sometimes needed, but it is best not to exceed a total dose of 600 to 800 mCi. Leukemia has developed in patients who received more than this. A rapidly fatal complication from a treatment for a disease which is relatively indolent is not acceptable.

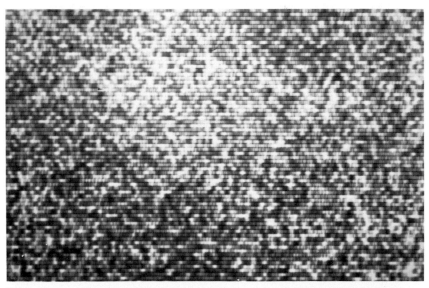

Figure 5–9. The lung scan after ^{131}I therapy shows only background activity.

Selected Current References for Case 5–3

1. Bonte FJ and McConnell RW: Pulmonary metastases from differentiated thyroid carcinoma demonstrable only by nuclear imaging. *Radiology* 107:585–590, 1973

This paper shows that imaging of the lungs with ¹³¹*I is more effective than radiography in the detection of pulmonary metastases from thyroid cancer.*

2. Harness JK, Thompson NW, Sisson JC, et al: Differentiated thyroid carcinomas: Treatment of distant metastases. *Arch Surg* 108:410–419, 1974

This is an excellent discussion of the problem of bad thyroid cancers. Too many papers deal almost exclusively with those that have such a good outlook that the treatment may have little to do with the outcome (other than to make it worse if the patient fails to survive the operation). Patients with distant metastases are uncommon; hence, this experience with 36 patients deserves careful reading.

3. Leeper RD: The effect of ¹³¹I therapy on survival of patients with metastatic papillary or follicular thyroid carcinoma. *J Clin Endocrinol Metab* 36:1143–1152, 1973

This is another important paper which deals with 46 patients with distant metastases, and the effects of ¹³¹*I on their survival. Forty-eight per cent of their patients died. Age was the most important factor in predicting response and survival after* ¹³¹*I therapy.*

CASE 5–4. A NONTOXIC AFTA

August, 1967. A 24 year old girl had had a thyroid nodule discovered 6 months earlier on a routine examination, and excision was advised. She delayed her decision until a second opinion could be obtained. She had received radiation therapy to the thymus at birth. She was clinically euthyroid. The nodule was about 1.5 cm in diameter at the lower pole of the right lobe of the thyroid gland. The nodule was no firmer than normal thyroid tissue. There were no other abnormalities and no palpable cervical lymph nodes. The FTI was 2.4, and the RAI was 15 per cent. The scan revealed a "hot" nodule with persistent contralateral lobe function. After 4 weeks' treatment with levothyroxine, 0.2 mg daily, the RAI fell to 8 per cent. The scan showed suppression of function in the left lobe with persistent nodular function, diagnostic of a nontoxic AFTA. Observation only was advised.

The patient was seen annually for 8 years. In this period the lesion gradually increased in volume.

September, 1975. The nodule was now 3 cm in diameter (a doubling of the diameter of an approximately spherical lesion is roughly equivalent to an eightfold increment in volume). The FTI was 2.9, the T_3 (RIA) 110 ng per 100 ml, and the RAI 13 per cent. The scan showed a "hot" nodule which was now completely

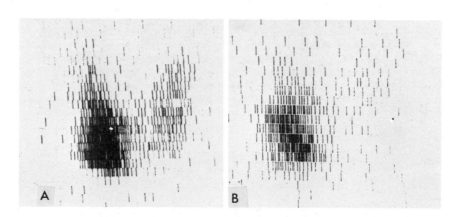

Figure 5–10. *A,* The baseline scan. *B,* The suppression scan.

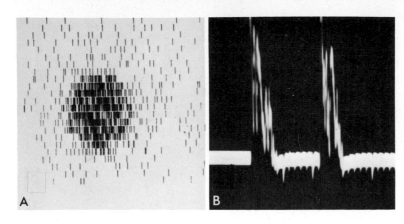

Figure 5-11. *A*, The followup scan. *B*, The ultrasound study.

suppressing function of the contralateral lobe. The ultrasound pattern was consistent with a predominantly cystic lesion.

With which of the following statements do you agree?

a. The increase in size makes excision mandatory.

b. In view of the history of radiation therapy the probabilities of thyroid cancer are too great to justify continued observation.

c. The increasing secretory activity as evidenced by the increased suppression of ENT function on the current scan indicates that toxicity is imminent. The nodule should be removed.

d. The ultrasound pattern suggests that the enlargement may in part reflect central hemorrhage or cystic degeneration.

e. Observation is still permissible.

f. The patient is now 32 years old, old enough for ^{131}I therapy.

g. The current RAI value of 13 per cent is unfavorable for ^{131}I therapy.

Case 5–4 — Followup

I am still following this patient. I was concerned about the history of radiation therapy in spite of the fact that the lesion was functional and autonomous. However, I had advised two other patients to have similar AFTA excised just because of a history of radiation therapy, and both nodules were benign. Hence, I felt that I might observe this patient in the hope of avoiding an unnecessary operation. The subsequent course is most consistent with central degeneration in conjunction with increasing secretory activity of the functioning remnant. The size is not such as to constitute a cosmetic problem, and the patient has been very reluctant to have an operation. I am not impressed with a need to ablate the functioning parenchyma in the absence of toxicity, and the rather low RAI value would increase the dose requirement if ^{131}I therapy were elected. All things considered, I am content for now to watch and wait.

The patient's most recent evaluation was in May, 1976. She was clinically euthyroid, but the T_3 (RIA) was slightly elevated. The AFTA was 3 cm in diameter, and no other nodules were palpable.

Selected Current References for Case 5–4

1. Hamburger JI and Meier DA: Cancer following treatment of an autonomously functioning thyroid nodule with sodium iodide I[131]. *Arch Surg* 103:762–764, 1971

2. Meier DA and Hamburger JI: An autonomously functioning thyroid nodule, cancer and prior radiation. *Arch Surg* 103:759-761, 1971

These two papers cover our experiences with the relationship of AFTA, thyroid cancer and radiation therapy. The message is that prior radiation therapy may predispose to the development of AFTA as well as thyroid cancer, and in some cases both lesions.

CASE 5-5. A NODULE IN A PREGNANT WOMAN

September, 1974. A 32 year old woman had a 2.5 cm nodule in the right lobe of the thyroid that had been discovered on routine examination 4 months earlier. She was treated with levothyroxine, 0.2 mg daily, and Lugol's solution, 5 drops three times a day. The nodule was firm. There were no palpable cervical lymph nodes. The patient was euthyroid. She was asked to discontinue the Lugol's solution and to return in 6 weeks for further study.

October, 1974. The FTI was 4.0. The RAI (while the patient was taking levothyroxine) was 33 per cent. The scan showed the nodule to have slightly less activity than the symmetrical contralateral area of the thyroid gland. Since the nodule was about twice as thick as the contralateral area, function per unit mass was reduced. The ultrasound study was consistent with a solid nodule.

Seven days after these studies, the patient called to report that she was pregnant. Her last menstrual period had been 4 weeks earlier.

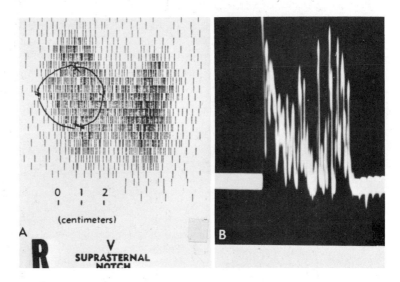

Figure 5-12. *A*, The scan. *B*, The ultrasound study.

With which of the following statements do you agree?

a. The patient should have a therapeutic abortion because of the radiation from the tracer dose of [131]I.

b. This patient may have thyroid cancer. The nodule should be removed now.

c. This patient has not only a suspicious nodule but also diffuse non-suppressible function — i.e., Graves' disease, although possibly in an inactive stage.

d. Continue treatment with thyroid hormone for the balance of the pregnancy and then proceed with an operation.

e. The finding of diffuse nonsuppressible function reduces concern for the malignant potential of the nodule.

f. The finding of diffuse nonsuppressible function increases concern for the malignant potential of the nodule.

Case 5–5 — Followup

Fetal radiation from a tracer dose of ^{131}I is insignificant, and there is no need to consider therapeutic abortion.

The patient may have thyroid cancer and indeed has diffuse nonsuppressible function, which indicates Graves' disease. The FTI is not very much elevated, and without supplemental thyroid hormone she will undoubtedly be euthyroid. However, it is possible that the secretory activity of this thyroid may increase, leading to hyperthyroidism. Nevertheless, there is no need to panic. It is safe to observe until the pregnancy is over and then take care of the problem surgically by means of a right lobectomy, isthmectomy, and subtotal left lobectomy.

If it were not for the nonsuppressible function, I would treat a pregnant patient with a nodule with thyroid hormone. In this instance, thyroid hormone, if continued, could produce thyrotoxicosis because of the combined effects of the exogenous hormone and the continuing endogenous secretion.

The nonsuppressible function neither increases nor decreases concern for the nodule with respect to its malignant potential. The nodule must be dealt with as an independent problem.

The balance of the pregnancy was uneventful.

August, 1975. A subtotal thyroidectomy was performed. The nodule proved to be benign.

The discovery of a nodule in a pregnant patient is always cause for concern, not only by the patient but also by the obstetrician. Having faced this problem many times, I am quite comfortable simply observing until the pregnancy is over. I generally order thyroid hormone, unless contraindicated as in this patient. I have had three such patients in whom thyroid cancer was found when thyroidectomy was performed after the delivery. For none of them was there any detectable growth of the lesion during the observation period, and all appear to have been cured surgically.

IN THE FOLLOWING EIGHT CASES DECIDE WHETHER TO ADVISE OPERATION OR OBSERVATION

CASE 5–6. A 16 year old girl was referred for evaluation of a 2 cm nodule found on routine examination. She had received x-ray therapy for an enlarged thymus gland at birth. The nodule was firm on palpation, hypofunctional on scanning, and solid on ultrasound (Fig. 5–13). There were several large, firm, anterior cervical lymph nodes on the side of the nodule.

CASE 5–7. A 19 year old girl reported that a nodule "popped out" about 6 months ago and has enlarged subsequently. There has been no pain or tenderness. The lesion was firm to palpation, hypofunctional on scanning, and solid on ultrasound (Fig. 5–14).

CASE 5–8. A 33 year old woman discovered a 3-cm, firm nodule 3 weeks ago. There were no palpable adjacent lymph nodes. The nodule was hypofunctional on scanning and solid on ultrasound (Fig. 5–15).

CASE 5–9. A 36 year old woman reported an enlarging nodule, first noted

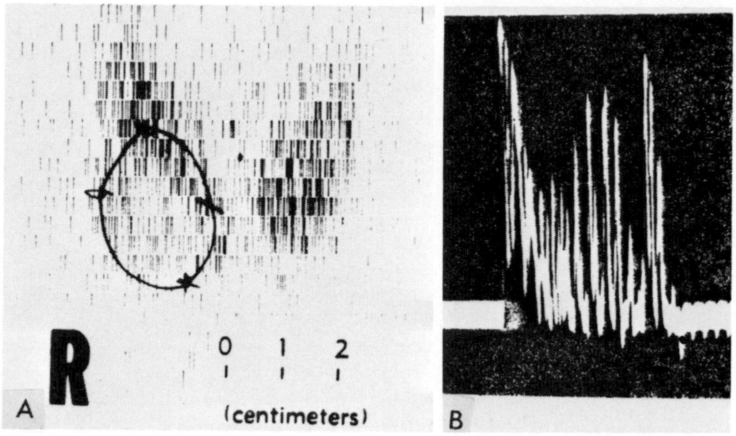

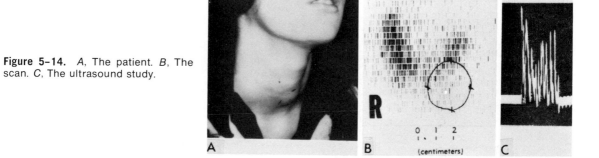

Figure 5–13. *A*, The scan. *B*, The ultrasound study.

Figure 5–14. *A*, The patient. *B*, The scan. *C*, The ultrasound study.

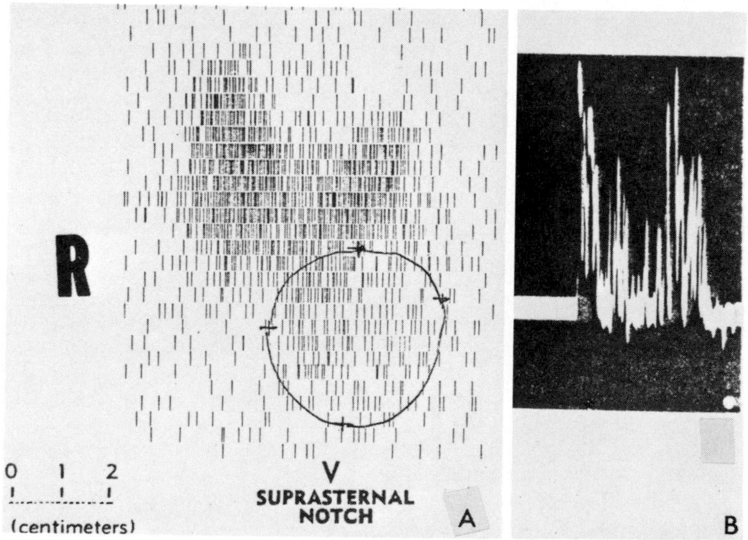

Figure 5–15. *A*, The scan. *B*, The ultrasound study.

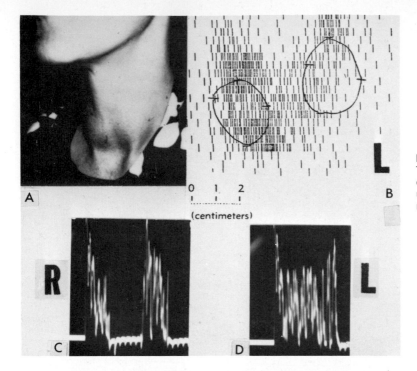

Figure 5–16. *A*, The patient. *B*, The scan. *C*, The ultrasound study on the right lobe nodule. *D*, The ultrasound study on the left lobe nodule.

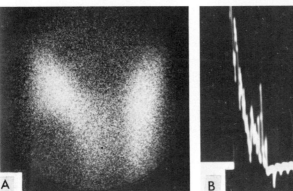
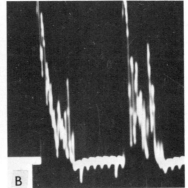

Figure 5–17. *A*, The gamma camera image. *B*, The ultrasound study.

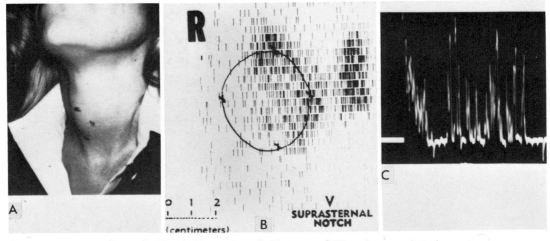

Figure 5–18. A, The patient. B, The scan. C, The ultrasound study.

2 months earlier, on the right side of the neck. On examination there were two nodules, one on the right and one on the left. Both were about 2.5 cm in diameter. Both were hypofunctional on scanning. The right sided lesion was cystic on ultrasound, and the left sided lesion was solid (Fig. 5–16).

The patient was treated with levothyroxine, 0.2 mg daily, for 3 months with no change in the nodules.

CASE 5–10. A 43 year old woman reported that a nodule "popped out" 1 week earlier. It was slightly tender to palpation, but there was no spontaneous pain. The nodule was in the lower pole of the right lobe, 2 cm in diameter. It was very firm and smooth on examination, hypofunctional on the gamma camera image, and cystic on ultrasound (Fig. 5–17).

CASE 5–11. A 53 year old woman had been taking desiccated thyroid hormone, 2½ grains daily, for over 20 years. A nodule was discovered by the patient 6 months earlier. Subsequent to its discovery, the patient had noted no obvious change in size. The nodule was in the right lobe, 4 cm in diameter, and firm. There were no palpable cervical lymph nodes. On scanning the nodule was hypofunctional, and on ultrasound it was predominantly solid with a minor cystic component (Fig. 5–18).

CASE 5–12. A low-lying nodular lesion was discovered on the left side of the neck in a 50 year old woman.

She was euthyroid clinically and biochemically. The scan is shown in Figure 5–19.

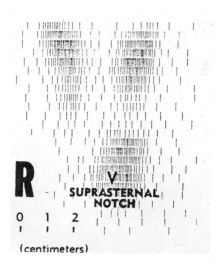

Figure 5-19. The scan.

CASE 5–13. A 75 year old woman was referred for evaluation of a rock-hard nodule in the right lobe of the thyroid. The nodule was hypofunctional on scanning. A radiograph revealed a solid ring of calcium outlining the nodule (Fig. 5–20).

Cases 5–6 to 5–13 — Followup and Comment

CASE 5–6. Obviously this nodule was a papillary cancer with lymph node metastases. The primary lesion was multifocal and involved both lobes of the

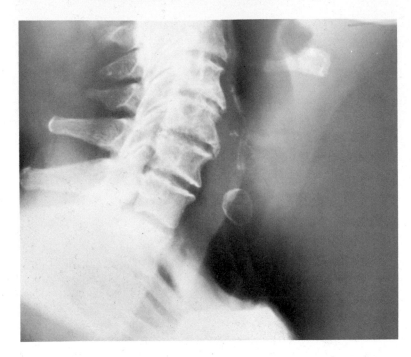

Figure 5-20. A soft tissue x-ray of the neck reveals a calcified shell in the area of the nodule.

thyroid. These are the usual findings in patients with radiation-induced thyroid cancer. The interval from the therapy to the detection of the cancer, 16 years, is somewhat less than the more usual 20 to 30 years. Fortunately, the prognosis for these cancer patients is excellent and is not materially worsened by the presence of lymph node metastases.

CASE 5-7. Once again we have a young patient with a firm nodule, and the scan and ultrasound data are consistent with a diagnosis of a neoplastic lesion. Excision was advised. The lesion was benign.

CASE 5-8. Same as Case 5-7. Thus, among the first three patients in this series the incidence of cancer was about 33 per cent, the same incidence I have found in that group of nodule patients I consider to have the highest risk of thyroid cancer.

CASE 5-9. I was less suspicious of the lesions in this patient; hence, I decided to give her a trial of treatment with thyroid hormone. I was partly influenced by the clear-cut cystic pattern shown on the ultrasound examination on the right sided lesion. This suggested that this might be a basically degenerative process. The failure to obtain any response in 3 months was disappointing but not unusual. Since the patient was in good general health and relatively young, excision was advised. The lesions proved to be degenerating benign thyroid nodules. Needle biopsy might have provided evidence for benign disease and saved this patient from an unnecessary operation.

CASE 5-10. The history and physical findings were characteristic of hemorrhage into a thyroid nodule. The patient was given levothyroxine, 0.15 mg daily, and observed. In 1 month the lesion had regressed by 75 per cent, and in 3 months there was no palpable abnormality. The gamma camera image was now normal. The patient was advised to continue thyroid hormone and to return for annual evaluation.

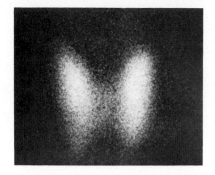

Figure 5-21. The gamma camera image for Case 5-10.

CASE 5-11. The development of a nodule in a woman who is taking a reasonably generous dose of thyroid hormone is worrisome. The fact that the hormone was the obsolete animal product whose potency must be suspect might bear upon our judgment. However, the lesion was firm and discrete, and the laboratory findings were consistent with a neoplasm. The cystic area on the ultrasound study was small, and the lesion was predominantly solid. Tumors may have some areas of either bleeding or degeneration and need not be solid throughout. In this patient there is no obviously correct course. If there were anything in her health history to suggest that surgical management might carry an increased risk, observation might be satisfactory, preferably with supplemental thyroid hormone (e.g., levothyroxine, 0.1 mg daily). On the other hand, the patient's preference for risks may make a difference in the decision — i.e., is she more concerned about the risk of the nodule or the risk of the operation? In this case, she was concerned about the nodule. It was removed, and it was a benign follicular adenoma.

CASE 5-12. This is an example of what has been called sequestered thyroid — i.e., a portion of normal thyroid tissue that became partially separated from the main mass of the gland. These lesions are, of course, benign and require nothing more than observation. Thyroid hormone may be given if the nodule enlarges.

CASE 5-13. Soft tissue radiographs of the neck occasionally are helpful in elderly patients with very hard nodules. The radiographic findings in this patient suggested a calcified degenerated nodule and practically excluded a diagnosis of malignancy. Fine spicules of calcium occasionally may be seen in papillary cancer. (See p. 279 for the surprise ending of this case.)

Selected References for Cases 5–6 Through 5–13

1. McKenney JF, Petty FC and Peterson RF: The variable nature of the thyroid nodule. *Surg Clin N Am* 52:383–396, 1972

   This paper illustrates a wide variety of causes of nodular thyroid lesions. The emphasis on operation for most seems inappropriate.

2. Staunton MD and Greening WP: Clinical diagnosis of thyroid cancer. *Brit Med J* 4:532–535, 1973.

   This paper deserves recognition if for no other reason than that the authors follow my approach to classifying thyroid nodules in three categories: cancer probable, cancer suspected, and benign. The clinical features upon which this classification is based are discussed. Most important is the degree of hardness of the mass.

3. Miller JM, Zafar S and Karo JJ: The cystic thyroid nodule: Recognition and management. *Radiology* 110:257–261, 1974
4. Blum M: Enhanced clinical diagnosis of thyroid disease using echography. *Am J Med* 59:301–307, 1975
5. Thijs LG and Weiner JD: Ultrasonic examination of the thyroid gland. *Am J Med* 60:96–105, 1976

These three papers discuss the contribution of diagnostic ultrasound to the evaluation of thyroid nodules. Miller also finds that aspiration offers an additional dimension to the workup as well as the treatment of cystic lesions.

6. Crile G, Jr, and Hawk WA, Jr: Aspiration biopsy of thyroid nodules. *Surg Gynecol Obstet* 136:241–245, 1973

These authors claim that needle biopsy could reduce the number of operations for thyroid nodules by a factor of 10. I think that figure is too high, but the procedure seems to deserve further attention.

7. Heimann P: Needle aspiration biopsy for thyroid cancer (editorial). *Arch Surg* 110:1517–1518, 1975
8. Frable WJ, and Frable MA: Thin-needle aspiration biopsy in the diagnosis of head and neck tumors. *Laryngoscope* 84:1–9, 1974

These authors use thin-needle aspiration of thyroid nodules. The technique is simple and apparently exceedingly safe. I am doubtful that the material will be adequate for most pathologists.

9. Sisson JC, Schmidt RW and Beierwaltes WH: Sequestered nodular goiter. *New Eng J Med* 270:927–932, 1964

This is the classic description of this entity. The physicians postulate that the mechanical action of neck muscles sequesters portions of the thyroid from the parent gland.

10. DeGroot L and Paloyan E: Thyroid carcinoma and radiation: A Chicago endemic. *JAMA* 225:487–491, 1973
11. Favus MJ, Schneider AB, Stachura ME, et al: Thyroid cancer occurring as a late consequence of head-and-neck irradiation. *New Eng J Med* 294:1019–1025, 1976
12. Refetoff S, Harrison J, Karanfilski BT, et al: Continuing occurrence of thyroid carcinoma after irradiation to the neck in infancy and childhood. *New Eng J Med* 292:171–175, 1975
13. Wilson SM, Platz C and Block GM: Thyroid carcinoma after irradiation. *Arch Surg* 100:330–337, 1970

These four articles contain the meat of the issue of thyroid cancer that occurs years after radiation therapy to the upper body. The lesions are usually papillary, characteristically multifocal, often involve cervical nodes, and carry a good prognosis. Therapy to the tonsils and adenoids may produce a higher incidence of thyroid cancer than thymic radiation. In the lay media the urgency of immediate diagnosis has been overemphasized, as have the life-threatening implications of these lesions. These patients should be screened. Careful physical examination by a physician experienced in the examination of the thyroid gland will be adequate to detect almost all clinically significant lesions. Administration of thyroid hormone to patients younger than 40 to 50 years old who are known to have had radiation therapy and have no thyroid abnormalities on examination, makes sense from the theoretical standpoint.

14. Foster RS, Jr: Thyroid irradiation and carcinogenesis: Review with assessment of clinical implications. *Am J Surg* 130:608–611, 1975

This article summarizes the principles of radiation dosimetry with respect to the potential for thyroid cancer induction. Of particular significance is the call for avoidance of ^{131}I for thyroid scanning, especially in young people, in whom the radiation dose to the thyroid may easily reach that which has been implicated in the induction of thyroid cancer. Although this point may be argued, the availability of suitable tracers that deliver much less radiation leaves the burden of proof upon those who fail to heed the warning.

15. Ju DMC: Salivary gland tumors occurring after radiation of the head and neck area. *Am J Surg* 116:518–523, 1968
16. Becker FO and Economou SG: Parotid tumor and thyroid cancer: Simultaneous occurrence after irradiation of the neck in childhood. *JAMA* 232:512–514, 1975

These two articles remind us that salivary gland tumors as well as thyroid tumors may be seen after radiation therapy to the upper body.

CASE 5–14. AN ELDERLY WOMAN WITH A HARD NODULE

September, 1967. A 73 year old woman was referred from a nursing home because a mass in the neck had been discovered. A 3.5-cm hard nodule was present in the left lobe of the thyroid. The lesion was hypofunctional on scanning. In view of the patient's age and the rather marked general debility, observation was advised. Over the next 3 months the mass doubled in size. There was no evidence of inflammatory disease.

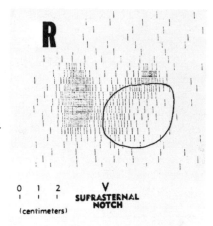

Figure 5–22. The scan.

With which of the following statements do you agree?

a. This could be an anaplastic cancer.

b. Occult subacute thyroiditis must be considered.

c. The rapid growth is an indication for biopsy.

d. A suitable biopsy specimen can be obtained under local anesthesia.

e. If this is an anaplastic cancer, prompt surgical excision may be curative.

f. If this is an anaplastic thyroid cancer, local palliative radiation therapy is all that is indicated.

g. The survival of patients after a diagnosis of anaplastic cancer has been established is usually no longer than 6 months regardless of treatment.

Case 5–14 — Followup

An open biopsy under local anesthesia revealed anaplastic thyroid cancer. Radiation therapy produced a marked reduction in the mass, but regrowth was rapid, and the patient succumbed to the disease in 6 months. This is the usual course of anaplastic thyroid cancer. No treatment is effective.

Occult subacute thyroiditis may present in similar fashion, but after the initial enlargement, progressive growth would be very unlikely.

In a case of this type there is no alternative to a tissue diagnosis. Needle biopsy is gaining attention in the literature. If one is practicing in a location in which pathologists are experienced with the interpretation of small samples, needle biopsy may prove satisfactory. However, with little extra effort and inconvenience an open biopsy under local anesthesia will provide a much more desirable specimen. This has been our choice in most cases.

Selected Current References For Case 5–14

1. Kyriakides G and Sosin H: Anaplastic carcinoma of the thyroid. *Ann Surg* 179:295–299, 1974.
2. Nishiyama RH, Dunn EL and Thompson NW: Anaplastic spindle-cell and giant-cell tumors of the thyroid gland. *Cancer* 30:113–127, 1972.

> *These two papers tell the grim story of anaplastic thyroid cancer. Of interest is the high frequency with which these lesions are associated with differentiated types of cancer, suggesting to these authors that the concept of transformation from differentiated to anaplastic cancer of the thyroid has merit.*

CASE 5–15. AN ELDERLY WOMAN WITH A FIRM NECK MASS

May, 1974. A 70 year old woman reported a mass on the left side of the neck that had been enlarging over the past few months. It was very firm, painless, and nontender. She had noted that she had less pep and some muscular cramps. There was no fever. No abnormal cervical lymph nodes were noted.

The FTI was 0.8, the TSH(RIA) 120 μU/ml and the RAI 8 per cent. Antithyroid antibodies were positive in high dilution, and the scan revealed that almost all of the tracer was concentrated by the nodular mass.

A diagnosis of Hashimoto's disease with hypothyroidism was made. The patient was treated with levothyroxine, 0.15 mg, every other day for 2 weeks and then daily.

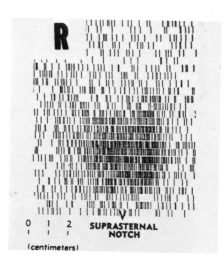

Figure 5–23. The scan.

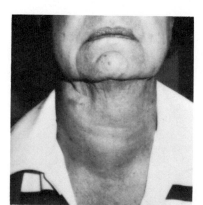

Figure 5–24. The patient.

October, 1974. The mass was unchanged. The FTI was 3.4 and the TSH(RIA) 2.5 μU/ml. Treatment was continued.

December, 1974. The patient returned complaining of a marked diffuse swelling of the lower neck that was painful and tender. The patient had low grade fever, night sweats, malaise, loose bowels, and palpitation.

The FTI was 3.6, and the ESR 52 mm/hr.

With which of the following statements do you agree?

a. This patient has subacute thyroiditis superimposed upon Hashimoto's disease. Adrenal steroids should bring about prompt relief of symptoms and regression in the goiter.

b. The patient may have anaplastic cancer — biopsy is urgent.

c. This patient could have a lymphoma, and a response to adrenal steroids may not be definitive.

d. For this flare-up of subacute thyroiditis only aspirin is needed.

e. This is a classic example of acute suppurative thyroiditis. Antibiotics and incision and drainage are urgently needed.

f. This is an acute phase of Hashimoto's disease. No action is needed. It will subside spontaneously in a few weeks. Reassure the patient.

Case 5–15 — Followup

The patient was treated with prednisone, 60 mg daily. The swelling decreased by about 50 per cent. The patient's symptoms rapidly cleared. However, it then became evident that there were pathologically enlarged cervical lymph nodes bilaterally. Biopsy revealed a lymphoma as well as Hashimoto's disease.

I really did think that this patient had subacute thyroiditis superimposed upon Hashimoto's disease. In retrospect, this was not overly bright thinking with respect to a woman of this age. This case demonstrates that a response to adrenal steroids need not be definitive. Complete regression of the lesion would be reassuring, but in this instance one could not expect complete regression in the swelling, for there was a nodular goiter to begin with. However, the regression was adequate to permit examination of the neck, which the previous pain and tenderness had limited. The enlarged lymph nodes were then discovered, and these, of course, suggested the necessity for biopsy.

Anaplastic cancer is not likely to produce such generalized swelling but would more likely appear as a localized mass. The constitutional symptoms are also not characteristic. Nevertheless, this was an important consideration.

Once again, this is not the picture of acute suppurative thyroiditis. High fever is uniformly present in this disease. Also, it is a localized process and leads to abscess formation.

The possibility that Hashimoto's disease, advanced to the point of hypothyroidism, would suddenly flare up in an acute exacerbation of this type is too unusual for serious consideration.

Selected Current References for Case 5–15

1. Woolner LB, McConahey WM, Beahrs OH, et al: Primary malignant lymphoma of the thyroid: Review of 46 cases. *Am J Surg* 111:502–523, 1966

   This is the classic reference on the subject.

2. Rayfield EJ, Nishiyama RH and Sisson JC: Small cell tumors of the thyroid: A clinicopathologic study. *Cancer* 28:1023–1030, 1971

   The difficulty of differentiating small cell anaplastic lesions from lymphoma is discussed. The suggestion is offered that the rare survivors of small cell anaplastic cancer may have had lymphoma.

3. Bisbee AC and Thoeny RH: Malignant lymphoma of the thyroid following irradiation. *Cancer* 35:1296–1299, 1975

Here is a case of lymphoma occurring in a 19 year old patient who had received radiation therapy to the thymus at the age of 4½ months.

CASE 5–16.   RECURRENT PAPILLARY CANCER

April, 1970.   A 67 year old woman was referred for the evaluation of a 4- by 8-cm mass in the left side of the neck. In 1960 she had undergone partial thyroidectomy for papillary thyroid cancer. No thyroid hormone was given postoperatively. The patient was euthyroid clinically and biochemically. The mass was hypofunctional on scanning and obviously represented recurrent papillary thyroid cancer. A second attempt at surgical ablation, consisting of a total thyroidectomy and a modified dissection of the left neck, was undertaken. Postoperatively, the patient was treated with levothyroxine, 0.2 mg daily, after scanning revealed no significant tracer concentration in the neck and chest. A 72-hour urinary collection contained 96 per cent of the administered tracer.

February, 1973 to March, 1975.   The patient returned for an annual checkup, and a 1-cm mass was detected in the left neck. Observation was advised. Over the next 2 years the mass gradually increased to 2 cm in diameter. Excision was advised. The lesion proved to be an enlarged cervical lymph node, which contained papillary cancer. No other nodes were found in the left side of the neck during the operation.

March, 1976.   Another 2.5 cm neck mass was discovered, this time on the right side. The patient was now 73 years old. The mass failed to concentrate ^{131}I after TSH stimulation. The chest radiograph was normal. The patient was in good general health.

With which of the following statements do you agree?

a.   Further operative therapy is futile and risky in this 73 year old woman. It is best to leave well enough alone and observe.

b.   External radiation therapy is the only additional treatment indicated.

c.   Chemotherapy is indicated.

d.   This is the last time that excision should be advised.

e.   Excision followed by external radiation therapy should be the recommendation.

f.   The patient may die of the disease, but she is more likely to die of her treatment if we continue to risk her life with general anesthesia.

g.   Papillary cancer in patients more than 60 years old is significantly more aggressive than in patients less than 40 years of age.

h.   The survival of patients with papillary cancer is significantly less in patients over 40 years of age than in those less than 40 years old.

Case 5–16 — Followup

The patient was subjected to another attempt at surgical excision, even though I was beginning to be concerned that the treatment might be a greater risk than the disease. Nevertheless, I was influenced by the fact that she was rather sturdy, and only a minimal surgical procedure would be needed. Postoperatively, she was given external radiation therapy in the hope of preventing another recurrence.

This is a classic example of the berry-picking procedure that is sometimes necessary in patients with papillary thyroid cancer. Her initial operation was inadequate, and the second procedure was long delayed; thus, time for multiple seedings in cervical nodes to take place was perhaps permitted.

Chemotherapy was not advised in the absence of known, inoperable, widespread metastases. Even then I am not convinced that there is much chance for any real benefit.

Papillary cancer does seem to be more aggressive in older patients than in younger ones. However, I have yet to have any patient die of this disease. A number have failed to survive for very long because of other illnesses, principally cardiac disease and other malignancies. This bears upon the last statement (h). This is the kind of useless truism that fills the literature. The absurdity of it is exposed when it is changed to read: Most people less than 40 years old will survive longer than people more than 40 years of age. What else is new?

Death after a diagnosis of thyroid cancer is far from the same thing as death from thyroid cancer, particularly if one excludes death directly attributable to the treatment for the disease, treatment which may be of questionable propriety.

Selected Current References for Case 5–16

1. Holmquest DL and Lake P: Sudden hemorrhage in metastatic thyroid carcinoma of the brain during treatment with iodine-131. *J Nucl Med* 17:307–309, 1976

   This is another example of the poorer outlook for differentiated cancer in older people.

2. Tollefsen HR, Shah JP and Huvos AG: Papillary carcinoma of the thyroid: Recurrence in the thyroid gland after initial surgical treatment. *Am J Surg* 124:468–472, 1972

   These authors found only a 5 per cent rate of clinical recurrence after unilateral lobectomy for papillary thyroid cancer, in spite of a 38 per cent incidence of occult carcinoma in the opposite lobe. They give no data on the relationship of age to recurrence rate, unfortunately.

CASE 5–17. HÜRTHLE CELL CANCER

April, 1974. A 53 year old man gave a history of thyroidectomy for non-malignant disease in 1963. A subtotal thyroidectomy was performed in October of 1973 for a recurrent mass in the left lobe. This proved to be a Hürthle cell cancer. In February of 1974 a third surgical procedure was undertaken in an attempt to remove all thyroid tissue, along with a left modified radical neck dissection. Two lymph nodes from the upper mediastinum contained tumor. During the hospitalization, a chest radiograph revealed an 8-mm nodule in the right midlung field and an 11-mm nodule in the right lower lung field. It was presumed that these represented pulmonary metastases.

Scans of the liver and skeleton were negative.

Six weeks after the last operation the RAI was 6 per cent; a scan of the neck revealed uptake of the tracer in the pyramidal lobe and an area consistent with a small remnant of normal thyroid tissue in the lower pole of the right lobe. There

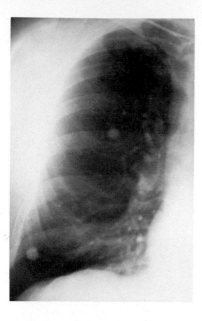

Figure 5-25. The chest x-ray reveals two coin lesions in the right lung.

was no concentration of the tracer in the chest. A 72-hour collection of urine contained 88 per cent of the tracer.

Treatment with levothyroxine, 0.2 mg daily, was advised, with reevaluation at 3-month intervals.

November, 1974. The patient was clinically euthyroid. The serum TSH was less than 1 μU/ml. There was no evidence of recurrent cancer in the neck. The nodules increased in size from 11 to 16 mm and from 8 to 11 mm, respectively.

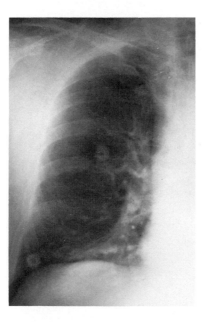

Figure 5-26. The chest x-ray shows that the coin lesions had enlarged between April, 1974 and November, 1974.

With which of the following statements do you agree?

a. These two isolated lesions, in the absence of any evidence of cancer elsewhere, might be amenable to surgical excision.

b. Therapy with ^{131}I is mandatory.

c. Radiation therapy (external beam) is needed.

d. The prognosis for a 10-year survival is poor.

e. The prognosis for a 1-year survival is poor.

f. The thyroid hormone dosage should be increased.

g. Chemotherapy offers a good chance for arresting the growth of this cancer.

h. The pulmonary nodules are coincidental and not related to the thyroid cancer.

Case 5–17 — Followup

I had hoped that I might find a thoracic surgeon willing to excise these two pulmonary lesions, presumably metastatic Hürthle cell cancer. The patient was referred to a nearby university hospital and discussed in conference. It was decided to employ Cytoxan. The patient has tolerated the medication well, and for 9 months the pulmonary lesions have been stable.

I am not happy with this decision. I know of no data to suggest that chemotherapy is of any lasting value for patients with metastatic thyroid cancer. Therefore, I suspect that the arrested growth of these lesions will be only temporary. My experience with Hürthle cell cancer, which has metastasized to the lungs (three patients) has been that the patients all die within a period of 5 years. In view of this dismal experience, even admitting that there is no guarantee that the pulmonary lesions represent the only metastases, I would have preferred an attempt at resection. There is very little to lose and perhaps a chance to be a winner.

In the absence of proof that these nodules represent metastatic thyroid cancer, the diagnostic value of the excisional biopsy is also worth considering. Wouldn't it be something if the lesions were coincidental?

These lesions do not concentrate ^{131}I in therapeutically useful amounts; therefore, ^{131}I therapy would be futile. External radiation therapy is generally not useful except for palliation in patients with thyroid cancer but may warrant consideration if the tumors continue to grow.

Increasing the dose of thyroid hormone will not be of value after there is evidence that the serum TSH level has been fully suppressed, as was the case with this patient.

October 11, 1977. As this book was in the final stages of preparation I learned that between 1975 and 1977 the pulmonary lesions had increased in size substantially, and new lesions were detected bilaterally in spite of continued chemotherapy. Because of radiographic evidence of bronchial compression, the thoracic surgeons undertook a two-stage bilateral resection of these Hürthle cell metastases.

CASE 5–18. HÜRTHLE CELL CANCER

July, 1961. A 57 year old woman had a relatively soft 1.5 cm nodule in the left lobe of the thyroid that was hypofunctional on scanning. A 6-month trial of treatment with thyroid hormone was advised.

June, 1968. The patient returned for reevaluation because of the development of a painful, tender, visible swelling on the left side of the anterior neck. In the intervening years the patient had seen another physician for various minor problems, and review of his records indicated that a thyroid nodule about 2 cm in diameter had been noted in 1966 and had gradually enlarged to about 3 cm by early 1968 in spite of treatment with desiccated thyroid hormone, 2 grains daily. The patient reported no fever, chills, night sweats or weight loss. There was some hoarseness. She was clinically euthyroid.

The left thyroid lobe was replaced by a hard irregular mass about 6 cm in diameter. There was also a 1-cm firm nodule in the right lobe.

The T_4 by column chromatography was 3.6 μg per 100 ml (normal), the ESR was 18 mm/hr, the RAI (while taking 2 grains of desiccated thyroid daily) was 2 per cent, and there was no response to TSH stimulation. Antithyroglobulin antibodies were negative. The chest radiograph was negative.

The possibility of SAT in a resolving phase was considered, and the patient was given levothyroxine, 0.2 mg daily, and asked to return in 1 month.

July, 1968. The mass was unchanged. Observation was continued.

August, 1968. The mass seemed slightly larger. A left total lobectomy, isthmectomy, and right subtotal thyroidectomy were performed. Except for the nodules, most of the thyroid had been replaced by fibrous tissue. The nodular lesions were initially thought to be benign Hürthle cell adenomas. On review by an experienced thyroid pathologist, the diagnosis was: Hürthle cell carcinoma of the angioinvasive or malignant adenoma variety.

Postoperative scanning revealed only a small focus of tracer uptake in a remnant of the right lobe. No uptake was demonstrated elsewhere in neck or chest.

With which of the following statements do you agree?

a. The duration of this lesion, with little growth and nothing to suggest aggressiveness in terms of distant metastases, makes the prognosis excellent for long-term survival.

b. Local recurrences of these lesions are common, and distant metastases rare.

c. External beam radiation therapy to the neck should be considered.

d. This case proves that it is best to remove all thyroid nodules.

Case 5–18 — Followup

August, 1968. Consultation was held with another thyroidologist and the thyroid pathologist with regard to the desirability of radiation therapy to the neck. The decision was to treat with levothyroxine, 0.2 mg daily, and observe. This decision was based upon the presumption that the danger to the patient was from growth of distant metastases which were not yet evident. Local radiation therapy could not prevent this. On the other hand, local recurrences could be dealt with surgically.

November, 1970. The patient had been seen at 2- to 3-month intervals for minor problems and also to watch for recurrent cancer. For the first time a small (less than 1 cm) nodule was discovered beneath the right sternocleidomastoid muscle. A chest radiograph was negative. Observation was elected.

March, 1971. The nodule had enlarged slightly but definitely, and removal was advised. It proved to be Hürthle cell cancer, and another small recurrence on the left was also removed. Postoperatively, a course of cobalt therapy was given to the neck in the hope of preventing local recurrences.

June, 1971. A recurrent nodule was noted on the left. Observation was advised.

March, 1972. The neck nodule was unchanged. However, 2.5-cm mass was seen in the left mediastinum on chest radiograph.

August, 1972. Chest radiography revealed enlargement of the left mediastinal mass to 4 cm; in addition, there were multiple nodules at the right lung base. The patient then moved to Akron, Ohio. The cancer continued to grow in the chest in spite of chemotherapy. The patient ultimately succumbed with widespread metastases in June of 1973.

This is the story of Hürthle cell cancer. One must anticipate a protracted but inexorably downhill course, extending over many years; regardless of treatment it is ultimately fatal. Perhaps the patient could have been saved if the nodule had been removed when first discovered in 1961. Unfortunately, the nodule had a very innocent physical appearance at that time. Even more unfortunate was the failure of the patient to return for regular rechecks as initially requested. Growth of the nodule in spite of treatment with thyroid hormone probably would have made the necessity for surgical intervention obvious much earlier than was the case. The confusing clinical features that suggested SAT led to a slight delay in recommending operation in 1968, but the delay was minor.

This case does not provide support for the conclusion that all thyroid nodules should be removed. This case is presented because of its exceptional features. The hundreds of patients with nodules that are judged probably benign and followed without incident are not reported because they aren't news.

It is admitted that selective removal of thyroid nodules exposes patients to some risk. But there are risks no matter what one does. I have had two otherwise healthy patients who died from thyroidectomies. Everyone else who sends any sizeable number of patients to the surgeon will sooner or later have similar experiences. Therefore, it makes sense to advise thyroidectomy only for patients with suspicious nodules. However, patients for whom observation is recommended must understand that reexamination at regular intervals is necessary and that unfavorable future events may necessitate a change in the advice.

Selected Current References for Cases 5–17 and 5–18

1. Tollefsen HR, Shah JP and Huvos AG: Hürthle cell carcinoma of the thyroid. *Am J Surg* 130:390–394, 1975

   The authors found no difference between Hürthle cell cancer and follicular cancer.

2. Lam CR: Malignant intrathoracic Hürthle-cell tumor. *Henry Ford Hosp Med J* 22:85–90, 1974

   This case of inexorable progression and recurrences leading to death is more in keeping with my bad experience with this tumor.

3. Gottlieb JA and Hill CS, Jr: Chemotherapy of thyroid cancer with adriamycin: Experience with 30 patients. *New Eng J Med* 290:193–197, 1974

   They found adriamycin "promising" on the basis of "partial" remission. I suppose anything may be better than nothing. Anyway, two of the five patients with Hürthle cell cancer exhibited a "partial response."

CASE 5-19. PERSISTENT MEDULLARY CANCER

December, 1973. A 26 year old man was referred after a total thyroidectomy that revealed a multifocal medullary carcinoma with bilateral multiple lymph node metastases. An incidental finding was a parathyroid adenoma. There was no history of diarrhea or flushing and no evidence of mucosal or cutaneous lesions. His mother had died at the age of 25 of a stroke, and at postmortem examination a pheochromocytoma was found.

Examination of the neck revealed no palpable evidence of residual tumor. A neck scan revealed no residual thyroid tissue and the chest radiograph was negative. Urine vanillylmandelic acid and metanephrine values were not elevated. The patient had hypoparathyroidism, which was controlled with calcium lactate and vitamin D. Serum calcitonin assays were performed before and during calcium infusion and reached elevated levels of 7.7 ng/ml, indicating that the cancer had not been completely excised. Selective blood samples were taken by venous catheter from the inferior vena cava, the hepatic veins, the superior vena cava, the internal jugular veins, and the larger cervical veins. Calcitonin assays provided no evidence of any tumor outside the neck.

June, 1974. The patient was subjected to a two-stage bilateral neck dissection, which revealed residual cancer on the right side involving cervical lymph nodes and connective tissue in the anterior triangle.

November, 1974. A postoperative random calcitonin assay remained elevated at 6 ng/ml. Observation was elected and there was no evidence of recurrent cancer by physical examination or chest radiography.

July, 1975. The serum calcitonin level 5 minutes after administration of pentagastrin was 130 ng/ml — distinctly elevated.

Now what do you do?

(It is of interest that the patient's two brothers were also studied; both had elevated calcitonin levels, and medullary cancer was found at surgery. The postoperative calcitonin assays were negative for both.)

Case 5-19 — Followup

There is no attractive therapeutic option available. Further surgical treatment did not seem promising after a bilateral radical neck dissection. External beam radiation therapy might be considered, but I could not really generate much enthusiasm for this without knowing where the residual cancer might be. Chemotherapy has not been shown to be of any real value for this disease. Our decision was to wait and see. The disease is sluggish in its development. If we are lucky and it is confined to the neck, a recurrent mass may yet develop which conceivably might be resectable. We will follow the calcitonin levels. If the tumor undergoes spontaneous necrosis and degeneration (by some miracle), falling values may provide us with some encouraging information. Rising levels (which are more likely) would have a more ominous prognostic implication.

Selected Current References for Case 5–19

The calcitonin–medullary cancer story is fascinating to follow, beginning with the description of the familial syndrome and its association with pheochromocytoma and parathyroid adenoma.

1. Paloyan E, Scanu A and Straus FH: Familial pheochromocytoma, medullary thyroid carcinoma, and parathyroid adenomas. *JAMA* 214:1443–1447, 1970
2. Catalona WJ, Engelman K, Ketcham AS, et al: Familial medullary thyroid carcinoma, pheochromocytoma, and parathyroid adenoma (Sipple's syndrome): Study of a kindred. *Cancer* 28:1245–1254, 1971
3. Hill CS, Ibanez ML, Samaan NA, et al: Medullary (solid) carcinoma of the thyroid gland: An analysis of the M.D. Anderson Hospital experience with patients with the tumor, its special features and its histogenesis. *Medicine* 53:141–171, 1973

Next comes the recognition of the value of the serum calcitonin assay, both to diagnose medullary cancer in advance of its clinical presentation and also to assess the completeness of the excision of the lesion.

4. Melvin KE, Miller HH, Tashjian AH, Jr: Early diagnosis of medullary carcinoma of the thyroid gland by means of calcitonin assay. *New Eng J Med* 285:1115–1120, 1971
5. Block MA, Jackson CE and Tashjian AH, Jr: Medullary thyroid carcinoma detected by serum calcitonin assay. *Arch Surg* 104:579–586, 1972
6. Goltzman D, Potts JT, Jr, Ridgway EC, et al: Calcitonin as a tumor marker: Use of the radioimmunoassay for calcitonin in the postoperative evaluation of patients with medullary thyroid carcinoma. *New Eng J Med* 290:1035–1039, 1974

Finally, there is a report of the recognition of C-cell hyperplasia as a premalignant lesion diagnosed by elevated calcitonin levels.

7. Wolfe HJ, Melvin KE, Cervi-Skinner SJ, et al: C-cell hyperplasia preceding medullary thyroid carcinoma. *New Eng J Med* 289:437–441, 1973

CASE 5–20. A MIDLINE MASS

April, 1970. A 65 year old man was referred for evaluation of a rock-hard mass at the base of the neck; it had been present for 2 to 3 months and was gradually enlarging. The mass was fixed to internal neck structures. There were no symptoms suggesting thyroid dysfunction. The FTI was 2.6. The scan revealed a mass that involved the inferior portion of the thyroid gland and had poor uptake of the tracer.

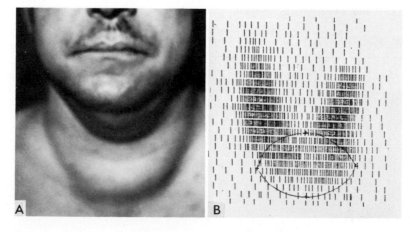

Figure 5-27. *A,* The patient. *B,* The scan.

With which of the following statements do you agree?

    a.   Biopsy is necessary.

    b.   This is Hashimoto's disease.

    c.   A chest radiograph is needed.

    d.   This is an anaplastic cancer.

    e.   Rule out subacute thyroiditis.

    f.   Rule out lymphoma.

Case 5–20 — Followup

The patient had bronchogenic carcinoma metastatic to the thyroid gland. An enlarging rock-hard mass in a patient this old suggests cancer, and biopsy was obviously appropriate. Metastatic cancer to the thyroid is exceedingly rare in the ambulatory population. It is not so rare in terminal cancer patients, but under such circumstances it is the least of their problems.

The cancers that metastasize to the thyroid most often include melanoma and renal, breast, and lung carcinoma.

Obviously, there is no specific treatment from the standpoint of the thyroidologist. This patient was dead in 6 months.

Selected Current Reference for Case 5–20

1. Wychulis AR, Beahrs OH and Woolner LB: Metastasis of carcinoma to the thyroid gland. *Ann Surg* 160:169–177, 1964

> *There are very few papers dealing with this rare situation. Of course the Mayo Clinic has the largest experience, 14 cases. It is interesting that eight cases involved metastasis from the kidney and four from the breast. There were none from the lung.*

CASE 5–21. AN ELDERLY WOMAN WITH A FIRM NECK MASS

February, 1971. A 63 year old woman had a 3-cm, firm mass on the left side of the neck that had been detected 3 weeks earlier. There was no pain or tenderness. There had been low grade fever. An RAI was 1 per cent, the FTI 4.6, and the ESR 51 mm/hr. A repeat RAI after TSH stimulation was 5 per cent, and the scan revealed no tracer concentration by the mass. The ultrasound pattern was consistent with a solid lesion.

With which of the following statements do you agree?

    a. This is probably an anaplastic cancer. An attempt at excision should be made, followed by radiation therapy, but the patient probably will not survive for a year.

    b. This may be subacute thyroiditis. A trial of adrenal steroids may be useful to confirm the diagnosis.

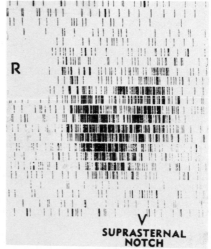

Figure 5-28. *A*, The scan. *B*, The ultrasound study.

    c.   This is the typical picture of acute suppurative thyroiditis. Incision and drainage and antibiotics are urgently needed.

    d.   Do not ignore the high FTI. She has hyperthyroidism with an unknown chemical block interfering with the RAI. The nodule is of no consequence.

Case 5–21 — Followup

The patient was treated with prednisone, 30 mg daily, and within 3 weeks the mass had completely regressed. Prednisone was gradually withdrawn. Three months later, all thyroid function tests were normal, and so was the thyroid scan.

The patient was referred with a presumptive diagnosis of thyroid cancer, and I was concerned about the possibility of an anaplastic lesion. However, the low baseline RAI in conjunction with a subnormal response to TSH stimulation suggested a more diffuse abnormality of which the mass was simply the area of maximum involvement. Hence, I elected a trial of prednisone with gratifying results.

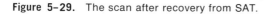

Figure 5-29. The scan after recovery from SAT.

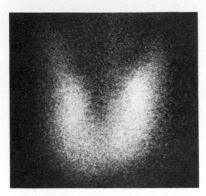

Figure 5-30. The gamma camera image in 1976.

The picture was not that of acute suppurative thyroiditis. This disease presents with much more pronounced evidence of acute inflammatory reaction, including high fever and local heat, erythema, and fluctuance. The disease is a medical emergency.

May, 1976. The patient was euthyroid, with no evidence of thyroid nodularity. The gamma camera image was normal.

CHAPTER 6

INFLAMMATORY THYROID DISEASES

PART I. PATHOPHYSIOLOGIC CONSIDERATIONS RELATIVE TO INFLAMMATORY DISEASES OF THE THYROID

ACUTE SUPPURATIVE THYROIDITIS (AST)

The acute suppurative form of thyroiditis is caused by bacterial infection (rarely fungal). The disease is localized to a portion of the thyroid and usually progresses to abscess formation. All of the classical local features of inflammation are present, including warmth, swelling, redness, tenderness, and ultimately fluctuation. This disease is very rare. I have not seen a single example in the last 10 years, during which I have evaluated more than 20,000 patients for thyroid disease.

Reference

1. Szego R, and Levy RP: Recurrent acute suppurative thyroiditis. *Can Med Assoc J* 103:631–633, 1970

RIEDEL'S STRUMA

Equally rare, or perhaps even more so, is Riedel's struma. This disease is characterized by an invasive fibrous involvement which extends beyond the thyroid capsule into the adjacent strap muscles, obliterating all lines of demarcation. The disease usually begins unilaterally and may or may not spread to involve the entire gland. Even when there is bilateral involvement, there are often areas of normal tissue, and hypothyroidism is not inevitable. The presenting complaints referable to the neck include goiter, but more important is obstruction of the trachea and esophagus. Apparently this disorder is not uniquely thyroidal but represents a process that may involve other areas, principally the mediastinum and retroperitoneal tissues, parotid glands, and even the orbital area.

References

1. Mitchinson MJ: Bowlby's disease? *Brit Med J* 2:46–47, 1971
2. Hines RC, Schuemann HA, Royster HP and Rose E: Invasive fibrous (Riedel's) thyroiditis with bilateral fibrous parotitis. *JAMA* 213:869–871, 1970

HASHIMOTO'S DISEASE

Having dispensed with the rare birds, we can now proceed to consider the more common inflammatory disorders of the thyroid. The inflammatory process in Hashimoto's disease is chronic, diffusely atrophic, and fibrotic, and leads ultimately to the destruction of the functional parenchyma. Earlier in the course of the illness lymphocytic infiltration is apparent. The abundant large, pale, eosinophilic epithelial cells (Hürthle cells) are characteristic. These epithelial cells are packed with mitochondria, showing the picture of intensive cellular activity. However, the output of thyroid hormone is reduced. Although the cells are working overtime, they are merely spinning their wheels futilely because of a defective synthetic apparatus.

The detection of elevated titers of serum antibody to thyroglobulin and thyroid microsomes has given rise to the theory that Hashimoto's disease is an autoimmune process. The implication is that the antibodies play a causative role in the progression of the disease until it reaches the end stage of fibrous atrophy. However, it is still possible that these antibodies, like many other antibodies, are only a reflection of the disease and that there is a more obscure etiologic agent or process.

SUBACUTE THYROIDITIS (SAT)

Subacute thyroiditis is less common than Hashimoto's disease by a factor of about 1 to 10. The cause of subacute thyroiditis appears to be viral infection. A number of viruses have been implicated, including mumps, influenza, coxsackie virus, and adenovirus. It seems possible that any virus may be involved, but those that invade the respiratory tract are more likely. The response of the thyroid is nonspecific.

Subacute thyroiditis characteristically presents with the picture of inflammatory disease. This includes local features such as pain, tenderness, and swelling, as well as systemic evidence of inflammation such as fever, sweats, and malaise. Depending upon the stage of the disease when the patient is first seen and the degree of involvement, the clinical features vary in severity. About 30 per cent of the patients we see have neither significant pain nor tenderness.

In addition to the typical local and systemic features reflecting the inflammatory process, there are also local and systemic consequences with respect to the thyroid malfunction. There is a temporary shutdown of thyroid hormonal synthesis and a discharge of stores of preformed hormone. Thus, there may be a mild temporary hyperthyroidism, which diminishes as the circulating thyroid hormone is metabolized. Since the recovery of the thyroid capacity for further hormonal synthesis may be delayed, there may be a period of hypothyroidism, beginning usually 2 to 3 months after the onset of the disease and lasting for a few weeks to a month or two.

The histological picture is one of edema, focal abscess and infiltration with polymorphonuclear leukocytes, disappearance of colloid, epithelial cell destruction, and later, fibrosis and infiltration with round cells and giant cells. As with Hashimoto's disease, the extent of involvement usually is diffuse, but there may be spared areas, and the disease may be sharply circumscribed within a small portion of the gland. In some cases, subacute thyroiditis begins as a localized process, but gradually extends throughout the gland over a period of several weeks. Ultimately, there is complete spontaneous recovery in almost all patients. For some there may be persistent goiter and, rarely, permanent hypothyroidism.

References

1. Hamburger JI: Subacute thyroiditis: Diagnostic difficulties and simple treatment. *J Nucl Med* 15:81–89, 1974
2. Hamburger JI: Subacute thyroiditis—Evolution depicted by serial ^{131}I scintigram. *J Nucl Med* 6:560–565, 1965.

PART II. CLINICAL EVALUATION OF NECK PAIN

The differential diagnosis of neck pain includes two thyroid diseases, subacute thyroiditis (SAT) and acute suppurative thyroiditis (AST); and a host of nonthyroidal diseases. The following outline summarizes the principal considerations in the differential diagnosis of neck pain.

    I. Thyroid diseases
        A. Subacute thyroiditis
        B. Acute suppurative thyroiditis (rare)
    II. Nonthyroidal conditions
        A. Musculoskeletal disorders
            1. Inflammatory
            2. Traumatic
        B. Pharyngeal-laryngeal inflammation
        C. Hysterical or neurotic (globus phenomenon)

The principal thyroidal cause of neck pain is SAT. The acute suppurative form of thyroiditis (caused by bacterial infection) is exceedingly rare. Pain or discomfort in the neck also may occur on the basis of nonthyroidal disorders; hence, the initial objective of the differential diagnosis is to learn whether the pain is related to the thyroid gland itself. Comparison of the response to pressure on the thyroid with compression of the sternocleidomastoid or other neck muscles may differentiate generalized neck sensitivity from tenderness localized to the thyroid gland.

TABLE 6–1. CORRELATION OF PHASE OF DISEASE, PATHOPHYSIOLOGIC PROCESSES, AND CLINICAL FEATURES OF SAT

PHASE	PATHOPHYSIOLOGIC PROCESS	CLINICAL FEATURES
Prodrome (up to 1 mo. before active phase)	Incipient inflammation	History of respiratory infection, malaise, painless goiter
I. Active (acute or subacute)	Inflammation, variable severity	
	A. Local inflammatory reaction	Painful, tender goiter, tachycardia
	B. Systemic inflammatory reaction	Malaise, night sweats, chills, fever, tachycardia
	C. Discharge of thyroid hormone into circulation	Tachycardia, weight loss, nervousness, tremor
II. Beginning resolution (2–4 mo. after active phase)	Resolving inflammation; beginning recovery of thyroid function	Painless goiter; possible hypothyroidism
III. Recovery (3–6 mo. after active phase)		
A. Complete	None	None
B. Incomplete	Chronic inflammation	Persistent painless goiter, or hypothyroidism, or both
IV. Relapse	Same as phase I	Same as phase I
V. Remote (years after active phase)	None,[a] or chronic inflammation[b]	None, or painless goiter, or hypothyroidism, or both

[a]Usual
[b]Uncommon

CLINICAL FEATURES OF SUBACUTE THYROIDITIS

The usual bout of subacute thyroiditis evolves through a series of phases. The severity of the active phase varies from what might properly be termed acute (uncommon) to the relatively more mild subacute form (most common) to the occult form (common), which is relatively free of the characteristic local manifestations of inflammation. Thus, it should be obvious that the clinical findings will depend upon two independent variables: (1) the phase of the disease when the patient is evaluated, and (2) the severity of involvement.

Table 6–1 correlates the phases of the disease with the underlying pathophysiologic processes and the clinical features that might be expected.

PART III. LABORATORY DIAGNOSIS OF SUBACUTE THYROIDITIS

Laboratory findings during the active stage of SAT directly reflect the underlying pathophysiologic events. The inflammatory reaction produces a discharge of preformed thyroid hormone into the circulation — hence the elevated FTI value. In addition, the inflammatory process impairs thyroid function. The characteristically suppressed RAI value — usually less than 5 per cent — is the result of *both* the inflammatory reaction per se upon the thyroid tissue *and* the suppressant effects of

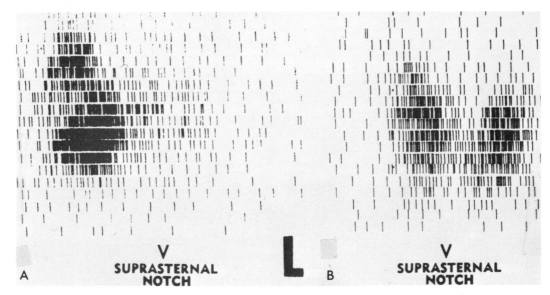

Figure 6-1. Subacute thyroiditis. *A,* Active phase after TSH. *B,* Recovery.

the discharged thyroid hormone upon the pituitary. The response to a TSH stimulation test will be negligible when the involvement is diffuse and uniform; however, if there is a sizeable amount of uninvolved tissue, an appreciable increase in RAI may occur in response to TSH stimulation, and the location of the responsive tissue may be identified by imaging. Figure 6–1 shows the patchy unilateral function following TSH stimulation in a patient with SAT (Fig 6–1 *A*). Four months later the disease had completely cleared, and a normal scan (Fig. 6–1 *B*) was obtained without TSH stimulation.

The characteristic elevation in ESR is, of course, a nonspecific index of the inflammatory process.

As the disease progresses toward recovery, the initial change in the laboratory data is a fall in the FTI as the discharged thyroid hormone is metabolized. If the ability of the thyroid gland to synthesize and secrete thyroid hormone remains impaired for more than a few weeks, there will be a temporary phase of hypothyroidism, during which the FTI and RAI values will both be low, whereas the TSH(RIA) level will be elevated. As recovery proceeds the FTI and RAI values gradually rise to normal, unless the disease has been so severe that permanent impairment of function develops (a very uncommon result). Table 6–2 correlates the pathophysiology and laboratory data in various phases of SAT.

OCCULT SAT

About 30 per cent of patients with SAT seen at the Northland Thyroid Laboratory do not have pain as the principal presenting manifestation. Painless goiter is the most common complaint in these patients. Other findings include a thyroid nodule or confusing abnormal laboratory data — i.e., usually an elevated serum thyroxine concentration in conjunction with a suppressed RAI value. The alert physician should consider the possibility of SAT under these circumstances, even if pain or tenderness is lacking. An elevated erythrocyte sedimentation rate and a subnormal or asymmetrical response (as visualized on the scan) to TSH stimulation

TABLE 6-2. CORRELATION OF PATHOPHYSIOLOGY AND LABORATORY DATA IN SAT

PHASE OF DISEASE	PATHOPHYSIOLOGIC PROCESS	LABORATORY DATA
I. Active	Local inflammatory reaction	Suppressed RAI Subnormally responsive to TSH stimulation
	Systemic inflammatory reaction Discharge of thyroid hormone	Elevated ESR Elevated FTI Suppressed RAI
II. Subsiding	Inflammation regressing Thyroid function still impaired	RAI suppressed FTI normal or low ESR normal
III. Recovery complete Recovery incomplete	None Hypothyroidism	Normal FTI low TSH(RIA) elevated

provide support for the diagnosis. Final confirmation depends upon both regression of clinical features and spontaneous return of laboratory values to normal.

In some cases a nodule that is caused by SAT might raise the possibility of thyroid cancer because of the appearance of hypofunction on scanning and the solid characteristics of the nodule on ultrasound evaluation. If SAT is suggested by other clinical or laboratory findings, a brief trial of adrenal corticosteroid therapy

TABLE 6-3. A COMPARISON OF CLINICAL AND LABORATORY FEATURES OF SAT AND AST

FEATURE	SAT	AST
General appearance	Variable, but at worst uncomfortable from moderately severe pain	Severely ill, often totally incapacitated
Pain	Minimal to moderate, rarely severe	Severe
Fever	Low grade or absent	High fever
Local findings	Firm, diffuse or unilateral enlargement. Minimal to moderate tenderness. At times nontender	Exquisite local tenderness with heat, fluctuance and overlying erythema
FTI	Usually elevated, at times normal	Normal
ESR	Elevated	Elevated
WBC	Normal or slightly elevated	>20,000
RAI	Decreased, with subnormal response to TSH stimulation	Normal
Imaging	Generalized nonfunction, or unilateral or patchy moth-eaten appearance after TSH stimulation	Localized functional defect at site of involvement

(prednisone, 50 mg daily) may prove to be of diagnostic and therapeutic value if there is complete resolution of the lesion within a few days.

The only important differential diagnosis for SAT is acute suppurative thyroiditis (AST). The clinical and laboratory features of SAT and AST are compared in Table 6–3. The differential diagnosis is usually not difficult.

PART IV.   TREATMENT OF PAINFUL THYROID DISEASES

AST

Acute suppurative thyroiditis is exceedingly rare (I have seen a total of two patients). Treatment includes incision and drainage and appropriate antimicrobial therapy.

References

1. Kirtland RT, Kirkland JL, Rosenberg HS, Harberg FJ, Librik L and Clayton GW: Solitary thyroid nodules in 30 children and report of a child with a thyroid abscess. *Pediatrics* 51:85–90, 1973
2. Perez Comas A: Acute suppurative thyroiditis. *Pediatrics* 42:308, 1973

SAT

Subacute thyroiditis is the usual painful disorder of the thyroid gland. It is an acute, self-limited disease that almost always subsides spontaneously regardless of treatment. Recovery is complete in more than 90 per cent of patients; however, some have persistent goiter, hypothyroidism, or both.

Treatment is directed at relief of pain. In my experience simple analgesics coupled with large doses of reassurance are all that is needed for the majority of patients. Reassurance cannot be overemphasized. Most of these patients are convinced that this sudden onset of a painful swelling in the neck means cancer. Immediate recognition of the true state of affairs, provision of a diagnosis, and emphasis on the benign implications of that diagnosis are very effective therapeutic weapons. Aspirin with codeine for the more uncomfortable patient is often adequate treatment. Adrenal corticosteroids may be needed occasionally, and even though their use may be followed by a higher relapse rate, they should be given when the patient finds no relief from simpler measures. Ordinarily, 40 to 80 mg of prednisone for the first 3 weeks followed by graded reductions over 6 to 8 weeks is satisfactory. Flare-up of the condition upon withdrawal requires resumption of the previously satisfactory dose and more prolonged weaning of the patient.

Extensive radiation therapy has been advised for persistent or recurrent forms of the disease. I have never used this treatment.

Another agent that may be employed effectively is propranolol if tachycardia is a prominent feature. A dose of 20 to 40 mg four times daily produces dramatic relief, and the drug can be progressively reduced over a 2- to 4-week period.

Almost all patients experience complete spontaneous recovery from SAT in about 3 months. For some there is a more prolonged course. Others pass through a temporary hypothyroid phase. A small proportion may be left with permanent residual goiter, hypothyroidism, or both. I advise permanent annual reevaluation of SAT patients to rule out late onset hypothyroidism. I have observed elevated TSH(RIA) values in three such patients in the absence of a reduction in serum levels for the FTI and T_3 (RIA). Augmented responses of the TSH(RIA) value after TRH administration have been observed in three additional patients.

References

1. Hamburger JI: Subacute thyroiditis: Diagnostic difficulties and simple treatment. *J Nucl Med* 15:81–89, 1974
2. Greene JN: Subacute thyroiditis. *Am J Med* 51:97–108, 1971
3. Torekai T and Kumaoka S: Subacute thyroiditis treated with salicylate. *New Eng J Med* 259:1265–1267, 1958
4. Cassidy CE: The diagnosis and treatment of subacute thyroiditis. In Astwood EB and Cassidy CE (eds): *Clinical Endocrinology II*. New York, Grune and Stratton, 1968, pp 220–231

PART V.   EXPERIENCE WITH SUBACUTE THYROIDITIS

In the 6-year period from 1968 to 1974, 100 patients with SAT were seen at Northland Thyroid Laboratory. There were 84 females and 16 males. They ranged in age from 14 to 69 years old. Only 4 patients were less than 20 years of age.

In 71 patients neck pain and thyroidal swelling and tenderness were prominent clinical features. The presentation was considered typical in these. However, in 29 patients the pain and tenderness were negligible or nonexistent, and the clinical presentation was therefore considered atypical.

Table 6–4 lists the principal presenting complaints in the 100 patients.

The most characteristic physical findings relative to the thyroid gland were firmness, tenderness, and diffuse enlargement. Unilateral enlargement was present in 23 patients, and seven patients presented with solitary nodules. In nine patients there was no appreciable thyroid enlargement.

TABLE 6–4. PRINCIPAL PRESENTING COMPLAINT IN 100 SAT PATIENTS

COMPLAINT	NUMBER OF PATIENTS
Neck pain	62
Painless goiter	17
Thyroid nodule	7
Confusing laboratory data	6
Suspected hyperthyroidism	6
Atrial fibrillation with goiter	1
Hair loss	1
Total	100

TABLE 6–5. FINDINGS ON INITIAL EXAMINATION OF THE THYROID GLAND IN 100 SAT PATIENTS

FINDINGS	PATIENTS (PER CENT)
Firmness	84
Tenderness	68
Diffuse enlargement	56
Unilateral enlargement	23
Solitary nodule	7
Multinodular	9
No enlargement	9

TABLE 6–6. RESULTS OF FOLLOWUP EVALUATION IN 55 SAT PATIENTS

FINDINGS		NUMBER OF PATIENTS
Complete recovery		44
Transient hypothyroidism	3	
Recurrence 2½ years later	1	
Hypothyroid at 3 months, no further followup		2
Hypothyroidism persistent for more than 1 yr		3
Goiter persistent more than 1 year		1
Euthyroid with elevated TSH(RIA)		3
Persistent nodule (probably antedated SAT)		2
Total		55

The RAI value was less than 5 per cent in all but three patients with SAT. The mean increment in RAI in response to TSH stimulation was 5.8 per cent ($\pm$SD 4.8 per cent). The mean $T_4(D)$ value was 13.1 μg per 100 ml($\pm$SD 3.3 μg per 100 ml). The mean ESR was 44.9($\pm$SD 9.8) in patients with tender thyroid glands, and significantly less (p $<$ .001) at 31.4 ($\pm$SD 15.2) for patients without pain or tenderness.

Table 6–6 gives the results of followup evaluation performed to assess the completeness of recovery in 55 SAT patients.

PART VI.   SELF-ASSESSMENT

CASE 6–1.   A PAINFUL NODULE

October, 1975.   A 41 year old nurse complained of mild neck pain in the thyroid area for about 4 to 6 weeks. There had been no fever, but she had experienced some malaise and nervousness. There had been a weight loss of 6 pounds and mild palpitation. She said that she had been taking no medication.

Examination revealed a normal temperature, a heart rate of 104, and moderately active reflexes. The thyroid gland was one and a half times normal size. It was

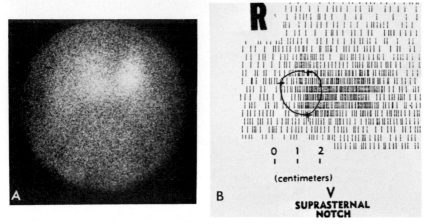

Figure 6-2. *A*, The gamma camera image. *B*, The fluorescent scan.

firm and contained a slightly tender nodule in the right lobe about 2 cm in diameter.

The FTI was 4.5, the T_3(RIA) 210 ng per 100 ml, and the RAI 3 per cent. A repeat RAI after TSH stimulation was still 3 per cent. A ^{99m}Tc gamma camera image revealed very poor concentration of the tracer. A fluorescent scan showed that iodine stores were generally reduced but more so in the area of the nodule. An ESR was 52 mm/hour.

With which of the following statements do you agree?

a. The nurse is malingering by taking high doses of thyroid hormone.

b. Prompt administration of adrenal steroids is indicated for both diagnosis and management.

c. This is a characteristic presentation of a hemorrhagic nodule.

d. The patient has hyperthyroidism.

e. The blocked RAI results from some source of iodine of which the patient is unaware.

f. Antithyroid drugs should be given, since the blocked RAI precludes the use of ^{131}I therapy.

g. Aspirin is all that is necessary.

h. No treatment is necessary.

i. In 3 months the thyroid will be normal. Reassurance is the treatment of choice.

j. This may be a very aggressive malignancy. A tissue diagnosis is mandatory.

k. One cannot exclude lymphoma in view of the elevated sedimentation rate.

l. Antibiotics and incision and drainage are indicated.

m. Antibiotics and analgesics are all that is necessary.

Case 6-1 — Followup

This is a rather characteristic example of subacute thyroiditis. The clinical features were typically rather low grade, with only minimal pain and tenderness. No treatment was necessary. Reevaluation in 3 months was advised.

March, 1976. The patient was asymptomatic. The FTI was normal. A normal ^{99m}Tc gamma camera image was obtained.

The negative response to TSH stimulation rules out self-administration of thyroid hormone. Patients taking thyroid hormone will have an increase in the RAI after TSH stimulation.

Adrenal steroids are unnecessary in view of the mild symptoms. Adrenal steroids do produce the most prompt and complete relief of the pain of SAT, but when the patient is not too sick, the simplest course is the best — i.e., reassurance and observation.

At this point I would like to emphasize the value of reassurance. Patients with neck pain, especially when there is a swelling or lump, and the characteristic malaise of SAT, are very often concerned that they might have cancer. A few moments of very positive reassurance by a physician often leads not only to remarkable relief of tension but a prompt willingness to tolerate the symptoms, which no longer seem so unpleasant.

Hemorrhagic nodules are usually not painful or tender. Furthermore, they are not associated with abnormal thyroid function tests.

The patient did have hyperthyroidism, as manifested by an elevation in the circulating levels of both thyroid hormones, nervousness, weight loss, palpitation, and mild tachycardia. This is the hyperthyroidism which results from discharge of stored thyroid hormone in response to the inflammatory reaction of SAT. In some instances, the manifestations of hyperthyroidism may be more severe and require some temporary therapeutic measures. In this case, the hyperthyroidism was mild and subsided spontaneously.

Failure to think of SAT as a common cause of a "blocked" RAI value is a common error of radiologists who also attempt to do thyroid function testing. The "unknown chemical block" is an explanation I encounter several times every year. The emphasis upon the pain caused by SAT has distracted the inexperienced physician from the appreciation that in a substantial proportion of SAT patients, pain and tenderness are either lacking or so minimal that they will easily be overlooked unless specifically sought. The physicians who first applied the term "subacute" to this disease knew what they were talking about. Unfortunately, other less perceptive individuals have preferred to refer to the disease as "acute." Greater appreciation of the frequent mildness of this disease has been expressed in recent reports.

The absurd suggestion for the use of ATD is included only for condemnation. Every year I see at least one patient receiving such treatment. The last one was taking PTU, aspirin, and prednisone for a diagnosis of hyperthyroidism and SAT. Needless to say, she had neither disease. Aspirin was not needed for the same reason that adrenal steroids were not needed. Had the pain been more troublesome, aspirin or even aspirin with codeine might have been helpful.

Biopsy is performed more often than necessary in patients with SAT. This presentation does not suggest cancer. Thyroid function tests are regularly normal in patients with thyroid cancer. With these findings, observation was all that was needed.

Antibiotics are frequently given to patients with SAT, but the disease is not bacterial in origin, and this treatment is useless. A viral cause is generally accepted.

Antibiotics and incision and drainage are the treatment for the rare case of acute suppurative thyroiditis. However, the patients with that disease are extremely ill, with high fever and marked local signs of inflammation, including very severe pain.

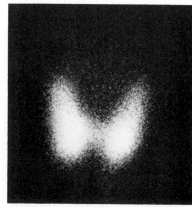

Figure 6-3. The gamma camera image after recovery.

CASE 6–2. SEVERE NECK PAIN FROM THYROIDITIS

November, 1974. A 48 year old man had a history of severe neck pain for over 2 months. A diagnosis of SAT had been made, and he had been treated with prednisone, 5 mg three times daily, without much relief. Also, he had been given levothyroxine, 0.3 mg daily. In addition to pain, his complaints included marked malaise, night sweats, chills, low grade fever, and palpitation.

Examination revealed a heart rate of 120, fine warm skin, a moderate hand tremor, and a diffusely enlarged, exquisitely tender thyroid gland, too tender to examine completely. The temperature was 99.6° F.

The FTI was 4.2, the RAI 1 per cent, and the ESR 38 mm/hr.

With which of the following statements do you agree?

a. Prednisone, 60 mg daily, should be given.

b. This degree of pain can be seen only in acute suppurative thyroiditis.

c. The prior adrenal steroid therapy aggravated the disease.

d. The condition is too severe for any treatment other than prompt surgical excision.

e. External radiation therapy will produce the most decisive relief.

f. Prednisone, if effective, will be needed only for 2 to 3 weeks.

g. Prednisone may be needed for 8 weeks or longer if a relapse after withdrawal is to be avoided.

h. The fact that prednisone failed to arrest the disease is convincing evidence against a diagnosis of SAT.

i. Thyroid hormone should be discontinued.

Case 6–2 — Followup

This patient, of course, had SAT. The absence of significant fever excludes the diagnosis of acute suppurative thyroiditis. Furthermore, that disease is usually a localized rather than a diffuse process.

Radiation therapy has been employed with good results in the past. I suggested to the patient that this might have to be given consideration if prednisone given in the proper dosage should fail. The earlier failure of prednisone simply indicates that the dose was inadequate.

Prednisone, 60 mg daily, produced prompt relief. The medication was gradually withdrawn over a 3-month period, during which there were two minor relapses of pain. By May of 1975 the patient was euthyroid and asymptomatic after taking no prednisone for 2 months.

Thyroid hormone is often given to patients with SAT without an understanding of its purpose. When the patient is in the acute phase of the disease, during which the plasma concentration of thyroid hormone is already elevated, it makes no sense to give additional thyroid hormone. This will only aggravate the hyperthyroid component of the disease.

Later in the course of the illness, thyroid hormone may be effective in hastening regression of the goiter, if present, especially if there is transient hypothyroidism that is characteristically seen 2 to 4 months after the onset of the disease. Usually, however, this is unnecessary.

Occasionally, if the patient presents with a localized nodule for which a diagnosis of cancer is under consideration, the use of combined levothyroxine and prednisone may be of diagnostic value if the lesion promptly and completely disappears. The contribution of thyroid hormone will be to suppress pituitary TSH, assuming that the stage of SAT is rather advanced.

CASE 6–3. SAT TREATED WITH PREDNISONE

June, 1973. A 37 year old woman had noticed the onset of typical clinical features of SAT 9 months earlier, including a painful, tender, enlarged thyroid gland. The diagnosis was confirmed by appropriate laboratory tests. Although her symptoms were not very severe, she was treated immediately with prednisone, 10 mg three times a day. The medication produced prompt and complete relief of her symptoms. Treatment was discontinued after 3 weeks, and a relapse occurred that was moderately worse than the initial episode. Prednisone was again administered with a good response. However, discontinuation of the drug was again followed by a relapse. This cycle of relief from prednisone followed by relapse after withdrawal was repeated five times over a period of 9 months. Consultation was then requested.

The patient had not had any treatment for 1 month prior to the examination and complained of tenderness and pain in the thyroid area, occasional night sweats, and mild malaise.

Examination revealed that the thyroid gland was enlarged to about twice the normal size and was firm and lobulated. Tenderness was definite but mild. The FTI was normal, the RAI 3 per cent, and the ESR 35 mm/hr.

With which of the following statements do you agree?

a.   This course is distinctly atypical for SAT.

b.   The repeated recurrences in spite of prednisone suggest that the diagnosis is not SAT.

c.   The prednisone, as administered, may have prolonged the course of the illness.

d.   Prednisone (or adrenal steroids of any type) is not the first choice of therapy for SAT.

e.   External radiation therapy is needed.

f.   Reassurance, analgesics, and patience will be best at this point.

Case 6–3 — Followup

The use of adrenal steroids for any patient with SAT is almost a reflex action on the part of many physicians. There is no doubt that prednisone produces prompt relief of the pain and tenderness and promotes regression of the goiter as well. However, adrenal steroids may have an important disadvantage in addition to their well-known potential side effects. Although I cannot prove it, it is my impression that relapses are more common when steroids are given. Whenever possible, I prefer to allow the disease to run its course, relying upon simple analgesics to maintain patient comfort.

I have successfully managed over 90 per cent of the patients I have seen with SAT without steroids. An essential component of the treatment is a large dose of positive reassurance. Only the unusual patient with severe pain (e.g., Case 6–2) must be given steroids.

When one finds it necessary to employ steroids he should follow the rule of enough and long enough. This disease runs a course of several months. The acute phase (during which pain is prominent) is usually a matter of 2 or 3 weeks. Nevertheless, when steroids are given, one should plan full dosage for 2 to 3 weeks and then gradually taper the drug over a period of at least 8 weeks. I begin with prednisone, 10 to 15 mg four times a day, depending upon the severity of the pain. (As an aside I should like to point out the obvious fact that the magnitude of pain that the patient appreciates and the intensity of his reaction to it is a function of the severity of the inflammatory reaction *and* the individual threshold for pain. In many instances, the latter is the more important consideration — hence, the extreme importance of high doses and repeat, reassurance.)

After 3 weeks of good control the dose can be tapered at 2-week intervals, with the plan of having the patient off the medication by 8 weeks. However, any flare-up of the pain requires either holding the dose level for a longer period of time (if the flare-up is mild) or reverting to the previously effective dose (if the flare-up is more severe) and holding at the level for 4 weeks.

A sudden withdrawal of the steroids will often be followed by a relapse.

Simple analgesics and high doses of reassurance were effective for this patient. In a few weeks she was free of pain and off all medication. Six months later she was euthyroid, and the thyroid gland was normal.

CASE 6–4. FACTITIOUS HYPERTHYROIDISM OR SAT?

February, 1976. A 37 year old nurse was referred for evaluation of possible hyperthyroidism. She had lost 30 pounds in the previous 3 months (from 167 to 137 pounds; she was 63 inches tall). She attributed this weight loss to dieting. She had increased nervousness and palpitation. Examination revealed a heart rate of 100 and a thyroid gland one and a half times normal size, firm, and slightly tender. The FTI was 4.2, the T_3(RIA) was 180 ng per 100 ml, and the RAI was 4 per cent. A repeat RAI after TSH stimulation was 14 per cent. The ESR was 47 mm/hr.

With which of the following statements do you agree?

a. This patient is malingering. The positive response to TSH makes the diagnosis.

b. She may have SAT. The high ESR is not seen in malingerers.

c. She has hyperthyroidism from an AFTA. The scan after TSH will be diagnostic.

d. The scan after TSH will be essential for a proper diagnosis.

e. The increase in RAI from 4 to 14 per cent is insignificant.

Case 6–4 — Followup

The gamma camera image after TSH stimulation shows that only the right lobe of the thyroid gland concentrates the tracer (Fig. 6–4).

The patient, of course, has SAT. Had she been malingering, the scan would have shown bilateral tracer concentration.

The TSH stimulation test is a very useful test but must be employed with full understanding of the underlying pathophysiology. There are two mechanisms whereby the RAI might be suppressed in patients with SAT:

1. The inflammatory reaction itself impairs follicular function and, if uniform, will preclude any trapping of the tracer.

2. In addition, the discharge of thyroid hormone by elevating plasma hormonal concentrations will suppress pituitary TSH release and thus suppress the RAI value.

If TSH is given, the response of the thyroid depends upon the extent of the inflammatory reaction. If this reaction is uniform or diffuse, there will be no increase in the RAI value. However, if the involvement is localized to one lobe or is nonuniform, then the lesser involved or noninvolved areas may retain the capacity to respond to TSH. Since the low baseline value in these patients is partly a reflection of suppression of endogenous TSH release, a scan after TSH stimulation will reveal the extent of the uninvolved tissue. Hence, this procedure is essential for proper diagnosis. The following scans are from three additional patients with SAT who responded to TSH stimulation.

The diagnosis of an AFTA producing elevated levels of thyroid hormone in the circulation is not very attractive in the absence of a palpable nodule. Hyperthyroidism from an AFTA is almost never seen unless the nodule is at least 2.5 to 3.0 cm in diameter. Furthermore, these nodules are not associated with a suppressed baseline RAI value.

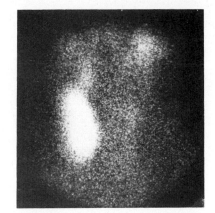

Figure 6-4. The gamma camera image after TSH stimulation.

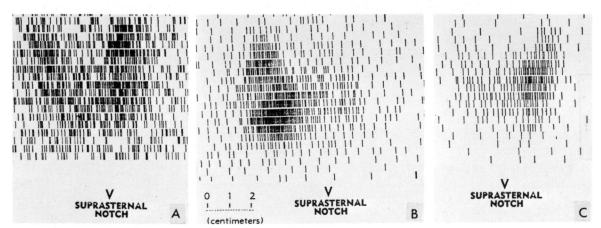

Figure 6-5. *Scans on patients with subacute thyroiditis who responded to TSH stimulation. A, A diffuse, patchy tracer distribution. B, Predominantly right lobe tracer uptake. C, Predominantly left lobe tracer uptake.*

CASE 6–5. TACHYCARDIA, CAUSE UNKNOWN

October, 1974. A 23 year old medical student was referred for tachycardia of 120 for which no cause was apparent. He was very uncomfortable because of the palpitation. In addition, he had lost 17 pounds in spite of no change in food intake. There had been no heat intolerance and no fever. A mild tremor was noted, and the thyroid gland was slightly enlarged, firm but not tender. The FTI was 11, the T_3(RIA) 265 ng per 100 ml, and the ESR 40 mm/hr. The RAI was 2 per cent and did not respond to TSH stimulation.

With which of the following statements do you agree?

    a. The patient has hyperthyroidism.
    b. The patient has been taking high doses of thyroid hormone.
    c. The patient has SAT.
    d. No treatment is needed.
    e. Give antithyroid drugs.
    f. Propranolol for a few weeks will be helpful.
    g. Lugol's solution will be helpful.

Case 6–5 — Followup

This is another patient with SAT, but the discharge of thyroid hormone was unusually great, causing a considerable cardiac response. Propranolol, 20 mg four times a day, slowed the heart rate to 90 and made the patient much more comfortable. After 2 weeks, the medication was gradually phased out over an additional 3 weeks. Reevaluation of thyroid function revealed normal values 3 months later.

This is the only patient for whom the cardiac features of SAT were so strong that we felt propranolol was indicated. However, this drug is something to keep in mind for the occasional patient for whom great relief may be provided so simply.

It does not seem necessary to review the reasons why the other suggestions are inappropriate.

CASE 6–6. HYPOTHYROIDISM AFTER SAT

August, 1974. A 43 year old woman presented with a 6-week history of malaise, neck pain, chills, palpitation, and low grade fever. The thyroid gland was diffusely enlarged to two and a half times normal size, firm, and moderately tender. The skin was moist and warm, the heart rate was 120, and the reflexes were hyperactive.

The FTI was 5.4, and the RAI was 1 per cent and unresponsive to TSH stimulation. The ESR was 54 mm/hr. A diagnosis of SAT was made. Observation was advised. Reevaluation was scheduled for 3 months.

November, 1974. The patient was feeling much better, although still lacking in pep. The heart rate was 72, and she had gained 9 pounds. The thyroid gland was twice the normal size and still firm. The FTI was 0.2, the TSH(RIA) 115 μU/ml, and the RAI 10 per cent.

With which of the following statements do you agree?

a. The patient had an acute case of Hashimoto's disease, which has now progressed to permanent hypothyroidism.

b. The patient had SAT but is one of the few who have permanent hypothyroidism afterward.

c. The patient had SAT and has only temporary hypothyroidism at this point.

d. Treatment with thyroid hormone is necessary.

e. Treatment with thyroid hormone is optional.

f. The reevaluation in 3 months will probably reveal recovery of normal function.

Case 6–6 — Followup

In the evolution of SAT there is often a period of transient hypothyroidism. The exact point in the course of the illness at which this should be anticipated is hard to fix. This is because the relatively vague clinical features make it difficult to pinpoint the onset of the disease, and the duration of the acute phase of the disease is variable.

If one measures the time interval from the end of the more severe acute manifestations, one might expect a mild episode of hypothyroidism 2 to 3 months later. I cannot say how often this occurs, because unless the patient is checked frequently, this period of hypothyroidism may be overlooked.

Thyroid hormone may be given if the symptoms are distressing, but usually it is unnecessary. In this patient observation was elected, and 2 months later she was symptom-free.

January, 1975. The FTI was 1.6, and the TSH(RIA) was still elevated at 86 μU/ml. The RAI was a rather high 44 per cent. Occasionally a high RAI value will be encountered during recovery from SAT. This should not be interpreted as an indication of hyperthyroidism.

November, 1975. The patient was completely well. The FTI was 2.1, and the TSH(RAI) was 7.2 μU/ml.

Selected Current References For Subacute Thyroiditis

1. Hamburger JI: Subacute thyroiditis: Diagnostic difficulties and simple treatment. *J Nucl Med* 15:81–89, 1974

   Most of the lessons I have included in this text were reviewed in this article.

2. Greene JN: Subacute thyroiditis. *Am J Med* 51:97–108, 1971

   This is a classic review article on the subject and has an exhaustive bibliography. It will be of most value to those with considerable experience, because almost every shade of opinion is recorded. This, of course, is a major defect. The good is included with the bad in totally nondiscriminatory fashion. The author either has no great experience or is too timid to advise the reader as to which of the myriad of conflicting concepts presented have practical utility, and which are better relegated to the status of historical curiosity.

3. Papapetrou PD and Jackson IM: Thyrotoxicosis due to "silent" thyroiditis. *Lancet* 1:361–363, 1975
4. Woolf PD and Daly R: Thyrotoxicosis with painless thyroiditis. *Am J Med* 60:73–79, 1976

   These two reports emphasize the importance of being aware of painless SAT.

5. Vagenakis AG, Abreau CM and Braverman LE: Prevention of recurrence in acute thyroiditis following corticosteroid withdrawal. *J Clin Endocrinol* 31:705–708, 1970

   This article tells us that we can avoid relapses after withdrawal of corticosteroids by maintaining treatment until the suppressed RAI value returns to normal. A close look at the data for the five patients treated suggests that steroids were unnecessary for two who had only moderate pain in the first place. In the few patients to whom I have given steroids, a gradual withdrawal over 6 to 8 weeks worked well without performing multiple RAI determinations.

6. Carney JA, Moore SB, Northcutt RC, et al: Palpation thyroiditis (multifocal granulomatous folliculitis). *Am J Clin Pathol* 64:639–647, 1975

   Palpation thyroiditis was present in over 83 per cent of thyroid glands removed surgically.

CASE 6–7. A NURSING MOTHER WITH HYPERTHYROIDISM

A 27 year old woman was referred for a goiter discovered 3 weeks earlier. Her complaints included fatigue, sweating, tremor, and a 24-pound weight loss (attributed to the delivery of her baby 6 weeks earlier). She was nursing the infant and was reluctant to stop because the baby would not feed from a bottle.

The heart rate was 116, the skin moist and warm, the hands mildly tremulous, and the thyroid gland firm and enlarged to about twice the normal size. There was no thyroid tenderness, and the patient had not noted any severe neck pain, although she had been aware of slight soreness for a few days 2 weeks previously.

The FTI was 5.6 and the T_3(RIA) was 280 ng per 100 ml. Antithyroid antibodies were strongly positive. The EST was 61 mm/hr.

With which of the following statements do you agree?

a. The patient has hyperthyroidism. Start treatment with ATD.

b. Although she has hyperthyroidism, both ATD and ^{131}I therapy are contraindicated because both would pass into her milk. She should be treated surgically.

c. Never make a diagnosis of hyperthyroidism without a radioactive iodine uptake. Insist that she stop nursing so this study can be done.

d. She has hyperthyroidism, but it may be "hyperthyroiditis," i.e., temporary hyperthyroidism of Hashimoto's disease, as recently reported by Gluck et al. The high antibody titers suggest this diagnosis.

e. SAT is a possibility. The high ESR suggests the diagnosis.

f. A needle biopsy will provide the diagnosis.

g. If this is SAT there should be spontaneous resolution of the hyperthyroidism in a few weeks.

Case 6–7 — Followup

We insisted that she stop nursing so a radioactive iodine uptake could be obtained. In 1 month she was able to wean the infant, and she returned for reevaluation. The goiter had increased in size by 25 per cent. The heart rate had slowed to 78, and she had gained 4 pounds. The reflexes were somewhat sluggish, and the skin was cool and dry. The FTI was 0.3, the TSH(RIA) 80 μU/ml, and the RAI was only 4 per cent. The ESR had fallen to 18.

In my opinion, this sequence of events fits best with a diagnosis of SAT in the hypothyroid phase of resolution. I suppose that a diagnosis of Hashimoto's disease does not preclude the development of SAT. The articles by Gluck et al and Jackson illustrate the confusion which can occur in the differentiation of various forms of inflammatory disease of the thyroid. Gluck et al felt content with their diagnoses of chronic thyroiditis (Hashimoto's disease) because they had obtained tissue by needle biopsy. However, Jackson, in a following editorial, noted that histologic findings are not necessarily diagnostic. In three of Gluck's patients the course from hyperthyroidism with a low RAI to spontaneous recovery suggested SAT to me. One of the three even had a mildly tender goiter initially. In any event, it seems reasonable to assume that there may be patients with both diseases who will have varying clinical features depending upon the stage of disease at the time the patient presents.

With respect to the other statements the following comments are offered.

a and b. Antithyroid drugs will be secreted in breast milk and should not be given to lactating women. Of course this patient was hyperthyroid, but if was the temporary hyperthyroidism of inflammatory disease (I think it was SAT). Obviously, surgical treatment was not indicated.

c. This is a "trick" question. One can make a diagnosis of hyperthyroidism without an RAI value. Hyperthyroidism is a clinical syndrome associated with elevated blood levels of thyroid hormone, which this patient had. Nevertheless, the RAI is essential to determine whether the hyperthyroidism is the result of a primary hypersecretory process (e.g., TDG, TMNG, toxic AFTA) or some other process (e.g., iatrogenic disease, SAT, or toxic ovarian struma). This differential diagnosis is essential for rational therapy. A paper presented at the 1976 meeting of the American Thyroid Association dealt with short-term ATD treatment of hyperthyroidism, pointing out that some patients go into remission after only a few months. The paper was criticized because the author failed to obtain pretreatment RAI values, and thus might have included some patients with SAT in his short-term success group.

f. Needle biopsy will not provide an unequivocal diagnosis and is therapeutically irrelevant.

g. Spontaneous resolution is one of the most important diagnostic features of SAT. I have not had the opportunity to determine whether this patient's subsequent hypothyroidism will be temporary or permanent. If it is temporary, then SAT is the best diagnosis. If the hypothyroidism is permanent, the diagnosis might be permanent impairment of thyroid function after an episode of SAT; or hypothyroidism following both SAT and Hashimoto's disease; or a more acute presentation of Hashimoto's disease, with rapid progression to hypothyroidism. These patients are relatively uncommon, and more data is needed before one can be too dogmatic. Fortunately, an etiologic diagnosis is not essential for proper management as long as one follows the patient, watching for changes in thyroid functional activity.

Selected Current References for Case 6–7

1. Gluck FB, Nusynowitz ML and Plymate S: Chronic lymphocytic thyroiditis, thyrotoxicosis, and low radioactive iodine uptake. *New Eng J Med* 293:624–628, 1975
2. Jackson I: "Hyper-Thyroiditis"—a diagnostic pitfall. *New Eng J Med* 293:661–662, 1975
3. Papapetrou PD and Jackson IMD: Thyrotoxicosis due to "silent" thyroiditis. *Lancet* 1:361–363, 1975

Supplemental References

Hyperthyroidism

1. Horn K, Erhardt F, Fahlbusch R, et al: Recurrent goiter, hyperthyroidism, galactorrhea and amenorrhea due to a thyrotropin and prolactin-producing pituitary tumor. *J Clin Endocrinol Metab* 43:137–143, 1976

   This is a report of a patient with the problems cited in the title; the onset of signs occurred at 16 years of age. The case is unique and well documented.

2. Hollingsworth DR and Mabry CC: Congenital Graves' disease. In Fisher DA and Burrow GN (eds): *Perinatal Thyroid Physiology and Disease.* Raven Press, New York, 1975, pp 163–183

   This long-term study and literature review challenges most of our concepts about neonatal thyrotoxicosis. In the first place, serious objections to LATS as the cause of this disease are raised. I never liked the idea that LATS caused anything, so I am easily persuaded to believe that it is blameless. The authors favor the idea that the disease reflects a genetically conditioned process. Furthermore, they show that neonatal thyrotoxicosis is often prolonged rather than transient and may be severe. Neonatal death was the outcome in 16 per cent of 74 infants whose records were reviewed.

3. Man EB and Serunian SA: Thyroid function in human pregnancy. IX. Development or retardation of 7-year-old progeny of hypothyroxinemic women. *Am J Obstet Gynecol* 125:949–957, 1976

   This report emphasizes the risk to the fetal intellect produced by untreated maternal hypothyroidism. Why do I include this reference under hyperthyroidism? It emphasizes the importance of avoiding overtreatment of the pregnant hyperthyroid patient with ATD.

4. Stanbury JB and Chapman EM: Nonoperative management of hyperthyroidism. In Varco RL and Delaney JP (eds): *Controversy in Surgery.* W.B. Saunders Co., Philadelphia, 1976, pp 555–564
5. Robertson JS and Gorman CA: Gonadal radiation dose and its genetic significance in radioiodine therapy of hyperthyroidism. *J Nucl Med* 17:826–835, 1976

   The above two papers are additional efforts to promote logical thinking in the selection of treatment for young adults with hyperthyroidism. The data indicate that the potential genetic risks of ^{131}I are too small to constitute a serious objection to the treatment. This lesson is not new but will undoubtedly fail to convince those who unhesitatingly prefer the vastly greater risk of anesthetic mortality that is unavoidable with thyroidectomy.

6. Haibach H: Hyperthyroidism in Graves' disease. *Arch Intern Med* 136:725–731, 1976

   This review article again reminds us of the risks of thyroidectomy and the poor results currently being reported with ATD. The author considers ^{131}I the primary therapy for this disease.

7. Buerklin EM, Schimmel M and Utiger RD: Pituitary-thyroid regulation in euthyroid patients with Graves' disease previously treated with antithyroid drugs. *J Clin Endocrinol Metab* 43:419–427, 1976
8. Martino E, Pinchera A, Capiferri R, et al: Dissociation of responsiveness to thyrotropin-releasing hormone and thyroid suppressibility following antithyroid drug therapy of hyperthyroidism. *J Clin Endocrinol Metab* 43:543–549, 1976

   These two papers provide additional evidence for a lack of agreement between T_3 suppression tests and TRH-testing after treatment of hyperthyroidism. The TRH test is no more reliable than T_3 suppression testing in predicting a sustained remission or relapse. It is still necessary to follow the patient.

9. Cihak RW and Beary FD: Elevated triiodothyronine and dextrothyroxine levels: A potential cause of iatrogenic hyperthyroidism. *South Med J* 70:256–257, 1977

   Since dextrothyroxine (DT_4) is metabolically weak, it is given in doses of 4 to 12 mg daily (compared to average LT_4 doses of 0.15 to 0.2 mg daily). Since DT_4, like LT_4, is converted to T_3 at the periphery, it is understandable that relatively larger amounts of T_3 may be derived from the usual doses of DT_4 than from those of LT_4. It is reasonable to think that DT_4 would give rise to DT_3, which is weaker than LT_3. The case reported by these authors suggests that DT_4 may be converted in part to LT_3 or that DT_3 may be more potent relative to LT_3 than DT_4 is to LT_4.

10. Teng CS and Yeo PBP: Ophthalmic Graves' disease: Natural history and detailed thyroid function studies. *Brit Med J* 1:273–275, 1977

These authors confirm the usefulness of the TRH test as a replacement for the T_3 suppression test in the diagnosis of the euthyroid stage of Graves' disease. It is of particular interest that very few of their patients subsequently developed hyperthyroidism. On the contrary, more of them became overtly hypothyroid. The hypothyroidism was attributed to the progression of associated autoimmune thyroiditis (Hashimoto's disease).

Hypothyroidism

1. Elewaut A, Mussche M and Vermeulen A: Familial partial target organ resistance to thyroid hormones. *J Clin Endocrinol Metab* 43:575–581, 1976.

This is another report of resistance at the tissue level to physiologic quantities of thyroid hormone. Cases as overt as this must be very rare. However, since we are employing the TSH(RIA) more often to check on the adequacy of replacement therapy, we do observe fairly often a failure of suppression of TSH levels with doses of levothyroxine that maintain normal serum concentrations of T_4. The lesson may be that the proper dose of levothyroxine is that which suppresses the elevated TSH(RIA) level. However, I would not accept elevated T_4 levels as necessary unless the elevated TSH levels were confirmed on more than one determination, preferably allowing an interval of a month or longer to be sure that the TSH value does not gradually decline.

2. Yamada T, Tsukui T, Ikejiri K, et al: Volume of sella turcica in normal subjects and in patients with primary hypothyroidism and hyperthyroidism. *J Clin Endocrinol Metab* 42:817–822, 1976

This is another report of the increased volume of the sella in an astounding 81 per cent of patients with hypothyroidism.

3. Vagenakis AG, Dole K and Braverman LE: Pituitary enlargement, pituitary failure, and primary hypothyroidism. *Ann Intern Med* 85:195–198, 1976

This is the same message in two patients.

4. Maeda M, Kuzuya N, Masuyama Y, et al: Changes in serum triiodothyronine, thyroxine, and thyrotropin during treatment with thyroxine in severe primary hypothyroidism. *J Clin Endocrinol* 43:10–17, 1976

This detailed and complicated analysis offers the suggestion that the 70 kg patient will require about 150 μg daily of levothyroxine for ideal maintenance. Somehow we came to the same conclusion empirically. The authors' suggestion that the ideal dose of levothyroxine may be related to patient weight does not sound right to me.

5. De Lean A, Ferland L, Drouin J, Kelly PA and Labrie F: Modulation of pituitary thyrotropin releasing hormone receptor levels by estrogens and thyroid hormones. *Endocrinol* 100:1496–1504, 1977

It is well established that patients with hypothyroidism respond to TRH with an augmented pituitary release of TSH. It has been concluded that an augmented response to TRH is the most sensitive diagnostic finding of hypothyroidism. Having personally administered TRH for about 6 months for some 3000 tests, I observed that modestly augmented responses occur at times in patients who by all other criteria are euthyroid. This article suggests that estrogens may potentiate the effect of TRH on the release of TSH. The following article confirms it, and our experience supports these observations.

6. Ramey JN, Burrow GN, Polackwich RJ and Donabedian RK: The effect of oral contraceptive steroids on the response of thyroid-stimulating hormone to thyrotropin-releasing hormone. *J Clin Endocrinol Metab* 40:712–714, 1975

The authors observed a rise of 19 ± 2.5 μU/ml (mean ± SEM) on serum TSH values in reponse to 100 μg of TRH in euthyroid women and a rise of 30 ± 2.5 μU/ml in euthyroid women receiving oral contraceptives.
The findings in these two papers permit two important inferences:
1. Patients who are receiving estrogens may have spuriously augmented responses to TRH. Unless the response is beyond that which may be attributed to estrogens, a diagnosis of hypothyroidism should not be considered supported by the data.
2. Since estrogens may overcome the blocking effects of thyroid hormone on TRH tests, it seems possible that some hyperthyroid patients who are receiving estrogens may respond normally to TRH. This requires further study.
Having noted the reports of augmented TRH responses in women who are taking estrogens, we

reviewed our data on 60 such patients. Forty-three had normal responses. Eight patients had post-TRH increments of between 16 and 20 μU/ml in TSH concentrations, and nine patients had greater increments, ranging from 21 μU/ml to 56 μU/ml. All patients had normal FTI values, and none had clinical evidence of hypothyroidism. Unfortunately, it is not possible to be certain that those patients who exhibited augmented responses to TRH did not have subclinical impairment of thyroid function. To settle this point it would have been necessary to study the patients before and after the administration of estrogen. In recent paper by Mishell et al* three patients were studied in this fashion. Two patients were less responsive to TRH while taking estrogen, and the third patient was more responsive; however, the differences in pre- and post-treatment responses were small in all three patients. Hence, we conclude that for most patients estrogen in conventional doses does not produce a significant alteration in the TRH response. The significance of this augmented response in the small proportion of patients who do respond more vigorously must await more extensive study.

Thyroid Cancer

1. Editorial. Irradiation of the thyroid gland. *Lancet* 1:1278–1279, 1976.

This editorial reviews the results from fallout in the Marshallese Islands. They conclude that low doses of ^{131}I for hyperthyroidism are bad (I agree) and that ^{131}I therapy should not be used in children (I am not so sure) or in young adults (I disagree). This conclusion disregards the risks of alternative treatments.

Of greater current interest to American thyroidologists is the issue of thyroid cancer occurring years after x-ray therapy to the thymus, tonsils, and other areas of the upper body. Physicians at the University of Chicago and the Michael Reese Hospital have published a series of reports suggesting a substantial incidence of thyroid cancer in these patients. The Michael Reese group has suggested that many of these cancers are impalpable but detectable by imaging with ^{99m}Tc pertechnetate as the tracer and a gamma camera with pinhole collimation as the imaging device. They acknowledged that the defects detected often did not correspond to the cancers, but claimed that the presence of these defects was a marker for cancer somewhere in the thyroid, and thus reason enough to consider surgical intervention.

A special conference was held at the University of Chicago, September 30th and October 1, 1976, for the purpose of assessing many controversial aspects of this general problem.

The matter which most concerned the participants was what to do about tiny occult cancers. Most of us were reinforced in our opinions that these lesions do not constitute a serious risk to the patient.

Dr. R. Nishiyama (pathologist at the University of Michigan) reported that careful serial sections of 100 thyroid glands obtained at autopsy revealed a 13 per cent incidence of tiny foci of cancer. Dr. R. Sampson (another pathologist) argued persuasively against the idea that these occult lesions were serious. He reported that they occurred with equal prevalence in the two sexes, whereas larger lesions are found three to four times more often in women. Although Switzerland has the highest mortality rate from thyroid cancer, the presence of occult cancer there is the lowest in the world. By contrast, Japan has the highest prevalence of occult thyroid cancer and the lowest mortality rate from thyroid cancer. Dr. Sampson cited a prevalence to mortality ratio of 100 to 1 for occult thyroid cancer.

The Mayo Clinic experience with occult cancer was reported by Dr. A. Edis. For 244 patients followed up to 40 years there were no deaths, no distant metastases, and only 12 local recurrences. These patients were treated with conservative operations.

Dr. R. Leeper (from Memorial Hospital, New York) added a further note of caution by reporting that 20 per cent of their deaths from papillary cancer and 29 per cent of the deaths from follicular cancer were attributable to the treatment.

At least one surgeon admitted having performed total thyroidectomies on two patients whose thyroid glands had defects on imaging but were normal when examined histologically.

By the conclusion of the meeting there was widespread agreement that it might be best to emphasize the detection of clinically evident thyroid cancer. Inappropriate overenthusiasm for the eradication of all occult lesions might lead to more patient injury than benefit. In this regard, I made a plea for caution in the interpretation of thyroid imaging studies. I emphasized that a defect on a thyroid image that does not correspond to a palpable nodule may be the result of many non-nodular abnormalities, including anatomical variations of no clinical significance. Dr. Gerald Burke (Mt. Sinai Hospital of Chicago) had shown examples of many of these variations that were reported in a recent paper by Hurley et al. (Hurley PJ, Strauss HW, Pavoni P, et al: The scintillation camera with pinhole collimator in thyroid imaging. Radiology 101:133–138, 1971).

Many other aspects of the diagnosis and treatment of thyroid cancer were covered. The proceedings will be published and undoubtedly deserve careful study. Dr. Leslie DeGroot and his associates deserve commendation for organizing such a fine program.

---

*Mishell DR, Kletzky OA, Brenner PF, Roy S and Nicoloff J: The effect of contraceptive steroids on hypothalamic-pituitary function. *Am J Obstet Gynecol* 128:60–74, 1977

2. Fernandez-Ulloa M, Maxon HR, Mehta S, et al: Iodine[131] uptake by primary lung adenocarcinoma. Misinterpretation of ^{131}I scan. *JAMA* 236:857–858, 1976

It is not surprising that tissue other than thyroid cancer can concentrate enough ^{131}I or any other tracer for visualization on imaging if a large enough tracer dose is given. I have long suspected that some examples of diffuse pulmonary metastases attributed to thyroid cancer demonstrated only by ^{131}I scanning after scan doses of 5 mCi or more might not represent anything more than temporary concentration by normal lymphatics. Technology can be dangerous.

3. Walfish PG, Miskin M, Rosen IB, et al: Application of special diagnostic techniques in the management of nodular goitre. *Can Med Assoc J* 115:35–40, 1976

This preliminary report supports Scandinavian claims that cytologic examination of fine needle aspirate is a simple and useful tool for the evaluation of thyroid nodules.

4. Boehm T, Rothouse L and Wartofsky L: Metastatic occult follicular thyroid carcinoma. *JAMA* 235:2420–2421, 1976

This "occult" cancer is not the type of occult cancer over which there was so much discussion in Chicago (see p. 277). This was a follicular lesion rather than the papillary tumor one generally thinks of as occult and unaggressive. Actually, there was a spirited debate in Chicago (rather silly in my opinion) over the definition of an occult thyroid cancer. The core of the dispute was how small a lesion had to be to be considered occult. I suppose it was thought that if agreement could be reached on the definition of an occult thyroid cancer, then one would be able to identify those cancers with low biologic potential for producing morbidity or mortality. To me it seems obvious that size is a criterion of limited use. After all, larger tumors were smaller before they grew up. On the other hand, a small tumor that has been completely excised will never get larger, and the determination of the size of a small tumor implies that it has been removed. Actually, the biologic potential for malignant behavior of any tumor is a retrospective determination. If the lesion fails to progress, whether because it is removed, or because some other disease kills the patient, or because it actually is not very aggressive, the net effect is the same for the patient. On the contrary, if the small lesion metastasizes distantly (as in this report) or gradually enlarges, even though tiny initially, calling it occult does not change its malignant behavior.

5. Bricout P and Kibler RS: Experience in the management of thyroid carcinoma by I-131. A report of 39 cases. *J Can Assoc Radiol* 24:323–327, 1973

These authors were rather aggressive with ^{131}I therapy. However, they were dealing predominantly with patients with disease that had extended beyond the neck. Their results seem to justify their approach.

6. Heitz P, Moser H and Staub JJ: Thyroid cancer. A study of 573 thyroid tumors and 161 autopsy cases observed over a thirty-year period. *Cancer* 37:2229–2337, 1976

This is a rather good review emphasizing the dangers of transition from follicular to anaplastic cancer. Their recommendation of removal of all nodules would not be acceptable in the United States. However, things may be different in Switzerland.

7. Shimaoka K, VanHerle AJ and Dindogru A: Thyrotoxicosis secondary to involvement of the thyroid with malignant lymphoma. *J Clin Endocrinol Metab* 43:64–68, 1976

The authors ask us to believe that a lymphoma invaded the thyroid, produced goiter, destroyed thyroid tissue so that the RAI was suppressed, and discharged thyroid hormone to produce a temporary hyperthyroidism, all of which regressed after treatment. One might ask what this remarkable treatment was. It included local x-ray therapy and nitrogen mustard (undoubtedly good for lymphoma), prednisone (good for a number of diseases), and PTU. (Although PTU is good for hyperthyroidism caused by hypersecretory diseases such as TDG, TMNG, and toxic AFTA, what possible rationale can there be for this treatment under these presumed circumstances?) In my opinion, in spite of this treatment, the most remarkable feature of this case was the restoration of the euthyroid state and partial recovery of the RAI value (probably only partial because of the x-ray therapy).

The authors note that the features of this case are remarkably similar to those attending an episode of SAT. At last I can find some basis for agreement. Although the patient had lymphomatous involvement of the thyroid, the hyperthyroid episode was most likely our old friend SAT. It is unfortunate that with all the studies she had, no one thought to do a TSH stimulation test when she was first seen. The combination of elevated serum thyroid hormone levels and a suppressed RAI value is an unequivocal indication for this procedure. A positive response suggests iatrogenic–factitious hyperthyroidism, struma ovarii, or possibly SAT. A negative response suggests SAT or hyperthyroidism in a patient who has received large quantities of iodide. A negative response might also be seen under the circumstances described by the authors. However, I find the suggestion of reversible destruction of the thyroid by infiltrating lymphoma less acceptable than simple old SAT. The authors are to be commended for their imagination but castigated for employing local x-ray therapy precipitously and not performing a TSH stimulation test. The editors of the Journal of Clinical Endocrinology and Metabolism *dropped the ball on this one.*

8. Wang C, Vickery AL, Jr, and Maloof F: Needle biopsy of the thyroid. *Surg Gynecol Obstet* 143:365–368, 1976

This paper provides data on 40 cancer patients diagnosed by needle biopsy. The authors emphasize that success improves with experience.

9. Park CH, Rothermel FJ and Judge DM: Unusual calcification in mixed papillary and follicular carcinoma of the thyroid gland. *Radiology* 119:554, 1976

Having presented a patient with a ring calcification of a nodule and postulated that this was a benign lesion (p. 241), I was chagrined to encounter this case report to the contrary. I was somewhat relieved to read the authors' conclusion that "The type of calcification seen in our case is rarely seen in patients with thyroid cancer."

As this book was on the way to the printer, Dr. Stoffer reported that he became worried when our patient (p. 241) developed a satellite nodule adjacent to the hard calcified lesion. He advised excision. The calcified nodule was indeed benign, but the adjacent nodule was a follicular carcinoma. Therefore, we can conclude that the benign features of a calcified nodule are not transferrable to other nodules in the same gland.

10. Miller JM, Kasenter AG and Marks DS: Disparate imaging of the autonomous functioning thyroid nodule with ^{99m}Tc pertechnetate and radioiodine. *Radiology* 119:737–739, 1976

This study shows that autonomously functioning thyroid nodules may have difficulty organifying iodide. Serial studies on one patient over 8 years showed that this defect may be temporary, perhaps representing an early stage in the maturation of a potentially toxic AFTA.

11. Lo Gerfo P, Stillman T, Colacchio D and Feind C: Serum thyroglobulin and recurrent thyroid cancer. *Lancet* 1:881–882, 1977

Scooped again. We were just in the process of setting up a thyroglobulin assay to assess this very point. It is clear that the thyroglobulin assay is not a reliable test for the diagnosis of thyroid cancer. However, it seems reasonable that, given a thyroid cancer patient with an elevated serum level of thyroglobulin, repeat levels after treatment might indicate whether the tumor had been eliminated and later might indicate the presence of a recurrence. This is in fact what these authors report.

12. Mazzaferri EL, Young RL, Oertel JE, Kemmerer WT and Page CP: Papillary thyroid carcinoma: The impact of therapy in 576 patients. *Medicine* 56:171–196, 1977

This detailed article on papillary thyroid cancer is worth careful reading. Only five patients out of 576 died from causes directly related to the cancer (less than 1 per cent). These five patients are described briefly, and it is clear that four of the five were grossly mismanaged. The treatment of the fifth patient (their patient 1) might be argued. Since this was a retrospective study it seems probable that a substantial number of other patients were treated with similar disregard for the principles generally accepted as important for good results. Therefore, it may be that these patients died because of unusually malignant disease and would have died no matter how they were treated. Nevertheless, the fact that for over 99 per cent of the patients papillary cancer did not prove fatal should promote an attitude of conservatism.

Painful Thyroid Diseases

1. Ginsberg J and Walfish PG: Post-partum transient thyrotoxicosis with painless thyroiditis. *Lancet* 1:1125–1127, 1977

Five cases of painless SAT are described. Symptomatic therapy was all that proved necessary. Two patients had persistent antibody elevations and needle biopsy findings consistent with chronic thyroiditis. One of them developed permanent hypothyroidism. It would seem that there may be some overlap in the clinical presentation of SAT and the more acute onset of chronic thyroiditis, the latter having a tendency to progress to hypothyroidism.

2. Weihl RB, Daniels GH, Ridgway EC and Maloof F: Thyroid function tests during the early phase of subacute thyroiditis. *J Clin Endocrinol Metab* 44:1107–1114, 1977

These authors observed the expected blunted responses for TRH testing in the early stages of SAT when serum T_4 levels were high. They also learned that the suppressed RAI might relate to both the inflammation per se and to the suppression of TSH by the discharge of T_4 (an observation I reported in 1974 — Hamburger JI: Subacute thyroiditis: Diagnostic difficulties and simple treatment. J Nucl Med 15:81–89, 1974). Their suggestion that Cytomel is of some specific value for SAT can be ignored.

INDEX

Page numbers in *italics* indicate illustrations. Page numbers followed by t indicate tables.